Neurotrauma and Critical Care of the Spine

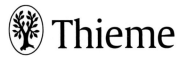

Neurotrauma and Critical Care of the spine

Jack Jallo, MD, PhD, FACS
Associate Professor
Department of Neurosurgery
Temple University School of Medicine
Philadelphia, Pennsylvania

Alexander R. Vaccaro, MD, PhD, FACS
Professor
Departments of Orthopaedics and Neurosurgery
Jefferson Medical College
Thomas Jefferson University
Vice Chairman
Department of Orthopaedic Surgery
Rothman Institute
Philadelphia, Pennsylvania

Thieme
New York • Stuttgart

Thieme Medical Publishers, Inc.
333 Seventh Ave.
New York, NY 10001

Executive Editor: Kalen Conerly
Associate Editor: Ivy Ip
Vice President, Production and Electronic Publishing: Anne T. Vinnicombe
Production Editor: Print Matters, Inc.
Vice President, International Marketing: Cornelia Schulze
Chief Financial Officer: Peter van Woerden
President: Brian D. Scanlan
Compositor: Thomson Digital Services
Printer: Maple Press

Library of Congress Cataloging-in-Publication Data

Neurotrauma and critical care of the spine / [edited by] Jack Jallo, Alexander Vaccaro.
     p. ; cm.
 Includes bibliographical references and index.
 ISBN 978-1-60406-033-1 (alk. paper)
 1. Spine—Wounds and injuries. I. Jallo, Jack. II. Vaccaro, Alexander R. III. Title: Spine.
 [DNLM: 1. Spinal Injuries—diagnosis. 2. Spinal Injuries—therapy. 3. Critical Care—methods.
 4. Spinal Cord Injuries—diagnosis. 5. Spinal Cord Injuries—therapy. WE 725 N4945 2008]
 RD533.N49 2008
 617.4'71059—dc22
                                                            2008018261

Important note: Medical knowledge is ever-changing. As new research and clinical experience broaden our knowledge, changes in treatment and drug therapy may be required. The authors and editors of the material herein have consulted sources believed to be reliable in their efforts to provide information that is complete and in accord with the standards accepted at the time of publication. However, in view of the possibility of human error by the authors, editors, or publisher of the work herein or changes in medical knowledge, neither the authors, editors, or publisher, nor any other party who has been involved in the preparation of this work, warrants that the information contained herein is in every respect accurate or complete, and they are not responsible for any errors or omissions or for the results obtained from use of such information. Readers are encouraged to confirm the information contained herein with other sources. For example, readers are advised to check the product information sheet included in the package of each drug they plan to administer to be certain that the information contained in this publication is accurate and that changes have not been made in the recommended dose or in the contraindications for administration. This recommendation is of particular importance in connection with new or infrequently used drugs.

Some of the product names, patents, and registered designs referred to in this book are in fact registered trademarks or proprietary names even though specific reference to this fact is not always made in the text. Therefore, the appearance of a name without designation as proprietary is not to be construed as a representation by the publisher that it is in the public domain.

Printed in the United States

5 4 3 2 1

ISBN 978-1-60406-033-1

Contents

IV Outcome

Foreword

To say that this is a timely work is an understatement. Spinal Cord injury (SCI) is a problem that can be viewed as particularly devastating, not only from the perspective of individual tragedy but from a broader societal perspective as well. SCI is the misfortune of youth. Thus, the ten to twelve thousand new cases of SCI annually strike not only at the humanity of society as it is, in the present, but as it was to have been, in the future.

Added to this substantial humanitarian burden is a large economic one. For a high tetraplegic patient, inpatient and outpatient costs approach one million dollars; this figure does not include the loss of productivity to society as comparative few patients with SCI return to the work force in their pre-injury capacity, if all[1]. Finally, the emotional cost to the patient and their loved ones is immeasurable.

As Dr. Dominique and colleagues point out in the first chapter in this volume, a patient with SCI was, in the past considered to be something of a lost cause. Given the tremendous advances in the understanding in the pathophysiology of injury, increased attention on timely prehospital management and critical evaluation of more aggressive intervention, treatment outcomes have improved significantly, and will, hopefully continue to do so.

Despite advances, many unanswered questions and frank controversies remain. Arguably the single greatest purpose of a text like this is to evaluate these issues in a balanced, critical way so as to help the practitioner make sense of the salient points, and, more importantly enable the reader to approach the body of knowledge with a demanding, perhaps even skeptical eye. In this regard, Drs. Jallo and Vaccaro have succeeded admirably.

As an example, consider the current classification schemes for the so-called "Hangman's fracture". This fracture is usually bony and canal expanding. Any subluxation is usually stable and any neurological deficit rare. Most will heal with nonoperative care. The first commonly used system to characterize these fractures was that of Pepin and Hawkins[2], who in a model of clarity and simplicity recognized only two types- displaced and nondisplaced with nonoperative treatment yielding acceptable results in most cases. The more contemporary system of Levine and Edwards[3] has four fracture types, with a recommendation for surgical stabilization for management of more displaced Type IIa and Type III fractures. In chapter 9 of this volume, Dr. Okonkwo and his co-authors note that no class I or II studies have been conducted to determine the optimal management of Hangman's fractures. Further, almost all fractures heal with traction and immobilization and 95% fuse in a halo. Unless clear data are forthcoming indicating the utility of a more complex classification in determining optimal treatment, one must wonder whether a simpler approach, keeping in mind the fundamental principles of fracture healing (displacement and bony versus soft tissue disruption) will serve just as well as a more comprehensive and complex one. The same point can be made for the approach to thoracolumbar trauma; while the newly proposed system of Vaccarro et al[4], is wonderfully comprehensive, will it have any practical advantages compared with the simple, elegant system of Denis[5]?

This is a text that will challenge and fulfill the reader. These are topics that demand active participation. Even in a comprehensive work such as this, more questions are raised than answered. And that is the essence of education.

F. Todd Wetzel, MD
Professor of Orthopaedic Surgery and Neurosurgery
Department of Orthopaedic Surgery and Sports Medicine
Temple University School of Medicine
Philadelphia, Pennsylvania

References

1. National Spinal Cord Injury Statistical Center. www. spinalcord.. uab.edu
2. Pepin JW, Hawkins RJ. Traumatic spondylolisthesis of the axis: Hangman's fracture. Clin Orthop Relat Res 1981;157:133–138.
3. Levine AM, Edwards CC. The management of traumatic spondylolisthesis of the axis. J Bone Joint Surg Am 1985;67: 217–226.
4. Vaccaro AR, Zeiller SC, Hurlbert RJ et al. The thoracolumbar injury severity score: a proposed treatment algorithm. J Spinal Disord Tech 2005;18: 209–215.
5. Denis F. Instability as defined by the three-column spine concept in acute spinal trauma. Clin Orthop Relat Res 1984;189:65–76.

Preface

Only as you do know yourself can your brain serve you as a sharp and efficient tool. Know your own failings, passions, and prejudices so you can separate them from what you see.

Bernard M. Baruch (1870–1965)

We are confronted again and again with injury that renders the "efficient tool" into varying levels of usefulness and uselessness. Our goal is to maintain the efficiency of this tool. Fortunately, our ability to treat brain and spinal cord injury continues to advance, allowing us to help our patients preserve the usefulness of this most precious tool. The ambition of this text is to provide a current and clear reference for the many physicians involved in the care of the patient with brain and spinal cord injury.

Despite significant advances in survival from severe head and spinal cord injury there is no miracle drug for treating these patients. Care of these patients depends wholly on applying the best available treatment in the field, upon arrival to the ER, in the ICU, the OR, and finally throughout their convalescence. While these elements have always been integral to the recovery of the patient, two major developments over the past decade are now affecting the care of the neurotrauma patient. Advances in critical care management and a push toward evidence based medicine with the development of treatment guidelines are evolving the care we provide care to the injured patient.

Charting these new developments in a comprehensive guide to the care of individuals with brain or spinal cord injury suggested a particular structure for this text. To that end, the material is presented in two volumes, one regarding head injury and the other spinal cord injury. Within each section there is an emphasis on the science underlying daily practices and acute care and critical care management. This is followed by chapters on non acute care, outcome and socioeconomics. There is a particular stress on accepted guidelines and the evidence based practice of medicine.

This will not yield a quick read, and yet it is my hope that it will be a help to my colleagues in the field as we confront the confounding problems associated with head and spinal cord injury.

Contributors

Neel Anand, MD, Mch Orth
Institute for Spinal Disorders
Cedars-Sinai Medical Center
Los Angeles, California

William S. Anderson, MD, PhD
Resident
Department of Neurosurgery
Johns Hopkins University School of Medicine
Department of Neurosurgery
Johns Hopkins Hospital
Baltimore, Maryland

Eli M. Baron, MD
Neurosurgeon, Spine Surgeon
Institute for Spinal Disorders
Cedars-Sinai Medical Center
Los Angeles, California

Darric E. Baty, MD
Resident
Department of Neurosurgery
Temple University School of Medicine
Temple University Health System
Philadelphia, Pennsylvania

Edward C. Benzel, MD
Chair
Department of Neurological Surgery
Director
Center for Spine Health
Neurological Institute
Cleveland Clinic
Cleveland, Ohio

Paul D. Campbell Jr., MD
Johns Hopkins Hospital
Baltimore, Maryland

John A. Carrino, MD, MPH
Associate Professor
Johns Hopkins University School of Medicine
Russell H. Morgan Department of Radiology and
    Radiological Science
Johns Hopkins Hospital
Baltimore, Maryland

Gordon K. T. Chu, MD, MSc, FRCSC
Department of Neurosurgery
St. Mary's Hospital
Decatur, Illinois

Kamal Dagly, MD
Resident
Department of Orthopedic Surgery
Long Island Jewish Medical Center
New Hyde Park, New York

Rob D. Dickerman, DO, PhD
Clinical Associate Professor
Department of Surgery
University of North Texas Health Science Center
Fort Worth, Texas
Presbyterian Hospital of Plano
Plano, Texas

Devanand A. Dominique, MD
Department of Neurosurgery
Temple University Health System
Philadelphia, Pennsylvania

Michael G. Fehlings, MD, PhD, FRCSC, FACS
Professor and Chair
Department of Surgery
Division of Neurosurgery
University of Toronto
Department of Neurosurgery
Toronto Western Hospital
Toronto, Ontario, Canada

Kevin T. Foley, MD, PhD
Associate Professor
Department of Neurosurgery
University of Tennessee Health Sciences Center
Memphis, Tennessee

Paul J. Ford, PhD
Assistant Professor
Department of Bioethics
Lerner College of Medicine of Case Western
  Reserve University
Clinical Bioethicist
Cleveland Clinic
Cleveland, Ohio

Alan S. Hilibrand, MD
Professor
Department of Orthopaedics
Jefferson Medical College
Thomas Jefferson University
Director
Department of Orthopaedic Surgery
Rothman Institute
Philadelphia, Pennsylvania

George I. Jallo, MD
Associate Professor
Department of Neurosurgery
Johns Hopkins University School of Medicine
Division of Pediatric Neurosurgery
Johns Hopkins Hospital
Baltimore, Maryland

Jack Jallo, MD, PhD, FACS
Associate Professor
Department of Neurosurgery
Temple University School of Medicine
Philadelphia, Pennsylvania

Michael Kessler, MD
Resident
Department of Orthopedic Surgery
Long Island Jewish Medical Center
New Hyde Park, New York

David H. Kim, MD
Assistant Professor
Department of Orthpaedic Surgery
Tufts University School of Medicne
New England Baptist Hospital
Boston, Massachusetts

Brian Kwon, MD
Clinical Instructor
Department of Orthpaedic Surgery
Tufts University School of Medicine
New England Baptist Hospital
Boston, Massachusetts

Howard B. Levene, MD, PhD
Chief Resident
Department of Neurosurgery
Temple University School of Medicine
Philadelphia, Pennsylvania

Adam S. Levin, MD
Resident
Department of Orthopedic Surgery
Long Island Jewish Medical Center
New Hyde Park, New York

Melissa Y. Macias, MD, PhD
Chief Resident
Department of Neurosurgery
Medical College of Wisconsin
Milwaukee, Wisconsin

Dennis J. Maiman, MD, PhD
Professor
Department of Neurosurgery
Medical College of Wisconsin
Veterans Affairs Medical Center
Milwaukee, Wisconsin

Stephen V. Nalbach Jr., MD
Resident
Department of Neurosurgery
Brigham & Women's Hospital
Boston, Massachusetts

David O. Okonkwo, MD, PhD
Assistant Professor
Department of Neurological Surgery
University of Pittsburgh School of Medicine
Pittsburgh, Pennsylvania

Michael O'Malley, MHMS
Philadelphia, Pennsylvania

F. Cumhur Oner, MD, PhD
Associate Professor
Department of Orthopedic Surgery
University Medical Center Utrecht
Utrecht, The Netherlands

Rod J. Oskouian Jr., MD
Swedish Neuroscience Institute
Seattle, Washington

Paul Park, MD
Assistant Professor
Department of Neurosurgery
University of Michigan Health System
Ann Arbor, Michigan

Eric P. Roger, MD, FRCS
Assistant Professor
Department of Neurosurgery
University at Buffalo, State University of New York
Buffalo, New York

Christopher I. Shaffrey, MD
Professor
Department of Neurosurgery
University of Virginia
Charlottesville, Virginia

Jeff S. Silber, MD, DC
Associate Professor
Department of Surgery
Albert Einstein College of Medicine
Great Neck, New York
Department of Orthopedic Surgery
Long Island Jewish Medical Center
New Hyde Park, New York

Kern Singh, MD
Assistant Professor
Department of Orthopedic Surgery
Rush University Medical Center
Chicago, Illinois

Tom Stanley, MD
Department of Orthopedic Surgery
Rush University Medical Center
Chicago, Illinois

Charles H. Tator, CM, MD, PhD, FRCSC, FACS
Professor
Department of Surgery, Division of Neurosurgery
University of Toronto
Department of Neurosurgery
Toronto Western Hospital
Toronto, Ontario, Canada

Eve Tsai, MD, PhD, CIP, FRCS
Division of Neurosurgery
Ottawa Hospital
Ottawa, Canada

Alexander R. Vaccaro, MD, PhD, FACS
Professor
Department of Orthopaedics
Jefferson Medical College
Department of Orthopaedic Surgery
Rothman Institute
Philadelphia, Pennsylvania

Bart Wojewnik
Resident
Division of Orthopaedics
Loyola University Medical Center
Chicago, Illinois

Steven C. Zeiller, MD
Tucson Orthopaedic Institute, P.C.
Tucson, Arizona

Jack E. Zigler, MD, FACS, FAAOS
Clinical Associate Professor
University of Texas Southwestern Medical School
Dallas, Texas

Introduction

1 Epidemiology of Spinal Injuries

Darric E. Baty, Howard B. Levene, Stephen V. Nalbach, Eli M. Baron, and Devanand A. Dominique

■ Historical Overview

Spinal cord injury (SCI) encompasses more than just the direct injury to the tissues of the spinal cord itself. The injury creates a range of disabilities and hurdles, encompassing everything from physical limitations to social embarrassment. In the United States, there are more than 200,000 people living with chronic SCI.[1] People with SCI suffer losses, physical and mental, with far-reaching impact on their ability to work and socialize. The effects of SCI involve families that now must care for a loved one with a potentially disabling neurologic condition; they most readily feel the costs, financial and personal, associated with SCI. Although not every injury is severe enough to make the injured person appear abnormal, the effects of SCI are felt by nearly all these families in the form of elevated health care costs, rising insurance premiums, and safety laws.[1]

It was not so long ago when SCI was considered a death sentence and a condition not worthy of treatment. Sir Ludwig Guttmann and Sir George Bedbrook were responsible for dramatically changing the way SCI was perceived by the medical community.[2]

Guttmann was a German who left his country for England in the 1930s when National Socialism gained favor in Germany. He was trained as a neurosurgeon and worked in basic science research at the beginning of World War II. He was therefore assigned the "hopeless" SCI cases in Stoke-Mandeville Hospital, because it was felt he could do "little harm." The hospital was actually separate from the other military hospitals, a place where SCI patients could "go to die." Guttmann used his neurologic and surgical knowledge to establish many of the principles of rehabilitative care; he is in fact considered one of the fathers of modern rehabilitation.[2]

Guttmann learned through experience and observation that laminectomies in the acute phase of SCI were indeed harmful, and thus he became a strong advocate of conservative management of SCI. He was referred patients from other hospitals and saw many complications, such as bed sores and infections; therefore, he insisted on direct admission of all SCI patients to his unit. With a team approach and insistence on 24-hour care, Guttmann emphasized avoidance of complications and therefore achieved astonishing results. Many of his patients returned to their homes and a productive life, taking up jobs that were suitable for their neurologic conditions.[2]

A short time later, Bedbrook, an orthopedist from Australia, also obtained excellent results from aggressive conservative care by utilizing a host of therapists and medical specialists devoted to complete care of the SCI patient. He, too, gained recognition as one of the fathers of modern rehabilitation and helped to further the emphasis on focused, quality care for those suffering with SCI.[2,3]

■ Data Sources and Adequacy

Much work has been done in recent years to understand and treat patients with SCI. The United States government has established model SCI care systems across the country to collect data, treat patients, and perform research; 25 such systems have been supported by federal funding since the inception of the National Spinal Cord Injury Database in 1973. Despite this emphasis, however, experts estimate that the database captures only 13% of patients with SCI. In addition, there have been no overall incidence studies of SCI in the United States since the 1970s.[4] These facts point to the inadequacy of current epidemiologic data and to the desperate need for expansion of ongoing research in the area.

Aside from the National Spinal Cord Injury Database, there is primarily one other large collection of data, located in Olmsted County, Minnesota, that provides historical clues to the trends of SCI epidemiology in the United States.[5,6] Several other, smaller studies from various parts of the country as well as from developing countries have also been published and provide some insight into the worldwide epidemiology of SCI.

■ Incidence

The incidence of SCI is the frequency with which new SCIs occur over a specified period of time (usually 1 year) in a designated population. In developed countries, the annual incidence of SCI varies from 11.5 to 53.4 cases per million population.[7,8] The National Spinal Cord Injury Statistical Center estimates the annual incidence of SCI in the United States to be 40 per million; this translates into approximately 11,000 cases per year.[4] A recent Canadian study showed the annual age-adjusted incidence in a tertiary referral center to be 42.4 per million for those 15 to 64 years old, and 51.4 per million for those 65 and older.[9] These numbers do not reflect patients who die at the scene of the accident or prior to arrival at the hospital.

Data collected from Olmsted County, Minnesota, between 1975 and 1981 established an age- and sex-adjusted incidence of 71 injuries per million; death prior to an SCI-injured patient's reaching the hospital was counted. The same study showed an incidence of 50 injuries per million for patients reaching the hospital alive.[5,6] These data demonstrate the importance of including those patients who do not make it to the hospital alive, as the mortality of SCI prior to arrival at a hospital ranges from 48.3 to 79%.[10] The rate of death after admission to a hospital ranges from 4.4 to 16.7%,[11] significantly less than the on-site and prior-to-hospital-arrival mortalities. In the Olmsted County data, 11% of SCI patients died during the first hospitalization.[10]

As mentioned previously, the overall incidence of SCI in the United States has not been studied since the 1970s; therefore, we cannot establish any recent trends. Again, the Olmsted County data give us earlier time points to analyze. The average annual age- and sex-adjusted SCI incidence rates rose steadily from 22 per million in 1935–1944, to 67 per million in 1965–1974, to 71 per million in 1975–1981, whereas the age-adjusted mortality declined slightly from 36 per million in 1965–1974 to 32 per million in 1975–1981 (**Fig. 1.1**). The incidence of those reaching the hospital alive increased from 17 (1935–1944) to 50 (1975–1981).[5,6] Data from New York provided an unadjusted incidence of SCI of 43 per million in 1982–1988.[8]

■ Prevalence

The prevalence of SCI is the percentage of a population that is directly affected by an SCI at one particular point in time. Various studies have given prevalence rates between 130 and 1124 per million.[12-15] Part of the difficulty in ascertaining prevalence is the lack of standardization of the definition of a prevalent case; lifelong SCI patients are generally counted, but those with mild injuries who

Table 1.1 United States Prevalence of Spinal Cord Injury (SCI)

Year	Prevalence (Number of People)
1980	132,000
2006	253,000

improve significantly may not be.[8] The Olmsted County data provided a prevalence of 583 per million in 1980,[5] which means that approximately 132,000 persons were living with SCI at that time. The National Spinal Cord Injury Statistical Center estimated the June 2006 United States prevalence to be 253,000 persons (**Table 1.1**).[4]

■ Etiology

The causes of SCI are variable. In some cases, traumatic injury directly transmits kinetic or shear energy to the substance of the spinal cord, causing damage to the sensitive tissues. Other causes of SCI come from gradual compression with vascular ischemia, such as seen with growing tumors and arthritis. Still other causes of SCI arise from systemic diseases such as multiple sclerosis, amyotrophic lateral sclerosis, infection, and thromboembolism.[16]

Industrial countries' etiologies of injury are naturally different from more agrarian or impoverished countries. Even within a country, however, there is variability from region to region and between primarily rural versus more urban populations. Nevertheless, on a global scale, about one half of all SCI cases can be attributed to accidents involving motor vehicles, bicycles, or pedestrians.[8]

The etiology of a country's SCI cases also changes with time.[8] In some developing countries where communal violence is becoming increasingly rampant, the number of SCIs secondary to penetrating injuries of an inflicted nature is on the rise.[17-19] On the other hand, in countries

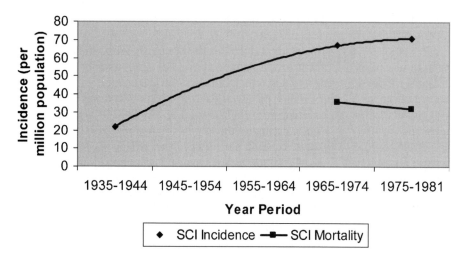

Fig. 1.1 Average annual age- and sex-adjusted spinal cord injury (SCI) incidence and mortality rates.

Table 1.2 Etiology of SCI since 2000

Injury Cause	Incidence
Motor vehicle accidents	46.9%
Falls	23.7%
Violence	13.7%
Sports	8.7%
Other/unknown	7.0%

Table 1.3 Violent Acts as an Etiology for SCI

Year Period	Proportion of Total SCI Cases
1990–1999	24.8%
2000–2006	13.7%

where there has been a focus on safe work practices, the number of SCIs taking place on the job is declining. Some countries' sports- and recreational-activity–related injuries are on the rise.[8]

Recent data from the United States indicate that motor vehicle accidents account for 46.9% of reported SCIs since 2000 (**Table 1.2**). The proportion of injuries caused by falls has increased, whereas the proportion of those attributed to sports has diminished. Acts of violence as a proportion of etiology for SCI peaked from 1990 to 1999 at 24.8% and declined to only 13.7% since 2000 (**Table 1.3**).[4]

Substance Abuse and Alcohol Use: Do They Play a Role?

Overall, evidence for substance abuse, apart from alcohol use, is found in only a small percentage of SCI patients. On the other hand, alcohol use is implicated as a causative or contributing factor to the incident, causing the SCI in approximately 25% of patients.[20]

Associated, Preinjury Conditions

In patients with SCI, the most common abnormality of the spine seen prior to the SCI is cervical spondylosis, with a prevalence as high as 10% in some studies.[8] Other acquired disorders such as rheumatoid arthritis, spinal arthropathy, and metastatic disease are also seen in patients with SCI. Congenital abnormalities like tethered cord, atlantoaxial instability, and congenital fusion may also be seen, and in some cases may exacerbate the injury.[17]

■ Neurologic Level

The neurologic level of injury as defined by the American Spinal Injury Association (ASIA) is the most caudal segment of the spinal cord with normal function on both sides of the body.[21] The need for precisely defining neurologic levels and the extent of incomplete SCIs led ASIA to publish *Standards for Neurological Classification of Spinal Injured Patients*[22] for the first time in 1982; subsequent revisions have been made, producing further refinements in the

definition of neurologic level, key muscle and sensory points, the Frankel scale (since modified to create the ASIA Impairment Scale), and the zone of partial preservation. The 1992 revision established sacral sparing as the basis for the definition of incomplete injuries and included recommendations for using an assessment of disability.[23] The international community endorsed these standards,[23] and they are now referred to as *International Standards for Neurological Classification of Spinal Cord Injury*.[21] The ASIA standards continue to serve as an important clinical and research tool and can aid in determining the prognosis of SCI patients.[24]

In general, the higher the neurologic level, the more devastating the injury. Therefore, the spine can be divided into three primary regions—cervical, thoracic, and lumbosacral—and two junctional zones—cervicothoracic and thoracolumbosacral.[8] Each region carries its own subset of clinical manifestations. For example, high cervical injuries may result in respiratory failure, along with tetraplegia, neurogenic bladder, and other symptoms, whereas lumbar injuries can present as bladder and rectal abnormalities, with or without lower extremity weakness. The degree of devastation for a particular injury also depends on its severity and the patient's clinical course, as a self-resolving cervical-level lesion would be less disabling than a permanent sacral-level injury.

The architecture of the cervical spine (C1 to C7-T1), including smaller vertebral bodies and greater relative mobility, makes it the most common location for SCI; indeed, cervical-level injuries account for approximately 55% of all injuries. The other regions of the spine, namely the thoracic (T1-T11), thoracolumbar (T11-T12 to L1-L2), and lumbosacral (L2-S5) levels, each account for approximately 15% of all SCI cases (**Table 1.4**).[8]

Injuries encountered during a specific activity sometimes have a predilection for a certain region of the spine, corresponding to a particular neurologic level of injury. For example, diving injuries have a propensity for the

Table 1.4 Percentage of SCI by Level

Neurologic Level	Percentage of SCI Cases
Cervical	55
Thoracic	15
Thoracolumbar	15
Lumbosacral	15

Table 1.5 Percentage of SCI Classified as Complete

Year/Period	Proportion of Total SCI Cases Considered Complete
1961	66%
2000–2006	52.4%

cervical spine, whereas injuries encountered in mining, logging, and some recreational activities tend to involve the thoracolumbar spine. It is interesting to note that the high lethality associated with cervical spine trauma is reflected in the striking difference between the incidence (52%) and prevalence (40%) of cervical-level injuries.[8]

■ Deficit Severity

Use of the terms *complete* and *incomplete* can be confusing, and, in fact, the definitions vary among individual physicians and specialist groups. In general, a *complete injury* is one in which there is no motor or sensory function below a specified level, whereas an *incomplete injury* describes abnormal, but present, function caudal to the area of discussion. The terms can give a sense of the severity of the injury, and have implications for recovery, but even the term *complete injury* should not be construed as meaning that improvement in neurologic function cannot occur. As discussed previously, the ASIA standards define the terms with a slightly different emphasis, in which a *complete injury* is any injury without sacral sparing.[21]

Since 2000, slightly more than half (52.4%) of all SCIs reported to the National Spinal Cord Injury Statistical Center have been complete.[4] This contrasts with 1961, when two thirds of injuries were reported as complete (**Table 1.5**).[20] The reasons for this are numerous (**Table 1.6**), including improved motor vehicle safety, increased awareness of the need for strict immobilization following injury, better initial care and retrieval systems, and implementation of the avoidance of hypotension and hypoxia. In addition,

Table 1.6 Reasons for Reduction in Number of Complete SCI Cases

Improved motor vehicle safety
Adherence to strict immobilization following injury
Better initial care
More sophisticated retrieval systems
Superior strategies for transporting patients
Advances in nursing care
Prevention/treatment of hypotension
Avoidance of hypoxia

strategies for transporting patients and nursing care in general have improved greatly.[25] Over time, incomplete tetraplegia has increased slightly as a percentage of cases, whereas both complete paraplegia and complete tetraplegia have shown a slight diminution.[4]

When the level of neurologic injury is correlated with the severity of the injury, thoracic injuries more commonly produce complete SCIs. The greatest neurologic recovery of complete injuries occurs in those with cervical-level injuries, followed by those with thoracic, and then those with lumbar injuries. For incomplete injuries, recovery is related to the severity of the neurologic deficit, regardless of level, with more severe initial injuries being associated with poorer neurologic recovery.[25] Overall, less than 1% of SCI patients experience complete recovery by hospital discharge.[4]

■ Vertebral Column Injuries

Bearing in mind the close proximity of the spinal cord and nerve roots to the bony elements of the spine, it is no wonder that SCI is often associated with some vertebral column abnormality. In fact, it is rather expected that there be radiographic evidence of injury or trauma. This is not always the case, as evidenced by the classification of some SCIs as *spinal cord injury without obvious radiologic abnormality* (SCIWORA) or *spinal cord injury without obvious radiologic evidence of trauma* (SCIWORET). The widespread availability of high-resolution computed tomography (CT) and magnetic resonance imaging (MRI) scanners has reduced the number of injuries that are classified in this manner, however. Underlying congenital abnormalities or spondylosis can often be identified when evidence of direct spinal cord trauma is lacking.[26]

The incidence for each type of vertebral column injury in adults is illustrated in **Fig. 1.2**.[27] Correlation of neurologic injury severity and vertebral column injury reveals that *complete* SCI is more likely to result from anterior dislocations and fracture dislocations compared with burst fractures and compression fractures.[8] Different types of vertebral column injury may be associated with similar neurologic-level injuries.

■ Systemic Injuries

Spinal cord injury occurs as the sole injury to a patient in approximately 20% of cases.[28-31] Other significant injuries occur 20 to 57% of the time.[17] Motor vehicle collisions are responsible for many of these multisystem traumas.[8] Traumatic brain injury patients have an associated SCI 5 to 10% of the time. Conversely, 25 to 50% of patients with acute SCI have a traumatic brain injury (**Fig. 1.3**).[30] Some data suggest that the multiplicity of injuries in SCI patients reduces the potential for neurologic recovery

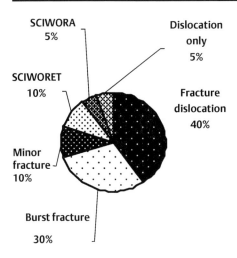

Fig. 1.2 Vertebral column injuries in adult SCI. SCIWORA, spinal cord injury without obvious radiologic abnormality; SCIWORET, spinal cord injury without obvious radiologic evidence of trauma.

Table 1.7 Reasons for Reduction in Neurologic Recovery in SCI Patients with Multiple Injuries

Causation or worsening of hypoxia
Increased likelihood of presence of hypotension
More severe initial SCI
More difficulty in treating other injuries
Challenges in diagnosing other injuries

and increases mortality.[8] There are more than likely several reasons for this (**Table 1.7**). First, hypoxia and hypotension may be caused, or worsened, by other injuries. These two physiologic aberrations have been implicated in secondary injury to the spinal cord. Second, multiple injuries may be associated with a more severe initial SCI. Third, treatment of the other injuries in an SCI patient becomes more challenging. For example, neurogenic shock may make hypotension difficult to treat. Furthermore, cervical injuries, especially higher injuries, can make the establishment of an airway more complicated and are associated with respiratory failure. In addition, SCI can disguise intra-abdominal pathology when a clinical assessment is being made.[32]

■ Demographics

Age

Spinal cord injury is primarily an injury of young men. As the median age of the general population has increased, the average age at injury has also steadily increased, from 28.7 years (1973–1979) to 38.0 years (since 2000) (**Table 1.8**). Historically, most injuries have occurred in the 16- to 30-year age group. The percentage of injuries occurring in those over 60 has increased from 4.7% (prior to 1980) to 11.5% (since 2000) (**Table 1.9**). Multiple factors probably account for this, including the aging of the population. Other factors might include changes in referral patterns, model systems' locations, improvements in elderly survival rates at the scene, and age-specific incidence rates.[4]

Gender

Among SCI patients, the ratio of males to females worldwide is typically 3:1 to 4:1. Males are consistently at greater risk for morbidity and mortality across all age groups.[8] Young men are more likely to sustain SCI in recreational and work-related accidents.[20] According to the National Spinal Cord Injury Statistical Center, there has been a trend toward a decreasing percentage of males in their study population. Prior to 1980, 81.8% of new SCI victims were males, whereas since the year 2000 that number has fallen to 77.8% (**Table 1.10**).[4]

Ethnicity

The ethnicity of patients sustaining SCI is also in flux. The potential reasons for this include changing locations of model systems, changing referral patterns to model systems, and true changes in the incidence of SCI among different

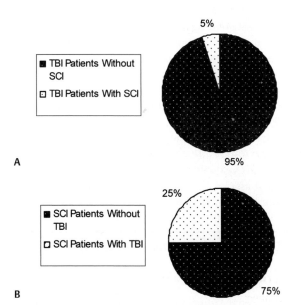

Fig. 1.3 (A) Percentage of traumatic brain injury (TBI) patients with SCI. **(B)** Percentage of SCI patients with TBI.

Table 1.8 Change in Average Age at Time of Injury

Year Period	Average Age (Years)
1973–1979	28.7
2000–2006	38.0

Table 1.9 Change in Percentage of Injuries Occurring in Those over 60 Years Old

Year Period	Proportion of Total SCI Cases Occurring in Those Older Than 60
Prior to 1980	4.7%
2000–2006	11.5%

races. The percentage of SCI patients who were Caucasians fell from 76.8% in the period 1973–1979 to 63.0% since the year 2000. During these same time intervals, the percentage of African Americans increased from 14.2 to 22.7%, the Hispanic percentage almost doubled from 6.0 to 11.8%, and the percentage from other ethnic groups fell slightly from 3.0 to 2.4%.[4]

Marital Status

Most (51.6%) patients who sustain an SCI are single at the time of injury. SCI patients are less likely than the general population to get married following their injury. They also have a higher divorce rate compared with the rest of the population, regardless of whether they married prior to or following their injury.[4]

Employment Status

At the time of injury, 64.2% of patients report gainful employment. For a plethora of reasons, finding a job after sustaining an SCI is difficult, especially for those with more substantial neurologic deficits. Only 24.2% of tetraplegics, compared with 32.4% of paraplegics, are employed by postinjury year 10.[4]

Overall employment rates range from 13 to 58%; this wide range may be reflective of differences in data acquisition rather than true differences in percentages of those working.[33,34] For example, one study reported that although 44% of the sample of SCI patients had worked at some point after their injury, only 27% were employed at the time of the survey.[35] The percentage of employed SCI patients does grow over time; in the first year following injury, 14% of SCI patients return to work. By year 10, 27% are employed, and by year 20, 40% are working.[4] Recovery, both physical and psychological, no doubt plays a role in this trend, as well as the fact that more severely injured patients tend to have reduced life expectancies. It is

Table 1.10 Change in Percentage of Injuries Occurring in Males

Year Period	Proportion of Total SCI Cases Occurring in Males
Prior to 1980	81.8%
2000–2006	77.8%

disturbing to note that 66% of patients with SCI have stopped working; many of them are no longer looking for a job. When asked why they had stopped looking for work, the most common reasons stated were "physically unable" (64%), "retired" (13%), and "in school" (8.5%).[35] Rates of employment were found to be dependent on several factors, including the level of education at the time of injury, preinjury employment in the white-collar sector, functional status after SCI, the ability to drive or use public transportation, and computer experience prior to injury.[33,35,36] In those with SCI who were employed, there was an interesting trend away from private sector jobs to not-for-profit, governmental, and self-employment jobs.[35] Four factors were found to predict employment in a group of patients who had SCIs before the age of 18 years (51% of whom were working): higher level of education, greater community mobility, greater functional independence, and fewer medical problems.[36] These results, once again, highlight the importance of having access either to a vehicle adapted for independent driving or to public transportation.[37]

Disposition

The overwhelming majority (88.1%) of patients who survive until discharge from the hospital are sent to private, noninstitutional settings, and in most cases the patients are sent home. Only 5.4% are discharged to nursing homes, whereas the rest are placed in hospitals, group living situations, or other facilities.[4]

Survival and Life Expectancy

Life expectancy is the average number of years remaining for an individual. Although the life expectancy for patients with SCI is increasing, even the most recent data provide evidence that sustaining an SCI diminishes one's life span. As expected, the older and the more severely injured patients have the least number of years remaining statistically. For example, a 20-year-old without SCI has a life expectancy of 58.4 years, whereas the same-aged person with SCI but with motor function at any level has, on average, 52.8 years, and a high-tetraplegic patient (C1-C4) has 36.1 years. Patients who survive the first year tend to have slightly longer life expectancies as well. As a comparison, the 20-year-old with SCI but with motor function preserved at any level who survives the first year has an average life expectancy of 53.3 years.[4]

■ Outcomes of Spinal Cord Injuries

Causes of Death after Injury

In the past, renal failure was the leading cause of death among SCI patients. Advances in urologic care have virtually eliminated this as a cause of death in modern treatment centers. Recent studies indicate that respiratory complications are presently at the top of the list. According to the most current data, pneumonia, pulmonary emboli, and septicemia are now the leading causes of death that appear to have a significant impact on reduced life expectancy.[4] Nonischemic heart disease, ischemic heart disease, suicide, and unintentional injuries are also listed among the leading causes of death in present-day SCI patients.[6]

Hospital Length of Stay

As anticipated, the length of stay is widely variable, depending on many factors such as the presence of other injuries, the severity of the initial neurologic injury, and complications that arise during hospitalization. The Olmsted County data from 85 patients showed that the length of stay ranged from 4 to 1000 days; the median was 67 days (inpatient rehabilitation included). In particular, 16 patients were discharged by 2 weeks, and 6 were hospitalized for more than 1 year.[38,39] Other data collected in the 1980s found the mean length of stay to be from 117.2 to 126.6 days.[40]

The average length of stay has decreased over time (**Table 1.11**). The National Spinal Cord Injury Statistical Center found that the average number of days hospitalized in the acute care setting declined from 25 days in 1974 to 18 days in 2004. The time in the rehabilitation unit similarly diminished from 115 to 39 days. SCI patients with neurologically complete injuries had longer acute-care and rehabilitation lengths of stay.[4]

Rehospitalization

Rehospitalization following SCI is an expensive and frequent occurrence and often takes place well after the initial injuries have been treated. A review of 88 consecutive, acute SCI patients who had completed initial rehabilitation revealed that 39% were readmitted at least once by the end of the first year. The mean length of stay was 11.9 days per admission, and the average hospital charge per admission was $9683. The readmitted patients were less educated and had longer initial rehabilitation lengths of stay.[8]

Estimates of Cost

The costs associated with SCI are immense. Direct costs such as the initial hospitalization, rehabilitation, home and vehicle modification, medical equipment and supplies,

medications, and attendant care are typically very high, especially during the first year after injury. These costs may be surmounted, however, by the indirect costs of lost wages and fringe benefits and lost productivity for un- or underemployment in the years following SCI. As expected, both direct and indirect costs increase with increasing severity of the injury; higher level injuries are also associated with greater costs.[4,37]

The direct costs of initial hospitalization and acute rehabilitation for the SCI patient averaged $232,245 in 2003.[4] Home modifications are important because most patients are ultimately discharged to their homes; these costs included building ramps, widening doorways, and remodeling bathrooms or other rooms in the home and averaged $21,000 (in 1996 dollars). Vehicle modification, important for reintegration of the patient into society, varied greatly, ranging from under $1000 to over $65,000. Cars tended to be less expensive to modify than minivans, but the modifications needed were also important in the final cost. The average yearly costs for attendant care for those requiring assistance with activities of daily living exceeded $21,000 (in 1996 dollars); paid assistants, as well as those providing care without direct payment, were included in this estimate. Obviously, the patients with more severe injuries required more care and incurred more costs.[37]

The direct costs for a high tetraplegic (C1-C4) patient are almost double those of a low tetraplegic (C5-C8) patient. In the first year alone, the direct costs for a high quadriplegic patient are $741,425, whereas those for a low quadriplegic patient are $478,782 (all values in 2006 dollars). For each subsequent year, the high tetraplegic patient incurs direct costs of $132,807, whereas the low tetraplegic patient has direct costs of only $54,400. The estimated direct lifetime costs of a 25-year-old with a high cervical (C1-C4) injury are almost $3 million.[4]

The indirect costs for an SCI patient are dependent on several factors, including the patient's education, the severity of the SCI, and the preinjury employment status.[37] Indirect costs average $59,212 per year (in 2006 dollars). After the first year, high tetraplegic patients are the only group with average annual *direct* costs greater than average annual *indirect* costs.[4]

Complications after Spinal Cord Injury

Spinal cord injury patients are subject to the typical medical complications seen in debilitated persons requiring lengthy hospitalizations and rehabilitation. These include pressure sores, chills, and fevers caused by urinary sepsis, pneumonia, atelectasis, and deep vein thrombosis.[41] Contractures, heterotopic calcification, cardiac arrest, and renal failure or insufficiency are other problems that commonly occur. Incidentally, tetraplegics have a higher incidence of urinary tract infections and pressure sores.[1]

Table 1.11 Decline in Acute Care and Rehabilitation Stays

Year	Average Days Hospitalized	Average Days in Rehabilitation
1974	25	115
2004	18	39

■ Trends in Spinal Cord Injury Epidemiology

Because of the varied sources available over time and the lack of recent studies on epidemiology, it is difficult to ascertain true trends in SCI epidemiology versus artificial trends from differences in patient population, data collection technique, or other factors; however, from the data at hand, it is instructive to review the trends seen in the United States. Although the overall incidence appears to be decreasing slightly, the prevalence of SCI is increasing.[4–6,10] The percentage of falls as an etiology of SCI is increasing, but the percentage of sports- and violence-related injuries are decreasing.[4] The percentage of complete SCIs has also decreased in recent years; incomplete tetraplegia has increased slightly, whereas both complete paraplegia and complete tetraplegia have shown a slight diminution.[4] The number of injuries that are classified as SCIWORA or SCIWORET has decreased.[26] The average age at the time of injury is increasing, and there has been a trend toward a decreasing percentage of males experiencing SCIs.[4] The percentage of SCI patients who are African Americans and Hispanics is increasing, whereas the percentage of SCI patients who are Caucasians, as well as those considered of "other" ethnicity, appears to be decreasing.[4] It is satisfying to note that the life expectancy for patients with SCI is increasing.[4] The leading causes of death that appear to have a significant impact on reduced life expectancy have changed from renal failure to pneumonia, pulmonary emboli, and septicemia.[4] The average length of stay in the hospital and the acute rehabilitation facility has decreased over time.[4]

■ Prevention Strategies

As there is currently no cure for SCI, and the costs to the individual and society are immense, the need for effective prevention strategies is paramount. The scientific literature has few studies on prevention, and most of the data available are several decades old. Further research into novel techniques that unveil successful methods, followed by industry and government involvement at all levels to aid in the implementation of data-driven results, is needed. Education of the public sector about SCI, its causes, and the steps that individuals can take to lower their risks is necessary. All strategies should be continuously analyzed for effectiveness, and intense study on the epidemiology and trends of SCI should be undertaken.

Motor Vehicle Accidents

Continued efforts in the manufacturing of safer vehicles will be important in the reduction of SCIs sustained in motor vehicle accidents. Likewise, safer roads and traffic laws that prioritize safety will help decrease the number of motor vehicle accidents. Continuing driver education and monitoring of individual safety records may help curtail the number of repeat offenders who have skills- and knowledge-related deficits in driving.

Drugs and Alcohol

There must be a zero-tolerance policy for driving or working with impairment related to drugs and alcohol. More severe and more effective penalties for those found and convicted may help deter hazardous behavior by others. In addition, methods of detecting and preventing intoxicated driv from reaching the steering wheel need to be addressed. Wider availability of public transportation for those who are impaired and wish not to drive may also be helpful.

Falls

Fall prevention applies mainly to the elderly population. Improved awareness, by elderly members of society and their families, of the risks of falls, including SCI, and the most effective prevention strategies will aid in reducing the incidence of those falls that cause SCIs. New legislation addressing the development of safer sidewalks, entrances to buildings, and living spaces for the elderly may make a marked difference as well. Recognition of those who would benefit from specific methods of preventing falls, as well as implementation of effectual prevention techniques, is also necessary to reduce the number of falls by the elderly.

Sports and Recreational Activities

Sports and recreational activities have become safer as personal protective gear has been developed and more widely used. Continued efforts at making sports less dangerous for the players and the fans are needed. The efforts should include improvements in safety gear, education for beginners and changes in rules and regulations.

Violence

A reduction in violence would be a major advance on many fronts, not the least of which is SCI prevention. Changing societal behaviors and educating the public on appropriate stress- and crisis-prevention methods would be difficult but extremely significant. Laws directed at modifying acceptance of violent acts may be one technique. More widespread availability of public counselors who guide patients and parents of children with violent tendencies might aid in the goal of preventing violence. Further research and monitoring are certainly needed in this arena.

■ Conclusion

The outlook for SCI patients has evolved greatly over the last century. Where SCI was once seen as a nonsurvivable injury, now there is great interest in treating and understanding this all-too-common entity. The importance of studying the epidemiology of SCI cannot be overstated. The data available enable lawmakers, scientists, and citizens alike to make informed decisions about where efforts should be directed to help prevent SCI; indeed, prevention is currently the only hope for "cure" for most patients. In addition, the continued collection of statistics enables monitoring of the effects of the changes that have been made. It also permits sharing of the societal impact of SCI, which opens the door for increased interest, financing, and research in the area.[3] The possibilities of properly treating or even curing SCI can only be realized with the allocation of sufficient resources. SCI epidemiology is a gateway to advancing knowledge and awareness of this most tragic of events, thereby providing hope for present and future SCI patients.

References

1. Anderson KD. Targeting recovery: priorities of the spinal cord-injured population. J Neurotrauma 2004;21:1371–1383
2. Kakulas BA. Neuropathology: the foundation for new treatments in spinal cord injury. Spinal Cord 2004;42:549–563
3. Kakulas BA. Problems and solutions in the rehabilitation of patients with progressive muscular dystrophy. Scand J Rehabil Med Suppl 1999;39:23–37
4. National Spinal Cord Injury Statistical Center. www.spinalcord.uab.edu
5. Griffin MR, O'Fallon WM, Opitz JL, Kurland LT. Mortality, survival and prevalence: traumatic spinal cord injury in Olmsted County, Minnesota, 1935–1981. J Chronic Dis 1985;38:643–653
6. Griffin MR, Opitz JL, Kurland LT, Ebersold MJ, O'Fallon WM. Traumatic spinal cord injury in Olmsted County, Minnesota, 1935–1981. Am J Epidemiol 1985;121:884–895
7. Botterell EH, Jousse AT, Kraus AS, Thompson MG, Wynne-Jones M, Geisler WO. A model for the future care of acute spinal cord injuries. Can J Neurol Sci 1975;2:361–380
8. Sekhon LH, Fehlings MG. Epidemiology, demographics, and pathophysiology of acute spinal cord injury. Spine 2001;26(suppl):S2–S12
9. Pickett GE, Campos-Benitez M, Keller JL, Duggal N. Epidemiology of traumatic spinal cord injury in Canada. Spine 2006;31:799–805
10. Kraus JF, Franti CE, Riggins RS, Richards D, Borhani NO. Incidence of traumatic spinal cord lesions. J Chronic Dis 1975;28:471–492
11. Kraus JF. Injury to the head and spinal cord: the epidemiological relevance of the medical literature published from 1960 to 1978. J Neurosurg 1980(suppl):S3–S10
12. Harvey C, Rothschild BB, Asmann AJ, Stripling T. New estimates of traumatic SCI prevalence: a survey-based approach. Paraplegia 1990;28:537–544
13. Ergas Z. Spinal cord injury in the United States: a statistical update. Cent Nerv Syst Trauma 1985;2:19–32
14. DeVivo MJ, Fine PR, Maetz HM, Stover SL. Prevalence of spinal cord injury: a reestimation employing life table techniques. Arch Neurol 1980;37:707–708
15. Anderson DW, Kalsbeek WD. The National Head and Spinal Cord Injury Survey: assessment of some uncertainties affecting the findings. J Neurosurg 1980(suppl):S32–S34
16. Kirshblum SC, Groah SL, McKinley WO, Gittler MS, Stiens SA. Spinal cord injury medicine: 1. Etiology, classification, and acute medical management. Arch Phys Med Rehabil 2002;83(suppl 1):S50–S57
17. Burney RE, Maio RF, Maynard F, Karunas R. Incidence, characteristics, and outcome of spinal cord injury at trauma centers in North America. Arch Surg 1993;128:596–599
18. Collins WF. A review and update of experiment and clinical studies of spinal cord injury. Paraplegia 1983;21:204–219
19. Sutherland MW. The prevention of violent spinal cord injuries. SCI Nurs 1993;10:91–95
20. Ho CH, Wuermser LA, Priebe MM, Chiodo AE, Scelza WM, Kirshblum SC. Spinal cord injury medicine: 1. Epidemiology and classification. Arch Phys Med Rehabil 2007;88(suppl 1):S49–S54
21. American Spinal Injury Association. International Standards for Neurological Classification of Spinal Cord Injury (revised 2000). Chicago: ASIA, 2002
22. American Spinal Injury Association. Standards for Neurological Classification of Spinal Injured Patients. Chicago: ASIA, 1982
23. American Spinal Injury Association, International Medical Society of Paraplegia (ASIA/IMSOP). International Standards for Neurological and Functional Classification of Spinal Cord Injury (revised 1992). Chicago: ASIA/IMSOP, 1992
24. Tator CH, Duncan EG, Edmonds VE, Lapczak LI, Andrews DF. Changes in epidemiology of acute spinal cord injury from 1947 to 1981. Surg Neurol 1993;40:207–215
25. Tator CH. Spine-spinal cord relationships in spinal cord trauma. Clin Neurosurg 1983;30:479–494
26. Eismont FJ, Clifford S, Goldberg M, Green B. Cervical sagittal spinal canal size in spine injury. Spine 1984;9:663–666
27. Fehlings MG, Rao SC, Tator CH, et al. The optimal radiologic method for assessing spinal canal compromise and cord compression in patients with cervical spinal cord injury: 2. Results of a multicenter study. Spine 1999;24:605–613
28. Exner G, Meinecke FW. Trends in the treatment of patients with spinal cord lesions seen within a period of 20 years in German centers. Spinal Cord 1997;35:415–419
29. Harris P. Acute spinal cord injury patients—who cares? Paraplegia 1985;23:1–7
30. Meguro K, Tator CH. Effect of multiple trauma on mortality and neurological recovery after spinal cord or cauda equina injury. Neurol Med Chir (Tokyo) 1988;28:34–41
31. Meinecke FW. Pelvis and limb injuries in patients with recent spinal cord injuries. Proc Veterans Adm Spinal Cord Inj Conf 1973;19:205–213
32. DeVivo MJ, Kartus PL, Stover SL, Rutt RD, Fine PR. Cause of death for patients with spinal cord injuries. Arch Intern Med 1989;149:1761–1766
33. Jang Y, Wang YH, Wang JD. Return to work after spinal cord injury in Taiwan: the contribution of functional independence. Arch Phys Med Rehabil 2005;86:681–686

34. Valtonen K, Karlsson AK, Alaranta H, Viikari-Juntura E. Work participation among persons with traumatic spinal cord injury and meningomyelocele1. J Rehabil Med 2006;38:192–200

35. Berkowitz M. Spinal Cord Injury: An Analysis of Medical and Social Costs. New York: Demos, 1998

36. Anderson CJ, Vogel LC. Employment outcomes of adults who sustained spinal cord injuries as children or adolescents. Arch Phys Med Rehabil 2002;83:791–801

37. Priebe MM, Chiodo AE, Scelza WM, Kirshblum SC, Wuermser LA, Ho CH. Spinal cord injury medicine: 6. Economic and societal issues in spinal cord injury. Arch Phys Med Rehabil 2007;88(suppl 1): S84–S88

38. DeVivo MJ, Rutt RD, Black KJ, Go BK, Stover SL. Trends in spinal cord injury demographics and treatment outcomes between 1973 and 1986. Arch Phys Med Rehabil 1992;73:424–430

39. Buchanan LE, Ditunno JF Jr, Osterholm JL, Cotler JM, Staas WE Jr. Spinal cord injury: a ten-year report. Pa Med 1990;93: 36–39

40. Davidoff G, Schultz JS, Lieb T, et al. Rehospitalization after initial rehabilitation for acute spinal cord injury: incidence and risk factors. Arch Phys Med Rehabil 1990;71:121–124

41. Young JS. Spinal cord injury: associated general trauma and medical complications. Adv Neurol 1979;22:255–260

II   Science

2 Pathophysiology of Spinal Injuries

Jeff S. Silber, Adam S. Levin, Michael Kessler, and Kamal D. Dagly

There are approximately 12,000 new cases of spinal cord injury (SCI) reported annually in the United States, and there are approximately 200,000 to 250,000 patients with various spinal cord injuries. Most involve males (82%) between 16 and 30 years of age and occur in the summer months on weekends involving motor vehicle accidents. The most common spinal level of injury reported is C5. SCIs produce devastating disabilities for the individual, the family, and society as a whole. SCI injury produces a decreased quality of life as well as a tremendous public health impact, with millions of dollars spent annually caring for these individuals along with lost productivity in this young affected population.

The spinal cord is a viscoelastic structure that has the potential to elongate at low applied tensile loads. It is protected by dura, cerebrospinal fluid, and epidural fat, and it is one of only two anatomical structures (the other is the brain) that is entirely encased and protected by bone. The vascular supply is mostly via segmental vessels through radicular arteries. There is an anterior and posterior spinal artery that runs longitudinally along the ventral and dorsal aspect of the spinal cord, respectively, supplying the entire spinal cord. There is a "watershed" area of blood supply located in the midthoracic level that is prone to ischemia in cases of hypotension and decreased blood flow.

■ Primary and Secondary Injury

Spinal cord injury can be divided into two separate injury events known as a primary and secondary injury (**Fig. 2.1; Table 2.1**). The primary event involves the immediate changes that take place following the initial SCI. Once the initial mechanical injury takes place (motor vehicle accident,

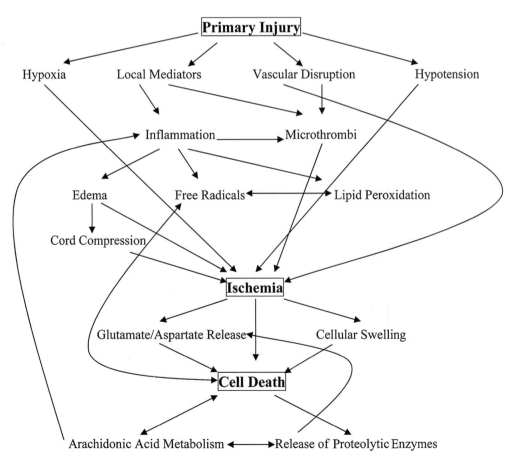

Fig. 2.1 Flow chart of the primary and secondary spinal cord injury pathways.

Table 2.1 Primary and Secondary Spinal Cord Injury Mechanisms

Primary injury

- Primary injury entails immediate changes following the initial SCI

- Once the initial mechanical injury takes place (motor vehicle accident, driving injury), subsequent events involve

  - Reduction of arterial blood flow to and venous flow from the cord

  - Decreased pO_2 supply

  - Decreased NA^+-K^+ ATPase activity

  - Capillary vessel rupture

  - Electrolyte shifts within the neural tissues

  - Cell membrane disruption with initiation of inflammatory cascades

Secondary injury

- Secondary injury cascade overlaps the primary injury

- Events involve

  - Local disruption of blood flow

  - Edema formation within and around the SCI

  - Loss of cellular and blood supply autoregulation

  - Overproduction of opiates, calcium ions, free radical production

  - Excitatory amino acid release

  - Infiltration of polymorphonuclear leukocytes (PMNs) into injured area

  - Hemorrhage/thrombosis

  - Axonal degeneration/demyelination

  - Cell death

diving injury), the subsequent events involve reduction of arterial blood flow to and venous flow from the cord, decreased pO_2 supply, decreased Na^+-K^+ adenosine triphosphatase (ATPase) activity, capillary vessel rupture, electrolyte shifts within the neural tissues, and cell membrane disruption with inflammatory cascades initiated. Following the initial primary injury is a secondary injury cascade. The secondary injury cascade overlaps the primary injury and is more of a continuum of the primary injury. During the secondary injury, there is edema formation within and around the SCI with loss of cellular and blood supply autoregulation. There is an overproduction of opiates, calcium ions, free radical production, excitatory amino acid release, and infiltration of polymorphonuclear leukocytes (PMNs) into the injured area.

A variety of pathophysiologic processes account for the secondary mechanisms of SCI: edema, inflammation, free radical production, hemorrhage/thrombosis, axonal degeneration/

demyelination, and cell death. Nearly all of these phenomena may be either directly or indirectly related to local ischemia at the site of injury. In experimental spinal cord models, ischemia appears to be more detrimental to the gray matter than the surrounding white matter, presumably due to increased metabolic demands of the gray matter. This ischemia can eventually spread vertically in the rostral and caudal directions from the site of initial injury.

The sequence of secondary events begins with a local disruption of blood flow, either as a result of direct microvascular trauma or from microthrombi at the site of initial SCI. As a result, local edema and release of inflammatory compounds from the structures of the damaged cells ensue. Reperfusion injury occurs as a result of the reintroduction of oxidative materials after a period of anaerobic metabolism, leading to a release of free radicals at the site of damage. All of these mechanisms further feed back on themselves, increasing the localized cell death through both necrosis and apoptosis, causing a further leakage from capillaries, an augmented release of cellular breakdown products and inflammatory/degradative enzymes. Significant research has been focused on the cascade of events involved in secondary SCI, as well as means of preventing further destruction. It is our increased understanding of these primary and secondary injury cascades that many therapeutic strategies target in an attempt to alter and decrease the potential negative effects and promote the potential positive effects involved in this complicated injury sequence.

■ Phases of Spinal Cord Injury

Spinal cord injury sequences can also be described in a temporal model known as phases. There are three phases described as the SCI site progresses over time: early, intermediate, and late (**Table 2.2**). During the early phase, from the initial traumatic event, central punctate hemorrhages develop with formation of edema within the spinal cord. Progressive blood vessel disruption occurs with thrombosis, further deceasing blood supply. Axon disruption begins with eventual neuron chromatolysis and cell death. Once this occurs, within days to weeks the intermediate phase continues with progression and longitudinal spreading of the edema in a caudad and cephalad direction within the spinal cord. There is an increased infiltration of PMNs with phagocytosis of the damaged neural tissue. Wallerian degeneration of the axons takes place, and granulation tissue formation starts to develop in place of the native neural tissue. In areas where granulation tissue has yet to develop, cystic cavities form from the phagocytic digestion of the damaged neural cells. The late phase takes place weeks to months following the initial injury. During this phase granulation tissue matures into scar formation, known as gliosis, and large cyst and syrinx formation takes place at and adjacent to the SCI site, progressing longitudinally along the spinal cord. During

Table 2.2 Temporal Model/ Phases of Spinal Cord Injury

Early phase

From the initial traumatic event:

- Central punctate hemorrhages develop with formation of edema within the spinal cord

- Progressive blood vessel disruption occurs with thrombosis, further decreasing blood supply

- Axon disruption begins with eventual neuron chromatolysis and cell death

Intermediate phase

Within days to weeks after the initial event:

- Progression and longitudinal spreading of the edema in a caudad and cephalad direction within the spinal cord

- Increased infiltration of PMNs with phagocytosis of damaged neural tissue

- Wallerian degeneration of axons

- Granulation tissue formation starts to develop in place of native neural tissue

Late phase

Weeks to months following initial injury:

- Granulation tissue matures into scar formation known as gliosis

- Large cyst and syrinx formation takes place at and adjacent to the SCI site, progressing longitudinally along the spinal cord

- Limited axonal sprouting from the damaged ends of injury

- Progressive loss of white and gray matter with atrophy of the spinal cord

this phase limited axonal sprouting occurs from the damaged ends of the injury, although there is a progressive loss of white and gray matter with atrophy of the spinal cord. It is the better understanding of these SCI phases that many therapeutic interventions target, and they are discussed below.

Demyelination/Remyelination

Once the spinal cord undergoes the initial trauma, oligodendrocytes suffer an apoptotic death, and demyelination accompanies wallerian degeneration. It is thought that the primary insult leading to the cascade of events associated with SCI revolves around the local vasculature. Decreased oxygen perfusion, edema, and the influx of inflammatory cells are related to the traumatic breakdown of the blood–spinal cord barrier.[1] Key inflammatory cells including the macrophage and activated microglia are found in close proximity to the traumatic lesion and segments of the spinal cord undergoing wallerian degeneration.[2] The microglia may lead to oligodendrocyte apoptosis

via inducible nitric oxide synthase and reduced nicotinamide adenine dinucleotide phosphate (NADPH) oxidase, both at the injury site and distally.[3] Demyelination and the subsequent delay in transmission of neural impulses are the key factors related to SCI patients' delayed physical advancement and functional recovery.

The traumatic SCI is only the first step in the loss of function. This initial attack on neuron integrity causes local axonal injury and oligodendrocyte death. As the wallerian degeneration occurs, distal axons succumb to the lack of nutrients and progressive demyelination.[4] As shown by Crowe et al,[5] it is likely that the oligodendrocytes are more susceptible to a traumatic injury, rather than the axons, because oligodendrocyte cell bodies are in closer proximity to the area of trauma, whereas the cell bodies of the axons may be significantly farther away. Once these axons have lost their myelin, they are rendered incapable of conducting action potentials, leaving distal motor units nonfunctioning. In the areas most distal to the site of injury, there is a greater quantitative loss of axons compared with glial cells. This is likely because the oligodendrocytes undergo apoptosis, whereas the axons degenerate and die due to necrosis.[6]

The loss of axons leads to a decrease in gray matter and the eventual creation of a glial scar at the site of injury, eventually forming a fluid-filled cyst. This cyst has a rim of intact axons that progressively become demyelinated. The cystic cavitation then advances symmetrically both rostrally and caudally from the initial area of injury.[6] The advancement of this central cavitation rostrally and caudally causes a significant hindrance to the benefits of therapeutic neural tissue transplantation at the site of injury.

Once the initial injury period has ended, progenitor cells, located at the site of the initial insult, begin remyelinating local axons. Because demyelinated areas lack migratory signals or matrix metalloproteinases, it is unlikely that distant progenitor cells will receive the proper signals to migrate to the injured area. Transplanting myelin-producing cells such as Schwann cells, or olfactory ensheathing glia, has been proposed; however, various complications including graft rejection have yet to be solved.[7,8]

Axonal Sprouting

Following a traumatic SCI, it is rare for the entire local population of axons to become completely devitalized at the injury site. Some axons remain viable, with the possibility of collateral axonal sprouting with potential filling of the void created during the trauma.[9] Unfortunately, there is no guarantee, even if the primary and collateral axons sprout appropriately and are nourished to grow, that the motor and sensory connections will be reestablished. This potential disconnect occurs from the traumatic event, precluding collateral axonal sprouting, and the

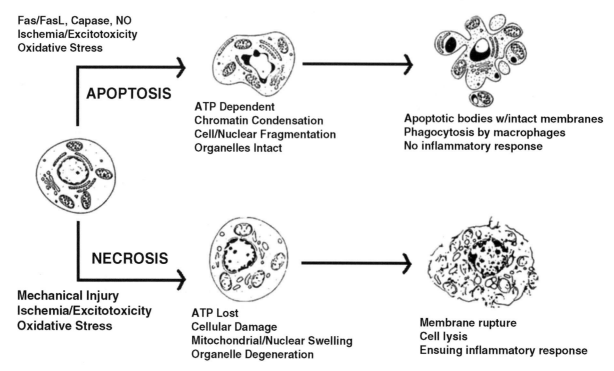

Fas/FasL, Capase, NO
Ischemia/Excitotoxicity
Oxidative Stress

APOPTOSIS

ATP Dependent
Chromatin Condensation
Cell/Nuclear Fragmentation
Organelles Intact

Apoptotic bodies w/intact membranes
Phagocytosis by macrophages
No inflammatory response

NECROSIS

Mechanical Injury
Ischemia/Excitotoxicity
Oxidative Stress

ATP Lost
Cellular Damage
Mitochondrial/Nuclear Swelling
Organelle Degeneration

Membrane rupture
Cell lysis
Ensuing inflammatory response

Fig. 2.2 Diagram comparing the similarities and differences between spinal cord cell necrosis and apoptosis.

myelin-associated growth inhibitor Nogo-A has been shown to inhibit growth-promoting proteins in the spinal cord.[10,11]

Although axonal sprouting and the formation of new neural connections distal to the site of injury are the goals after SCI, there are consequences. Aberrant sensory connections have the ability to form that lead to patients suffering from allodynia and various other forms of potentially devastating chronic pain symptoms. Sixty percent of patients with SCI suffer from some type of chronic pain and state that this pain is their primary complaint even if motor function is severely limited.[12] Furthermore, autonomic dysreflexia affects over half of the patients with chronic spinal cord injuries that occur at or above the T5-T6 level.[13]

Future work on the treatment of SCI will focus on reducing inhibitory molecules at the glial scar injury site, leading to increased sprouting from the affected axons. Also, having the ability to focus axonal sprouting toward motor neurons that will make functional connections distally and limit the sprouting of sensory fibers may prevent chronic pain syndromes associated with SCI while maximizing functional recovery.

Apoptosis and Necrosis

Spinal cord cells may undergo death by two mechanisms: (1) unintentional cell death or necrosis and (2) programmed cell death or apoptosis (**Fig. 2.2; Table 2.3**). Severe cell damage leads to cell death by necrosis, in which the cells passively swell, lose the potential to create energy, suffer intense mitochondrial damage, and

Table 2.3 Apoptosis and Necrosis

Necrosis

- Unintentional cell death
- During the process of necrosis:
  - Cells swell passively
  - Cells lose the potential to create energy
  - Cells suffer intense mitochondrial damage
  - Cells lose normal cell hemostasis
  - Intense secondary inflammatory reaction following cell membrane rupture and cell lysis
- Characterized by loss of ATP production

Apoptosis

- Programmed cell death
- Active programmed pathway in neuronal death, akin to suicide, where cell actively kills itself
- During the process of apoptosis:
  - Cells and nuclei characteristically shrink
  - Cellular organelles stay intact
  - Nuclear chromatin condenses
  - DNA fragmentation occurs
  - No inflammatory reaction because cells are autodigested and phagocytosed in a controlled, organized, and programmed sequence of events
- Characterized by ATP-dependent synthesis of proteins, which is required to carry out apoptosis

lose normal cell homeostasis. Following cell membrane rupture and cell lysis, an intense secondary inflammatory reaction ensues in response to the chemical release from the intracellular structures.[14] Apoptosis in contrast to necrosis is an active, programmed pathway in neuronal death, akin to suicide, where the cell actively kills itself. In apoptosis, the cells and nuclei characteristically shrink, cellular organelles stay intact, nuclear chromatin condenses, and DNA fragmentation occurs. Both apoptosis and necrosis can be triggered by exogenous factors such as excitoxins, hyperthermia, free radicals, and radiation. However, cells undergoing death by apoptosis do not produce an inflammatory reaction because they are autodigested by proteases and phagocytosed in a controlled, organized, and programmed sequence of events. Necrosis is characterized by the loss of adenosine triphosphate (ATP) production and energy failure, whereas ATP-dependent synthesis of proteins is required to carry out apoptosis. Although apoptosis and necrosis appear to be distinct and separate pathophysiologic pathways, it is likely that cell death actually occurs along a spectrum between the two mechanisms; however, a distinction is clinically relevant because there is increased potential for therapeutic intervention in the apoptosis pathway.

Emery et al[15] confirmed the existence of apoptosis after traumatic human SCI. Data from rat models of SCI have strengthened the notion that apoptosis significantly contributes to SCI and may occur for several weeks after the initial injury at locations that are significantly distant from the site of injury.[16-18] All cell types within the spinal cord, including axons/neurons, microglia, oligodendrocytes, and astrocytes, have demonstrated the ability to undergo apoptosis. Apoptosis in microglia leads to secondary injury by means of an inflammatory process.[19] Following the first several weeks after acute SCI, oligodendrocytes may begin to express receptors such as Fas and p75, initiating apoptosis and leading to postinjury demyelination. Neuronal apoptosis leads to cell loss that has a profound negative effect on long-term functional outcome and occurs via extrinsic and intrinsic pathways.[20] The extrinsic pathway (receptor-dependent) is mediated by Fas ligand and the Fas receptor or by inducible nitric oxide synthase production by macrophages.[21,22] This pathway is called the extrinsic pathway because it is activated by extracellular signals, mainly tumor necrosis factor, which is known to rapidly accumulate in the injured spinal cord and activates the Fas receptor. The intrinsic (receptor-independent) or caspase-mediated pathway occurs via direct caspase-3 proenzyme activation or mitochondrial damage, release of cytochrome *c*, and activation of the inducer caspase-9.[23,24] This intrinsic pathway is activated by intracellular signals. Current investigations are focusing on the intrinsic pathway specifically targeted at the caspase inhibitors as a potential therapeutic intervention against this known secondary SCI mechanism.

■ Types of Spinal Cord Injury

Complete Spinal Cord Injury

Complete SCI is defined as no motor or sensory function below the level of the spinal cord lesion after the resolution of spinal shock (**Table 2.4**). The usual prognosis of motor or sensory function is poor, and improvement may occur in one or two spinal levels. Spinal shock is defined as a state of physiologic spinal cord dysfunction with no motor or sensory function or autonomic reflexes. This state usually ends within 24 to 72 hours after the initial injury, with return of the most distal innervated reflex known as the bulbocavernosus reflex. The bulbocavernosus reflex is elicited by manually squeezing the glans penis or clitoris or tugging on a urinary catheter with reflex contraction of the anal sphincter. The entire reflex is innervated through the lowest sacral nerve roots, suggesting that spinal shock is over, as the distal end of the spinal cord is functioning enough to allow the reflex to return.

Incomplete Spinal Cord Injury

Incomplete SCI is defined as any remaining spinal cord tract function after the resolution of spinal shock (**Table 2.4**).

Table 2.4 Types of Spinal Cord Injury

Complete

- Defined as no motor or sensory function below the level of the spinal cord lesion after the resolution of spinal shock
- Usually prognosis is poor, and improvement may occur in one or two spinal levels

Incomplete

- Defined as any remaining spinal cord tract function after the resolution of the spinal shock
- Remaining function may be sacral sparing or any distal sensory of motor function
- Several incomplete SCI symptoms include
  - Central cord syndrome: follows hyperextension injury to the cervical spine with buckling of the ligamentum flavum and posterior vertebral body osteophytes impinging on the cervical spinal cord
  - Brown-Séquard syndrome: follows injury involving half of the spinal cord, usually from penetrating trauma
  - Anterior cord syndrome: rare SCI involving anterior two thirds of the spinal cord, leaving only the posterior columns functional
  - Posterior cord syndrome: isolated injury to the posterior columns
  - Autonomic dysreflexia: clinical syndrome related to sympathetic nervous dysfunction occurring in up to 85% of patients with a complete SCI above T6 level

This remaining function may be sacral sparing or any distal sensory of motor function. Additionally, there are several incomplete SCI syndromes described depending on the anatomical spinal cord area of involvement determining the clinical neurologic presentation. These include the syndromes discussed in the following subsections.

Central Cord Syndrome

Central cord syndrome is seen most commonly in older patients with cervical spondylitic changes resulting in stenosis. It follows a hyperextension injury to the cervical spine with buckling of the ligamentum flavum and posterior vertebral body osteophytes impinging on the cervical spinal cord.

The clinical findings in central cord syndrome consist of motor loss to a greater degree in the upper extremities as compared with the lower extremities with varying degrees of sensory loss below the level of the spinal cord lesion. Urinary retention and sacral sparing may also occur. The somatotopic organization of the spinal cord, with the cervical motor tracts located at a more central location within the spinal cord and the sacral tracts in a more peripheral location, is the anatomical basis for the clinical findings described above (**Table 2.5**).

Brown-Séquard Syndrome

Brown-Séquard syndrome results from an injury involving half of the spinal cord usually from penetrating trauma. The clinical presentation involves ipsilateral loss of motor function below the level of the lesion (lateral corticospinal tract); ipsilateral loss of fine touch, vibration, and proprioception below the level of the lesion (posterior columns); and contralateral loss of pain and temperature sense one to two levels below the level of the lesion (spinothalamic tract) (**Table 2.5**).

Anterior Cord Syndrome

Anterior cord syndrome is a very rare SCI involving the anterior two thirds of the spinal cord, leaving only the posterior columns functional. It most commonly occurs following a vascular insult of the spinal cord. Patients usually present with an acute loss of motor and most sensory function below the level of the injury. Sparing of the posterior columns preserves some deep pressure, vibratory, and light touch sensation. The prognosis for recovery is generally poor.

Posterior Cord Syndrome

Isolated injury to the posterior columns is unusual and may present with ipsilateral loss of fine touch, vibration, and proprioception with preservation of pain and temperature sense.

Autonomic Dysreflexia

A clinical syndrome related to sympathetic nervous dysfunction is autonomic dysreflexia, also known as hyperreflexia. This syndrome occurs in up to 85% of patients with a complete SCI above the T6 level. Symptoms include severe headache, sweating, pupillary dilation, bradycardia, and peripheral upper extremity vasodilation. Severe hypertension is the most dangerous manifestation and can lead to convulsions and may even result in intracranial hemorrhage, resulting in death. Autonomic dysreflexia is most commonly due to overdistention of the bladder or bowel viscera that may occur in the SCI patient. Symptoms may begin approximately 4 to 6 weeks after the initial injury. A distended bladder or rectum may cause an abnormal neural discharge of sympathetic afferent nerves, causing reflex activity of the sympathetic efferent outflow. This results in increased sympathetic tone, causing vasoconstriction in the lower extremities, resulting in overall systemic hypertension. The systemic hypertension stimulates the baroreceptors located in the carotid sinus in the neck and aortic arch, causing an increase in central vagal tone as a reaction to try to lower the hypertension. The increased vagal tone results in bradycardia and upper body vasodilation. This response is unable to influence lower body autonomic function

Table 2.5 Incomplete Spinal Cord Injury Syndromes

Injury/Syndrome	Region Etiology	Clinical Significance
Anterior spinal cord	Above cauda equina	Ipsilateral: upper motor neuron findings
Brown-Séquard	Spinal cord hemisection	Ipsilateral: motor, fine touch, and proprioception loss and contralateral pain and temperature loss
Central cord	Cervical spinal cord compression	Upper greater than lower: extremity motor loss, urinary retention, and sacral sparing
Autonomic dysreflexia	Bladder/bowel overdistention spinal cord lesion above T6 sympathetic nerves	Hypertension, bradycardia, headache, pupil dilation, and sweating

because this feedback information cannot descend past the injured spinal cord lesion. This results in a cycle of increased sympathetic discharge and continued extremely elevated systemic blood pressure. Management is rendered on an emergent basis and entails attempts to relieve a distended bladder or impacted bowel. Emergent bowel disimpaction and bladder catheterization along with antihypertensive medications are often necessary to control blood pressure and prevent possible recurrence of the condition (**Table 2.5**).

■ Current Therapies (Table 2.6)

Glucocorticosteroids (Methylprednisolone)

One of the most reproducible pathophysiologic changes in SCI is a localized edema and inflammatory response. The exact cascade of inflammatory markers has not been fully elucidated, though many theories have been developed. Since the National Acute Spinal Cord Injury Study (NASCIS)-2 and NASCIS-3 trials, the use of methylprednisolone in the setting of acute SCI has become the standard of care, although recently challenged, with evidence of improvement in long-term clinical outcomes. Proposed mechanisms of action of systemic corticosteroids include a decrease in localized edema, a decrease in microvascular damage with an increase in localized blood flow, stabilization of lysosomal membranes with a resultant decrease in degradative enzyme deposition, a decrease in necrosis in the early and intermediate phases, a decrease in lipid peroxidation and free radical production, and an immune suppression or decrease in inflammatory cytokines[25–27] (**Table 2.7**).

The NASCIS-2 trial was the first trial on human subjects to indicate that pharmacologic intervention after SCI

Table 2.6 Summary of Current Therapies

- Glucocorticosteroids (methylprednisolone)
- Other antiinflammatory agents
- Lipid peroxidation and reactive oxygen species
- Excitotoxicity
- Kallikrein
- EphA7
- Nitric oxide synthase inhibitor
- Inducible nitric oxide synthase (iNOS)
- Olfactory ensheathing cells
- Stat3/ Socs3
- 4-chloro-3-hydroxyanthranilate

Table 2.7 Glucocorticosteroids (Methylprednisolone)

Proposed mechanisms of action of systemic corticosteroids include

- Decrease in localized edema
- Decrease in microvascular damage
- Increase in localized blood flow
- Stabilization of lysosomal membranes with resultant decrease in degradative enzyme deposition
- Decrease in necrosis in early and intermediate phases
- Decrease in lipid peroxidation and free radical production
- Immune suppression or decrease in inflammatory cytokines

could affect outcomes. The study chose methylprednisolone because of its favorable profile as a corticosteroid that rapidly traverses the blood–brain barrier, with a decreased propensity for causing neutropenia.[28,29] It compared SCI patients administered methylprednisolone as a bolus of 30 mg/kg, followed by 5.4 mg/kg/hour over the next 23 hours, to those in a placebo group, as well as to a cohort receiving naloxone. Subjects were further stratified by the timing of initiation of therapy. The study concluded that patients with blunt SCI had improved motor and sensory function at 6 weeks, 6 months, and 1 year after injury in those initiating treatment within 8 hours of injury.[28,30]

After significant criticism of the NASCIS-2 trial, as well as consideration that the proposed effects of glucocorticosteroid therapy would affect components of secondary injury that may endure longer than 24 hours, the role of more prolonged methylprednisolone therapy was studied in NASCIS-3. This trial examined those patients treated with a bolus of 30 mg/kg followed by either 23 or 47 hours of 5.4 mg/kg/hour infusion of methylprednisolone. Findings suggested that for those patients in whom initiation of therapy began between 3 and 8 hours postinjury, the functional outcomes may be improved by prolonging therapy for a total of 48, rather than 24, hours.[31] Recently, the usage of methylprednisolone has been intensely challenged and is no longer the standard of care in many SCI centers.

Other Antiinflammatory Agents (Table 2.8)

Glucocorticoid therapy has the potential for a myriad of untoward side effects, including delayed wound healing, systemic immune suppression, gastrointestinal bleeding, and delayed axonal sprouting and repair postinjury. As a result, despite the clinical efficacy of glucocorticosteroids, significant research has focused on potential alternative therapies, with fewer side effects.

Both cyclooxygenases 1 and 2 (COX-1 and COX-2) are capable of converting arachidonic acid into inflammatory

Table 2.8 Other Antiinflammatory Agents

- Glucocorticoid therapy (side effects include delayed wound healing, systemic immune suppression, gastrointestinal bleeding, delayed axonal sprouting, and repair postinjury)

- Both cyclooxygenases (COX-1 and COX-2): recent studies suggest COX-2 inhibition results in improved functional outcomes[34–36]

- CM101, an antiangiogenic compound

- IL-10, an antiinflammatory cytokine

Table 2.9 Lipid Peroxidation and Reactive Oxygen Species

- Lazaroids, such as tirilizad mesylate: show some neuroprotective efficacy

- Immunosuppression agent: cyclosporin A demonstrated efficacy in animal models

- EPC-K1, a phosphate diester linkage of vitamins E and C: demonstrated efficacy in animal models

- Melatonin, vitamin E, and edaravone, a novel free radical scavenger: demonstrated efficacy in early animal studies

prostaglandins. Although both are normally expressed in the spinal cord, and it presently still remains unclear which may play a more important role in inflammation in the diseased state, COX-2 is rapidly upregulated after an SCI.[32,33] Studies of animal models have indicated that COX-2 inhibition resulted in improved functional outcomes after injury.[34–36]

Additional modalities for prevention of inflammation in the setting of acute SCI have included CM101, an antiangiogenic compound,[37] and the antiinflammatory cytokine interleukin-10 (IL-10), which has shown contradictory study results.[38,39] Also considered, as in brain injury patients, has been iatrogenic hypothermic therapy either to the entire body or localized to the spinal cord, which has been suggested to decrease edema and metabolic demand on the ischemic spinal cord. This may lead to the decreased release of excitatory amino acids, and ultimately cell death in the acute period after injury. Early trials with small cohorts have indicated favorable results after hypothermia, both systemically and locally.[40–43]

Lipid Peroxidation and Reactive Oxygen Species (Table 2.9)

Reactive oxygen species as a result of lipid peroxidation has been implicated as a major secondary mechanism of SCI.[44] Although the administration of methylprednisolone and other glucocorticosteroids have some action in the inhibition of lipid peroxidation, research into more specific inhibitors, without the adverse reactions of glucocorticosteroids, has shown some promise. Lazaroids, such as tirilizad mesylate, has been shown to have some neuroprotective efficacy with fewer side effects.[31,45] The majority of work with these chemicals has been with regard to vascular injury in the brain, but there have been recent encouraging results in spinal injury patients as well.[31]

Additional compounds such as the immunosuppressive agent cyclosporin A[46] and EPC-K1, a phosphate diester linkage of vitamins E and C, have demonstrated efficacy as antioxidants in animal models of SCI.[47,48] Melatonin,[48] vitamin E, and edaravone, a novel free radical scavenger,[49] are additional compounds shown to have equal or superior efficacy

compared with methylprednisolone in early animal studies of spinal cord contusions, again without the local and systemic side effects of glucocorticosteroids. Further investigation is required to determine their clinical applicability in humans.

Excitotoxicity (Table 2.10)

A reproducible pathologic process in the acutely injured spinal cord is the swelling of neurons at the site of injury, presumably from an alteration of ion gradients across the cellular membrane as a result of inflammation and ischemia. These changes in membrane potential, coupled with cellular swelling, lead to a release of excitatory amino acids, namely, glutamate and aspartate. The effects of the release of excitatory amino acids is augmented by an impaired ability for reuptake by the damaged and ischemic cells, resulting in an extracellular increase in glutamate to toxic levels as early as 15 minutes after injury, with levels approaching eight times its normal extracellular concentration compared with normal tissue.[50,51]

In the brain, it has been shown that intracellular stores of glutamate reach 10 mmol/L, with extracellular concentrations of around 0.6 μmol/L.[52–54] Because excitotoxicity can occur with extracellular concentrations of as little as 2 to 5 μmol/L, the potential exists for significant local injury

Table 2.10 Excitotoxicity

- Changes in membrane potential, coupled with cellular swelling, lead to a release of excitatory amino acids, namely, glutamate and aspartate

- This release, combined with an impaired uptake, results in extracellular increase in glutamate to toxic levels

- At toxic levels of glutamate, the following occurs:
  - Massive influx of calcium into neurons
  - Dysregulation of many cellular processes
  - Inflammation
  - Cytotoxicity
  - Eventually, cell death

with the death of even a single neuron.[50] Presumably, the concentrations in the spinal cord are similar to those measured in the brain with the same potential for excitotoxicity.

Glutamate acts on the N-methyl-D-aspartate (NMDA), alpha-amino-3-hydroxy-5-methyl-4-isoxazole-propionic acid (AMPA), and kainite receptors on the spinal cord cell surfaces. The NMDA receptor regulates calcium flux across the cell membrane, whereas the AMPA and kainite receptors mediate sodium influx. At toxic levels of glutamate, there is a massive influx of calcium into the neurons, causing a dysregulation of many cellular processes, as well as inflammation and cytotoxicity, resulting in eventual cell death.[50] Investigations using antagonists against NMDA receptors, such as MK-801[55,56] and gacyclidine,[57] and inhibitors against AMPA receptors, such as NBQX,[58] have shown improvements in functional outcomes in animal spinal cord contusion models.

Kallikrein (Table 2.11)

Kallikrein 6 (K6) is a member of the kallikrein gene family. The family compromises 15 structurally and functionally related serine proteases. This enzyme is expressed in neurons and oligodendroglia in the adult central nervous system and is also upregulated at sites of SCI. It is hypothesized that K6 may be a key contributor in the pathophysiology of traumatic SCI influencing neural repair and regeneration. Scarisbrick et al[59] have shown that in cases of human traumatic SCI, significant increased levels were identified at acute and chronic time frames after the injury. Furthermore, increased K6 levels were identified not only at the injury site, but also at segments above and below. The authors also investigated the potential effects of K6 on neural regeneration by exposing recombinant K6 to laminin, a growth-facilitatory substrate. K6 mediated proteolytic digestion of the growth enzyme, significantly decreasing neurite outgrowth. In contrast, K6 exposure produced hydrolysis of aggrecan, a growth inhibitory substrate, significantly increasing neurite extension. The authors concluded that K6 may influence enzymatic activities involved in secondary SCI, especially axonal outgrowth.

Table 2.11 Kallikrein

- Kallikrein 6 (K6): member of the kallikrein gene family
- May be a key contributor in the pathophysiology of traumatic SCI, influencing neural repair and regeneration
- Significantly increased levels in acute and chronic injury
- Increased levels found not only at injury site, but also at segments above and below
- Scarisbrick et al[59] concluded that K6 may influence enzymatic activities involved in secondary SCI, especially axonal outgrowth

Table 2.12 EphA7

- Eph receptor protein tyrosine kinase family and its ligands, the ephrins, have been identified in axonal outgrowth, synapse formation, and target recognition
- A recent study demonstrated increased expression of EphA7 1 week post-SCI[60]
- The study concluded that EphA7 receptors in early stages of SCI pathophysiology (first week) may play a significant role[60]

EphA7 (Table 2.12)

Functional impairment following SCI is partially attributed to neuronal cell death. Further degeneration is seen with apoptosis of central nervous system myelin-forming oligodendrocytes. The Eph receptor protein tyrosine kinase family and its ligands, the ephrins, have been identified in axonal outgrowth, synapse formation, and target recognition. A recent study investigated the effects of EphA7 after SCI.[60] The authors demonstrated an increase in the expression of EphA7 1 week postinjury. Receptor immunoreactivity was most prevalent in astrocytes of the white matter in the center of the injury. Furthermore, blocking the expression of EphA7 after SCI resulted in significant acceleration of hindlimb locomotor recovery at 1 week in treated animals, but at 2 weeks there was no difference as compared with controls. The authors concluded that EphA7 receptors in the early stages of SCI pathophysiology (first week) may play a functional role.

Nitric Oxide Synthase Inhibitor (Table 2.13)

The positive effects of nitric oxide synthase on neuronal survival are well known. Its effect on regeneration of neuronal tissue is now being explored. A recent study investigated the role of nitric oxide synthase on injured motoneurons in rats.[61] The investigators avulsed a ventral motor root from the spinal cord and transplanted a section of peripheral nerve directly into the spinal cord. The results showed that the rats treated with nitric oxide synthase inhibitor reduced the number regenerating motoneurons to 50% at 2 and 4 weeks as compared with sham controls. Only the total number of motoneurons regenerating was reduced as the rate of axonal regeneration of the existing motoneurons was not affected. The

Table 2.13 Nitric Oxide Synthase Inhibitor

- Positive effects of nitric oxide synthase on neuronal survival are well known
- Effect on regeneration of neuronal tissue being explored
- A recent study concluded that nitric oxide synthase is potentially beneficial to the amount of axonal regeneration in injured spinal cord motoneurons[61]

Table 2.14 Inducible Nitric Oxide Synthase (iNOS)

- One of three isoforms of nitric oxide synthase producing nitric oxide
- iNOS producing increased amounts of nitric oxide has been found to be a major contributor in initiation and promotion of inflammatory reactions following SCI
- On the other hand, complete removal of iNOS and the formation of nitric oxide can be more detrimental than protective
- The extracellular environment in which nitric oxide is produced determines whether it is detrimental of advantageous

authors concluded that nitric oxide synthase is potentially beneficial to the amount of axonal regeneration in injured spinal cord motoneurons.[61]

Inducible Nitric Oxide Synthase (iNOS) (Table 2.14)

Inducible nitric oxide synthase (iNOS) is one of three isoforms of nitric oxide synthase producing nitric oxide. Inducible nitric oxide synthase producing increased amounts of nitric oxide has been found to be a major contributor in the initiation and promotion of inflammatory reactions following an SCI. Therefore, iNOS and nitric oxide generation has become a therapeutic target in SCI patients. In contrast, it has been shown that the complete removal of iNOS and the formation of nitric oxide can be more detrimental than protective. Additionally, it is now believed that the cellular environment in which nitric oxide is produced determines whether it is detrimental or advantageous. This dilemma makes therapeutic interventions targeted against the formation of nitric oxide with iNOS a bit more complicated. Investigators are now trying to produce a pharmacologic strategy (nitric oxide synthase inhibitor) that, it is hoped, will produce a delicate therapeutic balance and therefore allow the production of a physiologic amount of nitric oxide.[62]

Olfactory Ensheathing Cells (Table 2.15)

Olfactory ensheathing cells (OECs) have been a recent area of intense interest and study. The cells are located in the olfactory bulb of the nose, and the nerve cells act as a conduit between the peripheral nervous system and the central nervous system. It is this unique anatomical situation that has been the center of interest. The theory is that these cells can be transplanted at an SCI site, aiding axonal growth across the defect. Recently, Moon et al[63] reported on the transplantation of OECs following complete spinal cord transection in rats. The authors reported an induced recovery of hindlimb function 14 weeks postinjury in rats placed in motor enrichment housing, which encouraged

Table 2.15 Olfactory Ensheathing Cells (OECs)

- Hypothesis that OEC, located in the olfactory bulb of the nose, can be transplanted at an SCI site, aiding axonal growth across the defect
- Lima et al[64] concluded that olfactory mucosa autograft transplantation into complete human SCI sites was potentially beneficial

hindlimb exercise, as compared with rats placed in a basic housing. which did not.

Lima et al[64] reported on seven patients with transplanted olfactory mucosa autografts following a complete SCI. The olfactory mucosal grafts contain olfactory ensheathing and stemlike progenitor cells for neural repair. All patients were American Spinal Injury Association (ASIA) class A and were between 18 and 32 years of age. They underwent an olfactory mucosal autograft transplantation as early as 6 months and as late as 6.5 years after injury. The spinal cord lesions ranged from 1 to 6 cm in length and were present between the C4 and T6 spinal levels. Posttransplantation magnetic resonance imaging (MRI) studies revealed moderate to complete filling of the SCI defects. Two of the seven patients went from ASIA class A to class C, and every patient had improvement in ASIA motor scores. The authors concluded that olfactory mucosa autograft transplantation into complete human SCI sites was potentially beneficial.

Stat3/Socs3 (Table 2.16)

In the injured central nervous system, including the spinal cord, over time reactive astrocytes form a glial scar, which is thought to be detrimental to the reformation and regeneration of axonal growth. Some researchers theorize that astrocytes may play a more crucial positive role following SCI in wound healing and ultimately functional recovery. Okada et al,[65] using a mouse model, following an iatrogenic spinal cord contusion selectively deleted either a protein signal transducer and activator of transcription

Table 2.16 Stat3/Socs3

- Over time, reactive astrocytes form a scar that is thought to be detrimental to reformation and regeneration of axonal growth
- Astrocytes may play a more crucial positive role following SCI in wound healing and ultimately functional recovery
- Stat3: protein signal transducer and activator of transcription 3
- Socs3: protein suppressor of cytokine signaling 3
- Okada et al[65] concluded that Stat3 may be a target strategy for a positive intervention following SCI

Table 2.17 4-Chloro-3-Hydroxyanthranilate

- Secondary mechanisms following SCI involve inflammatory response
- One mechanism involves activation of neurotoxins by activated macrophages and microglia
- Recently researcher evaluated QUIN (neurotoxin quinolonic acid) in adult guinea pig model
- Administration of 4-chloro-3-hydroxyanthranilate (4CL-3HAA) initiated 5 hour after injury attenuated local amount of QUIN production by 50% with reduction in severity of secondary functional deficits
- Hartley et al concluded that QUIN contributes to secondary functional deficits and its reduction with 4CL-3HAA can lead to improved functional outcomes following acute SCI

3 (Stat3) or a protein suppressor of cytokine signaling 3 (Socs3). The mice selectively deleted for Stat3 (without activator) showed limited migration of astrocytes with increased infiltration of inflammatory cells, neural cell disruption, and axonal demyelination leading to severe motor deficits. In contrast, the Socs3 (without suppressor) mice showed rapid migration of reactive astrocytes, decreased inflammatory cells, a smaller contracted contusion area, and improvement of motor recovery and functional outcomes. The authors concluded that Stat3 may be a target strategy for a positive intervention following an SCI.

4-Chloro-3-Hydroxyanthranilate (Table 2.17)

It is well documented that secondary mechanisms following SCI involve an inflammatory response. One mechanism involves activation of neurotoxins by activated

macrophages and microglia. Recently, researchers evaluated the role of endogenous tryptophan metabolite and neurotoxin quinolinic acid (QUIN). In an adult Hartley guinea pig spinal cord contusion model, QUIN accumulated at the site of SCI. Furthermore, on postinjury day 12, the amount of QUIN that accumulated was proportional to the severity of the functional neurologic deficits. The administration of 4-chloro-3-hydroxyanthranilate (4Cl-3HAA) initiated 5 hours after iatrogenic injury attenuated the local amount of QUIN production at the site of injury by 50%, with a reduction in the severity of secondary functional deficits. The authors found that cross-sectional microscopic evaluation of the SCI site revealed a 100% increase in surviving white matter tracts (both axons and myelin) as compared with the untreated group. The authors concluded that QUIN contributes to secondary functional deficits and its reduction with 4Cl-3HAA can lead to improved functional outcomes following an acute SCI.[66]

■ Conclusion

Spinal cord injury can lead to devastating loss of function, resulting in paraplegia and quadriplegia. We are continually gaining knowledge in the pathophysiology of the secondary mechanisms of injury and are developing interventions to either promote or diminish various cascades. Presently, there are no ideal or restorative treatments for patients suffering an SCI. Numerous cellular, molecular, and rehabilitative strategies have been used in animal and human studies, with many of them reaching clinical trials. To date there is no one therapy in sight that appears to be a panacea, but a combination of strategies may soon lead to better long-term functional outcomes for different types of SCI.

References

1. Bareyre FM, Schwab ME. Inflammation, degeneration and regeneration in the injured spinal cord: insights from DNA microarrays. Trends Neurosci 2003;26:555–563
2. Emery E, Aldana P, Bunge MB, et al. Apoptosis after traumatic human spinal cord injury. J Neurosurg 1998;89:911–920
3. Li J, Baud O, Vartanian T, Volpe JJ, Rosenberg PA. Peroxynitrite generated by inducible nitric oxide synthase and NADPH oxidase mediates migroglial toxicity to oligodendrocytes. Proc Natl Acad Sci U S A 2005;102:9936–9941
4. McDonald JW, Belegu V. Demyelination and remyelination after spinal cord injury. J Neurotrauma 2006;23:345–359
5. Crowe MJ, Bresnahan JC, Shuman SL, et al. Apoptosis and delayed degeneration after spinal cord injury in rats and monkeys. Nat Med 1997;3:73–76
6. Grossman SD, Rosenberg LJ, Wrathall JR. Temporal-spatial pattern of acute neuronal and glial loss after spinal cord contusion. Exp Neurol 2001;168:273–282
7. Santos-Benito FF, Ramon-Cueto A. Olfactory ensheathing glia transplantation: a therapy to promote repair in the mammalian central nervous system. Anat Rec B New Anat 2003;271:77–85
8. Tuszynski MH, Weidner N, McCormack M, Miller I, Powell H, Conner J. Grafts of genetically modified Schwann cells to the spinal cord: survival, axon growth, and myelination. Cell Transplant 1998;7:187–196
9. Hagg T, Oudega M. Degenerative and spontaneous regenerative processes after spinal cord injury. J Neurotrauma 2006;23:264–280
10. Raineteau O, Fouad K, Bareyre FM, Schwab ME. Reorganization of descending motor tracts in the rat spinal cord. Eur J Neurosci 2002;16:1761–1771
11. Zagrebelsky M, Buffo A, Skerra A, Schwab ME, Strata P, Rossi F. Retrograde regulation of growth-associated gene expression in adult rat Purkinje cells by myelin-associated neurite growth inhibitory proteins. J Neurosci 1998;18:7912–7929
12. Finnerup NB, Jensen TS. Spinal cord injury pain-mechanisms and treatment. Eur J Neurol 2004;11:73–82

13. Karlsson AK. Autonomic dysreflexia. Spinal Cord 1999;37:383–391

14. Cohen JJ. Apoptosis. Immunol Today 1993;14:126–130

15. Emery E, Aldana P, Bunge MB, et al. Apoptosis after traumatic human spinal cord injury. J Neurosurg 1998;89:911–920

16. Casha S, Yu WR, Fehlings MG. Oligodendroglial apoptosis occurs along degenerating axons and is associated with FAS and p75 expression following spinal cord injury in the rat. Neuroscience 2001;103:203–218

17. Crowe MJ, Bresnahan JC, Shuman SL, Masters JN, Beattie MS. Apoptosis and delayed degeneration after spinal cord injury in rats and monkeys. Nat Med 1997;3:73–76

18. Springer JE, Azbill RD, Knapp PE. Activation of the caspase-3 apoptotic cascade in traumatic spinal cord injury. Nat Med 1999; 5:943–946

19. Shuman SL, Bresnahan JC, Beattie MS. Apoptosis of microglia and oligodendrocytes after spinal cord contusion in rats. J Neurosci Res 1997;50:798–808

20. Li GL, Farooque M, Holtz A, et al. Apoptosis of oligodendrocytes occurs for long distances away from the primary injury after compression trauma to rat spinal cord. Acta Neuropathol 1999;98:473–480

21. Sakurai M, Hayashi T, Abe K, et al. Delayed selective motor death and Fas antigen induction after spinal cord ischemia in rabbits. Brain Res 1998;797:23–28

22. Satake K, Matsuyama Y, Kamiya M, et al. Nitric oxide via macrophage iNOS induces apoptosis following traumatic spinal cord injury. Brain Res Mol Brain Res 2000;85:114–122

23. Li M, Ona VO, Chen M, et al. Functional role and therapeutic implications of neuronal caspase-1 and -3 in a mouse model of traumatic spinal cord injury. Neuroscience 2000;99:333–342

24. Citron BA, Arnold PM, Sebastian C, et al. Rapid upregulation of caspase-3 in rat spinal cord after injury: mRNA, protein, and cellular localization correlated with apoptotic cell death. Exp Neurol 2000;166:213–226

25. Anderson DK, Means ED, Waters TR, Green ES. Microvascular perfusion and metabolism in injured spinal cord after methylprednisolone treatment. J Neurosurg 1982;56:106–113

26. Hall ED, Braughler JM. Non-surgical management of spinal cord injuries: a review of studies with the glucocorticoid steroid methylprednisolone. Acta Anaesthesiol Belg 1987;38:405–409

27. Bracken MB. Methylprednisolone and acute spinal cord injury: an update of the randomized evidence. Spine 2001;26(suppl):S47–S54

28. Bracken MB, Shepard MJ, Collins WF Jr, et al. Methylprednisolone or naloxone treatment after acute spinal cord injury: 1-year follow-up data. Results of the second National Acute Spinal Cord Injury Study. J Neurosurg 1992;76:23–31

29. Bracken MB, Holford TR. Effects of timing of methylprednisolone or naloxone administration on recovery of segmental and long-tract neurological function in NASCIS 2. J Neurosurg 1993;79: 500–507

30. Bracken MB, Shepard MJ, Collins WF, et al. A randomized, controlled trial of methylprednisolone or naloxone in the treatment of acute spinal-cord injury. Results of the Second National Acute Spinal Cord Injury Study. N Engl J Med 1990;322:1405–1411

31. Bracken MB, Shepard MJ, Holford TR, et al. Administration of methylprednisolone for 24 or 48 hours or tirilazad mesylate for 48 hours in the treatment of acute spinal cord injury. Results of the Third National Acute Spinal Cord Injury Randomized Controlled Trial. JAMA 1997;277: 1597–1604

32. Maihofner C, Tegeder I, Euchenhofer C, et al. Localization and regulation of cyclo-oxygenase-1 and -2 and neuronal nitric oxide synthase in mouse spinal cord. Neuroscience 2000;101:1093–1108

33. Hoffmann C. COX-2 in brain and spinal cord implications for therapeutic use. Curr Med Chem 2000;7:1113–1120

34. Resnick DK, Graham SH, Dixon CE, Marion DW. Role of cyclooxygenase 2 in acute spinal cord injury. J Neurotrauma 1998;15: 1005–1013

35. Lapchak PA, Araujo DM, Song D, Zivin JA. Neuroprotection by the selective cyclooxygenase-2 inhibitor SC-236 results in improvements in behavioral deficits induced by reversible spinal cord ischemia. Stroke 2001;32:1220–1225

36. Hains BC, Yucra JA, Hulsebosch CE. Reduction of pathological and behavioral deficits following spinal cord contusion injury with the selective cyclooxygenase-2 inhibitor NS-398. J Neurotrauma 2001;18:409–423

37. Wamil AW, Wamil BD, Hellerqvist CG. CM101-mediated recovery of walking ability in adult mice paralyzed by spinal cord injury. Proc Natl Acad Sci U S A 1998;95:13188–13193

38. Takami T, Oudega M, Bethea JR, Wood PM, Kleitman N, Bunge MB. Methylprednisolone and interleukin-10 reduce gray matter damage in the contused Fischer rat thoracic spinal cord but do not improve functional outcome. J Neurotrauma 2002;19:653–666

39. Bethea JR, Nagashima H, Acosta MC, et al. Systemically administered interleukin-10 reduces tumor necrosis factor-alpha production and significantly improves functional recovery following traumatic spinal cord injury in rats. J Neurotrauma 1999;16:851–863

40. Clifton GL, Miller ER, Choi SC, et al. Hypothermia on admission in patients with severe brain injury. J Neurotrauma 2002;19:293–301

41. Clifton GL, Choi SC, Miller ER, et al. Intercenter variance in clinical trials of head trauma—experience of the National Acute Brain Injury Study: Hypothermia. J Neurosurg 2001;95:751–755

42. Hansebout RR, Tanner JA, Romero-Sierra C. Current status of spinal cord cooling in the treatment of acute spinal cord injury. Spine 1984;9:508–511

43. Hayes KC, Hsieh JT, Potter PJ, Wolfe DL, Delaney GA, Blight AR. Effects of induced hypothermia on somatosensory evoked potentials in patients with chronic spinal cord injury. Paraplegia 1993;31:730–741

44. Barut S, Canbolat A, Bilge T, et al. Lipid peroxidation in experimental spinal cord injury: time-level relationship. Neurosurg Rev 1993;16:53–59

45. Clark WM, Hazel JS, Coull BM. Lazaroids, CNS pharmacology and current research. Drugs 1995;50:971–983

46. Diaz-Ruiz A, Rios C, Duarte I, et al. Lipid peroxidation inhibition in spinal cord injury: cyclosporin-A vs methylprednisolone. Neuroreport 2000;11:1765–1767

47. Iwasa K, Fukuzawa K, Ikata T. Protective effect of vitamin E on spinal cord injury by compression and concurrent lipid peroxidation. Free Radic Biol Med 1989;6:599–606

48. Fujimoto T, Nakamura T, Ikeda T, Taoka Y, Takagi K. Effects of EPC-K1 on lipid peroxidation in experimental spinal cord injury. Spine 2000;25:24–29

49. Ohta S, Iwashita Y, Takada H, Kuno S, Nakamura T. Neuroprotection and enhanced recovery with edaravone after acute spinal cord injury in rats. Spine 2005;30:1154–1158

50. Lipton SA, Rosenberg PA. Excitatory amino acids as a final common pathway for neurologic disorders. N Engl J Med 1994;330:613–622

51. Choi DW. Glutamate neurotoxicity and diseases of the nervous system. Neuron 1988;1:623–634

52. Kvamme E, Schousboe A, Hertz L, Torgner IA, Svenneby G. Developmental change of endogenous glutamate and gamma-glutamyl transferase in cultured cerebral cortical interneurons and cerebellar granule cells, and in mouse cerebral cortex and cerebellum in vivo. Neurochem Res 1985;10:993–1008

53. Bouvier M, Szatkowski M, Amato A, Attwell D. The glial cell gluta-mate uptake carrier countertransports pH-changing anions. Nature 1992;360:471–474

54. Benveniste H, Drejer J, Schousboe A, Diemer NH. Elevation of the extracellular concentrations of glutamate and aspartate in rat hippocampus during transient cerebral ischemia monitored by intracerebral microdialysis. J Neurochem 1984;43: 1369–1374

55. Faden AI, Lemke M, Simon RP, Noble LJ. N-methyl-D-aspartate an-tagonist MK801 improves outcome following traumatic spinal cord injury in rats: behavioral, anatomic, and neurochemical studies. J Neurotrauma 1988;5:33–45

56. Wada S, Yone K, Ishidou Y, et al. Apoptosis following spinal cord injury in rats and preventative effect of N-methyl-D-aspartate receptor antagonist. J Neurosurg 1999;91(suppl):98–104

57. Gaviria M, Privat A, d'Arbigny P, Kamenka J, Haton H, Ohanna F. Neuroprotective effects of a novel NMDA antagonist, gacyclidine, after experimental contusive spinal cord injury in adult rats. Brain Res 2000;874:200–209

58. Wrathall JR, Teng YD, Choiniere D. Amelioration of functional deficits from spinal cord trauma with systemically administered NBQX, an antagonist of non-N-methyl-D-aspartate receptors. Exp Neurol 1996;137:119–126

59. Scarisbrick IA, Sabharwal P, Cruz H, et al. Dynamic role of kallil-rein 6 in traumatic spinal cord injury. Eur J Neurosci 2006;24: 1457–1469

60. Figueroa JD, Benton RL, Velazquez I, et al. EphA7 up-regulation af-ter spinal cord injury reduces apoptosis and promotes locomotor recovery. J Neurosci Res 2006;84:1438–1451

61. Chu TH, Wu WT. Nitric oxide synthase inhibitor attenuates number of regenerating spinal motorneurons in adult rats. Neuroreport 2006;17:969–973

62. Pannu R, Singh I. Pharmacological strategies for the regulation of inducible nitric oxide synthase: neurodegenerative versus neuro-protective mechanisms. Neurochem Int 2006;49:170–182

63. Moon LD, Leasure JL, Gage FH, Bunge MB. Motor enrichment sustains hindlimb movement recovered after spinal cord injury and glial transplantation. Restor Neurol Neurosci 2006;24: 147–161

64. Lima C, Pratas-Vital J, Escada P, et al. Olfactory mucosa autografts in human spinal cord injury: a pilot clinical study. J Spinal Cord Med 2006;29:191–203

65. Okada S, Nakamura M, Katoh H, et al. Conditional ablation of Stat3 or Socs3 discloses a dual role for reactive astrocytes after spinal cord injury. Nat Med 2006;12:829–834

66. Yates JR, Heyes MP, Blight AR. 4-chloro-3-hydroxyanthranilate reduces local quinolinic acid synthesis, improves functional recovery, and preserves white matter after spinal cord injury. J Neurotrauma 2006;23:866–881

3 Spinal Cord Regeneration

Charles H. Tator

There are two broad categories of strategies to promote repair of the injured spinal cord: neuroprotection and regeneration (**Table 3.1**). To date, neuroprotection has not produced major recovery after spinal cord injury (SCI); treatment with agents such as steroids or antiinflammatory agents has been disappointing, especially for injuries of major severity, such as American Spinal Injury Association (ASIA) grade A injuries, with complete absence of voluntary motor function and sensation below the level of the injury. Even for less severe injuries, neurologic improvement in patients treated with neuroprotective agents has been minimal[1] and not without controversy.[2] Ideally, clinicians would like to have a variety of effective neuroprotective agents to counteract the many secondary injury mechanisms that are known to cause progressive damage to the injured spinal cord. Furthermore, it would be highly desirable to have effective neuroprotective strategies for patients with injuries of all severities. The secondary injury mechanisms that require treatment include ischemia, inflammation, excitotoxicity, major electrolyte shifts, and apoptosis. Patients with less severe injuries would benefit if these agents prevented further damage to the spinal cord, and patients with the most severe injuries would benefit from limiting the extent of the damage.

The pathologic effects of acute SCI spread centrifugally in all directions to cause ventral-dorsal, lateral, and rostrocaudal damage.[3] Ideally, effective neuroprotective agents would limit the pathologic spread and shorten the distance that regenerating axons would have to travel rostrocaudally in the cord. It is well known that the end result of this cascade of pathophysiologic events is major necrosis and cavitation, a process that has been termed posttraumatic infarction of the cord.[3,4] The cavity that forms can be up to several centimeters long rostrocaudally, and thus large portions of spinal cord tissue would have to be replaced by actual ingrowths from the stumps or replacement by transplantation to improve function. In general, it is highly likely that improvement of neurologic recovery after major cord injuries would require a combination of regenerative strategies designed to produce regeneration or replacement of lost tissue. The regenerative strategy that is most likely to be successful is transplantation of cells or tissues, but it is unlikely that this will be sufficient. The goal of functional recovery will require a combination of strategies that include neurotrophic factors and agents to minimize scarring and to counteract endogenous inhibitors that are known to be plentiful in the injured cord.[1] Also, combination therapy must include attention to rehabilitative measures such as gravity-assisted ambulation, and some of these rehabilitative measures have proven effectiveness.[5,6]

■ The Treatment Window at Various Stages of Spinal Cord Injury

Neuroprotective strategies such as surgical decompression, are designed to counteract the secondary mechanisms of injury. Each strategy has a specific time course and therapeutic window for effectiveness.[7] It is also apparent from experimental studies that regenerative strategies are subject to therapeutic time windows. For example, the acutely injured spinal cord is less amenable to the survival of transplanted cells. There is greater survival of transplanted cells in the subacute stage.[8–11] However, the chronic stage may be the most difficult with respect to

Table 3.1 Two Categories of Strategies Promoting Spinal Cord Repair

Neuroprotection	• Has not produced major recovery after spinal cord injury (SCI)
	• Includes treatments involving agents such as steroids or antiinflammatory agents
	• Ideally, future use may protect patient from secondary injury such as ischemia, inflammation, excitotoxicity, electrolyte shifts, and apoptosis and prevent necrosis and cavitation
	• Agents limit pathologic spread of injury and shorten distance for regenerating axons
Regeneration	• Likely that regeneration is needed for improvement in neurologic recovery
	• Strategy with greater chance of success is the transplantation of cells or tissues
	• Combination of strategies likely to be required

Table 3.2 Specific Mechanisms to Enhance Regeneration after Spinal Cord Injury

Promotion of endogenous regeneration	Includes:
	• Regeneration of axons
	• Collateral sprouting of axons
	• Renewal of astrocytic or oligodendrocytic cells
	• Blood vessels by angiogenesis
	• Neuronal somata
Regeneration by replacement with transplantation	Includes:
	• Oligodendrocytes or Schwann cells for myelination
	• Astrocytes for axonal guidance
	• Neurons to act as "relay stations"
	• Synthetic channels for axonal guidance and prevention of scarring
	• Hematopoietic cells
	• Microglia/macrophages

improving neurologic function because of the long distances that axons would have to regenerate. For example, axons continue to die back for several months after SCI. Also, the classic view is that the astrocytic scarring that develops progressively in the subacute and chronic stages will hinder axonal regeneration, although this is still controversial.

■ Types of Regeneration

There are a two main types of regeneration that can be accomplished (**Table 3.2**). The first depends on regrowth of endogenous cells, and here there are many cell types that need to be considered. The more severe the lesion, the greater the number of cell types that will have to be regrown to accomplish restoration of function. For example, with mild lesions, regeneration of axons or sprouting of collaterals may suffice, whereas more severe lesions may require regeneration of axons, glia, and blood vessels. Regeneration of neuronal cell bodies is possible, but it is extremely unlikely that they would establish useful functional relationships. Similar considerations relate to the specific aims of regeneration, as indicated in **Table 3.3**. It may be feasible to devise strategies to replace several cell types, and this may be possible with stem/progenitor cell transplantation.

With respect to axonal regeneration and collateral sprouting, there are several anatomical sites where this can occur, as shown in **Fig. 3.1**. Axonal regeneration is defined as occurring from the injured axon itself, either from the damaged end or from a more proximal location on the damaged axon. In contrast, collateral sprouting occurs from an undamaged axon, possibly a neighboring axon in the same tract or from an axon in a different tract. The collateral may grow at the injury site or from a remote site. As well, a new neuron at the origin of the tract in the cerebral cortex or brainstem may give rise to a replacement axon.

■ Aims of the Regenerative Strategies

The necrotic tissue or cavity left behind after acute and subacute/chronic injuries, respectively, have to be replaced with functioning living tissue, and there are many strategies

Table 3.3 Aims of Regenerative Strategies

Regrowth of surviving stumps	• Axonal regeneration: regrowth from damaged axon (axonal regeneration is more difficult but may result in more accurate functional connections)
	• Sprouting: regrowth from a nearby intact axon
Revascularization of restored tissue	• Prevent ischemia
	• Use of fibroblast growth factor-1 (FGF-1)

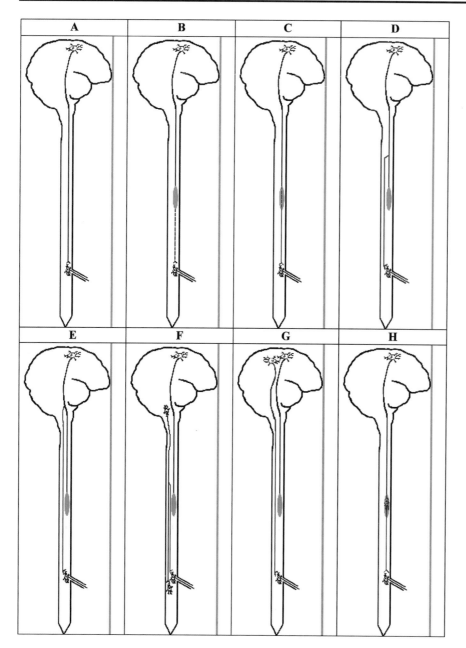

Fig. 3.1 Types of regeneration and regrowth after spinal cord injury (SCI), which may involve regeneration from the original damaged axon, at or remote from the injury site, or from another neuronal soma at the origin of the tract in the cerebral cortex or brainstem. In contrast, collateral sprouting is from a neighboring undamaged axon at or remote from the injury site. **(A)** Normal brain and spinal cord showing an axon from the corticospinal tract synapsing with an anterior horn cell in the lumbar cord. **(B)** Thoracic spinal cord injury (shaded area) has completely interrupted the axon, which then shows caudal wallerian degeneration. **(C)** Axonal regeneration from the original damaged axon. **(D)** Axonal regeneration from a rostral segment of the originally damaged axon in the thoracic cord. **(E)** Axonal regeneration from a proximal segment in the brainstem of the originally damaged axon. **(F)** Collateral sprouting from an adjacent undamaged axon of another tract, such as the rubrospinal tract, which then grows caudally to synapse with the original denervated anterior horn cell. **(G)** Collateral sprouting from an adjacent neuron in the cerebral cortex giving rise to an axon of the corticospinal tract, which then regenerates to synapse with the original denervated anterior horn cell. **(H)** Transplantation of a neuron into the injury site, which then gives rise to an axon that synapses with the original denervated anterior horn cell.

that have been designed in an attempt to accomplish this. Regrowth of tissue from the surviving stumps has been attempted in a variety of ways (**Table 3.3**). One such way is the promotion of axonal regeneration, which is described as regrowth from the stump of the original transected or otherwise damaged axon. This can be contrasted with sprouting, which is classified as regrowth of an axon from a nearby intact axon. The former is much more difficult to accomplish but might result in more accurate functional improvement. After very severe injuries that transect all the axons present at the site of injury, regeneration from transected axons and transplantation are the only ways to regenerate axons. Regrowth of the supporting tissue including astrocytes and oligodendrocytes would be possible from the stumps, although these cells do not appear to be very mobile, and even if they multiplied in the stumps, as astrocytes are known to do, it is unlikely that they could migrate the long distances necessary to bridge the two stumps. Thus, restoration of glial tissue may have constraints similar to axons, in that replacement by transplantation may be necessary to bridge the large cavities after major SCI.

It is also necessary to consider revascularization of the restored tissue because SCI causes major ischemia of the injured segment, and therefore it would be highly desirable to be able to stimulate regrowth of the vasculature in the area of injury (**Table 3.3**). Some agents, such as fibroblast growth factor-1 (FGF-1), promote angiogenesis. Other older, unproven strategies such as omental transplantation to restore blood supply[12] are not reviewed in detail here.

■ Overview and Classification of the Types of Regenerative Strategies for Spinal Cord Injury

Table 3.4 shows the broad variety of focused regenerative strategies that have been studied in experimental models of SCI. Many of these strategies have also been tried in

Table 3.4 Classification of Types of Regenerative Strategies

Neurotrophic factors	• Nerve growth factor (NGF)
	• Brain-derived growth factor (BDGF)
	• Neurotrophin 3 (NT-3)
	• Fibroblast growth factor-1 or -2 (FGF-1 or -2)
	• Epidermal growth factor (EGF)
	• Many others
Matrices and scaffolds	• Collagen
	• Matrigel
	• Millipore
	• Synthetic materials (hydrogels, polyesters)
	• Natural materials (chitosan)
Neuronal/axonal growth stimulation	• Cyclic adenosine monophosphate
	• Gangliosides
	• Inosine
Cell and tissue transplantation	• Spinal cord segments
	• Peripheral nerve grafts
	• Schwann cells
	• Macrophages
	• Porcine stem cells
	• Blood stem cells
	• Bone marrow stromal stem cells
	• Umbilical cord/blood stem cells
	• Olfactory ensheathing glia or bulb stem cells
	• Human embryonic stem cells
	• Many others
Stimulation of endogenous stem cells	• Growth factors
	• Erythropoietin

(Continued on page 32)

Table 3.4 *(Continued)* **Classification of Types of Regenerative Strategies**

Electrical stimulation	• Direct current fields
	• Alternating current
Reduction of scarring	• Enzymes (chondroitinase ABC)
Manipulation of extracellular matrix	• Tenascin
	• Many others
Neutralization of inhibitors	• Immunotherapy with antibodies
	• Anti-Nogo antibodies
	• Nogo receptor antagonists
	• Rho inhibition
Fusion molecules	• Polyethylene glycol
Manipulation of signaling molecules	• Ephrins
	• Semaphorins
Rehabilitation strategies	• Exercise
	• Functional electrical stimulation (FES)
	• Gravity-assisted ambulation
Immunomodulation	• Immunization
	• Macrophages

patients, including neurotrophic factors, cell and tissue transplantation, electrical stimulation, and neutralization of inhibitors. Most of the studies in experimental models of SCI have been in the acute and subacute stages, although some also have been in the chronic stage. The studies in patients have been mainly in the subacute and chronic stages and have mostly been phase 1 trials. There have been several comprehensive reviews of the experimental strategies[8,13–15] and several reviews of the clinical strategies.[1,16–18] Most of the recent clinical trials of regeneration have been phase 1 trials of the transplantation of cells or tissues involving patients in the subacute and chronic stages of SCI. Unfortunately, very few of these trials have been published in peer-review journals and are not available in any other format in the public domain. Issues regarding design of cell transplantation trials for central nervous system (CNS) diseases in general have been critically reviewed by Cesaro[19] and commented on by Sagen.[14] The need for great care in translation is evident from the study of Hofstetter et al,[20] who showed allodynia-like hypersensitivity of the forepaws due to aberrant axonal sprouting in rats after transplantation of adult neural stem cells into the injured thoracic spinal cord. Furthermore, Dobkin et al[21] recently issued a warning about poor trial design, complications, and lack of effectiveness of transplanted olfactory ensheathing glia (OEG) cells in seven patients treated in one very active transplant center. The present chapter provides the experimental background

for 25 main strategies and a brief description of any clinical trials of specific strategies.

Space does not permit detailed description of some of the other strategies listed in **Table 3.4**.

Neurotrophic and Growth Factors (Table 3.5)

Neurotrophic and growth factors have been major strategies in experimental SCI.[22,23] Many of these agents have produced remarkable growths of proliferating glial, fibrous, and Schwann cells. In our laboratory, direct injection of brain-derived neurotrophic factor (BDNF) produced the most remarkable proliferation of cells at the injury site, with virtually complete disappearance of the cavitation.[24] To date, these agents have not been used in SCI patients, except for the Cheng et al[25] application of FGF-1 in patients in whom peripheral nerve grafts were transplanted into the spinal cord. However, two of these agents have been used in patients with amyotrophic lateral sclerosis (ALS). Ciliary neurotrophic factor (CNTF) was delivered intrathecally through an indwelling catheter attached to a pump in a phase 1 trial in four patients with ALS. There was no improvement, but there were complications and side effects.[26] An initial study with BDNF delivered subcutaneously in ALS patients was not beneficial, and the subsequent trial of BDNF by intrathecal catheter and pump was a phase 3 randomized prospective controlled trial organized by Amgen,[27] but the final result has not been reported.

Table 3.5 Neurotrophic and Growth Factors

Brain-derived neurotrophic factor (BDNF)	• Produced the most remarkable cell proliferation at site of injury
	• Virtually complete disappearance of cavitation
	• To date, not used in SCI patients (except FGF-1 in Cheng study)
	• Used in amyotrophic lateral sclerosis (ALS) patients; delivered subcutaneously and no benefits seen
Ciliary neurotrophic factor (CNTF)	• Used in ALS patients
	• Delivered intrathecally via catheter
	• No improvement; complications and side effects present

Note: These factors have been major strategies in experimental SCI and have shown growth of glia, fibroblastic, and Schwann cells.

Manipulation of Endogenous Spinal Cord Stem Cells (Table 3.6)

The use of endogenous stem cells for regeneration of the spinal cord after SCI is a highly attractive method for enhancing regeneration of the spinal cord that theoretically could result in the regrowth of new glial cells and new neurons. This strategy is based on the relatively recent discovery by Reynolds and Weiss[28] in 1996, which noted the presence of endogenous stem cells in the adult mammalian spinal cord. This has now been confirmed in several laboratories, including mine, and has led to extensive experimentation on methods of stimulating these stem cells to proliferate, differentiate, and migrate into the injured area after SCI. One of the major problems is that the most multipotential cells are located in the ependyma region around the central canal, whereas those located in the parenchyma of the cord are progenitors with less potential.[29] Central hemorrhagic necrosis and posttraumatic infarction are cardinal features of the pathology of acute SCI and cause the destruction of the stem cells at the epicenter of the lesion and rostrocaudally for a considerable distance.[3,30] Most of the efforts to enhance the proliferation and migration of endogenous stem cells have been with growth factors such as epidermal growth factor (EGF) and FGF-2 and have been successful in increasing the proliferation of these cells but have resulted in only minimal improvement in functional recovery in experimental SCI.[29] There have also been efforts to enhance survival of these endogenous stem cells after injury, but mainly in brain injury.[31]

GM$_1$ Ganglioside (Table 3.7)

GM$_1$ ganglioside is present in neuronal membranes and was studied extensively in animal models of SCI and CNS ischemia, as reviewed by Geisler et al.[32] It is of interest that this agent also has neuroprotective effects. After an initial positive result in a small series of patients, a subsequent multicenter randomized prospective control trial in approximately 800 patients failed to show an overall significantly improved neurologic recovery, although the authors pointed to some improvement in the ASIA grade B incomplete injuries.[33,34] This was a landmark study and provided a great deal of useful information about the epidemiology and natural history of neurologic recovery in patients with SCI.

Transplantation of Whole Spinal Cord Segments (Table 3.8)

Reier et al[35] pioneered the implantation of fetal spinal cord in experimental SCI, and there have been some remarkable examples of the potential for this method in experimental studies. One of the best examples was produced by Iwashita et al,[36] who transplanted fetal spinal

Table 3.6 Endogenous Stem Cell Usage for Regeneration

Logic	Theoretically, can enhance regrowth of glial cells and new neurons, as precursors of these stem cells (progenitors) were discovered in adult mammalian spinal cord
Problems	Multipotential cells are located in ependyma regions around central canal (those in parenchyma of cord have less potential); necrosis and infarction associated with SCI will kill these cells at injury site, with some spread rostrocaudally
Growth factors	EGF and FGF-2 have been used successfully to increase proliferation of stem cells; however, functional recovery minimal

Table 3.7 GM₁ Ganglioside in Regeneration

Logic	• May be useful as it is located in neuronal membranes
	• May have neuroprotective effects as well
Geisler et al's randomized prospective controlled trial (RPCT)	• No overall improvement in neurologic recovery
	• Some improvements in ASIA grade B, incomplete SCI patients
Relevance	This study provided information on epidemiology and natural history of neurorecovery in SCI patients

cord into the completely transected spinal cord of newborn rats and showed impressive fusion of the transplant with the adjacent spinal cord stumps and excellent neurologic recovery. Patients with syringomyelia in Sweden[37] and the United States[38] were treated with implants of human fetal spinal cord in an attempt to obliterate the cavities and stop the progression of neurologic deterioration. It appears that the procedure can be performed without major complications, but the survival of the grafts and long-term benefit have not been proven.

Transplantation of Autologous Activated Macrophages (Table 3.9)

Schwartz et al[39] in Israel studied the effect of transplanting into spinal cords, and found homologous macrophages from the peripheral blood that had been incubated with peripheral nerves and found improved recovery in rats with experimental SCI. In a phase 1 trial in patients, autologous activated macrophages prepared from the peripheral blood of patients with SCI were incubated in tissue culture conditions in the presence of autologous skin, then injected at surgery into the injured spinal cord just caudal to the epicenter of the injury within 14 days of injury. Three of eight ASIA grade A thoracic cases showed improved neurologic recovery to ASIA grade C,[40] and a second publica-

tion about this strategy in 2005 reported that 5 of 14 patients treated had neurologic improvement.[41] A further trial is in progress.

Peripheral Nerve Grafts (Table 3.10)

Several clinical applications of peripheral nerve grafts have been reported based on the initial animal experiments of Richardson et al's group.[42] Cheng et al[43] then showed remarkable recovery in rats after complete transection of the thoracic spinal cord. In Olson's laboratory in Sweden, this group inserted peripheral nerves and FGF-1 in fibrin glue to bridge from white to gray matter.[43] Cheng et al[25] then applied this strategy to a patient in Taiwan with a chronic SCI from a stab wound at 4 years after injury and reported recovery of neurologic function; other patients have also been treated with this strategy in Taiwan (Cheng, personal communication). Peripheral nerve grafts have also been used in eight patients from Brazil without apparent benefit.[44] In one patient, Brunelli and von Wild[45,46] in Italy inserted autologous sciatic nerves into the corticospinal tract of the spinal cord rostral to the injury site and then anastomosed them to the femoral nerves to restore quadriceps function and directly to the gluteus muscles several months after injury; then reported improvement. Tadie et al[47] in France reported a

Table 3.8 Fetal Spinal Cord Implantation Method for Regeneration

Washita et al study	• Transplanted fetal spinal cord into completely transected stem cells of infant rats
	• Results:
	1. Fusion with adjacent stumps
	2. Excellent neurorecovery
Treatment for syringomyelia	• Goal: obliterate cavities and halt neurologic deterioration with transplants of human fetal spinal cord
	• Results:
	1. Procedure done without complications
	2. Survival of grafts and long-term benefits not yet proven

Table 3.9 Autologous Activated Macrophages in Regeneration

Autologous activated macrophages	• Autologous macrophages from peripheral blood, incubated with peripheral nerves of skin
Phase I trial (phase 2 trial started and then discontinued)	• Autologous macrophages injected caudal to injury site within 14 days of injury
	• Results:
	1. Three of eight ASIA grade A thoracic cases showed improved neurologic recovery
	2. Five of 14 (in another publication) patients had neurologic improvements

similar case in which peripheral nerve grafts bridged from the cord rostral to the injury site to the L2-L4 spinal roots. Several years earlier, Carlstedt et al[48] in Sweden reported recovery of upper limb function after brachial plexus injuries treated with implantation of the avulsed nerve roots directly into the spinal cord. In 10 patients with root reinsertion from 10 days to 9 months after injury, the results were beneficial in at least three cases. Thus, there is some evidence that peripheral nerve bridging is worth pursuing.

Transplantation of Bone Marrow Stem Cells (Table 3.11)

Whole bone marrow contains a mixture of hematopoietic cells, various mononuclear cells such as macrophages, and marrow stromal cells. The initial reports in animal studies showed that populations of bone marrow–derived stem cells showed neuronal and glial differentiation and improved neurologic recovery after transplantation into the injury site after SCI.[49] These studies generated a large number of other animal trials in experimental SCI models,[50] and now also in patients in several countries. The major attractions of this strategy are the ease of obtaining autologous tissue for transplantation and the possibility that bone marrow cells have a "homing instinct" so that they may be effective after administration remote from the injury site, through either intravascular or intrathecal routes. In 2005, Park et al[51] in South Korea reported that whole

bone marrow transplantation into the injury site produced improvement in ASIA grades in all five patients in a phase 1 trial who received whole bone marrow transplants into the injured spinal cord within 7 to 14 days of injury. All five patients also received intravenous injections of granulocyte-macrophage colony-stimulating factor (GM-CSF), whereas a sixth patient who also recovered received only the latter. There are other trials of this strategy in China, the Czech Republic, and Russia, as noted in my recent review.[1]

Transplantation of Peripheral Blood Stem Cells (Table 3.11)

For reasons similar to those underlying the use of bone marrow–derived stem cells, peripheral blood–derived stem cells have been used in patients with spinal cord diseases. Janson et al[52] reported a trial of intrathecal administration in patients with ALS, but there were few details. There are also unreported trials of this strategy in Brazil and Russia.

Umbilical Cord Stem Cells (Table 3.11)

Currently, homologous umbilical cord blood stem cells are being transplanted into patients with chronic SCI in China. The transplantations are performed intravenously, intrathecally, or directly into the spinal cord. There are some published trials of the use of human umbilical cord

Table 3.10 Peripheral Nerve Graft Studies

Cheng et al[43]	• Inserted peripheral nerves and FGF-1 in fibrin glue, bridging white to gray matter in rats with neurorecovery
	• Neurologic recovery after stab wound in one patient with peripheral nerve grafts into cord
Barros et al[44]	• Nerve grafts into spinal cord showed no benefits
Brunelli and von Wild	• Autologous sciatic nerve inserted in corticospinal tract and anastomosed to femoral nerve and gluteus muscles; showed improved muscle function
Tadie et al[47]	• Peripheral nerve graft bridging from spinal cord rostral to injury to L2-L4 roots; improved muscle function
Carlstedt et al[48]	• Implantation of avulsed nerve roots directly into spinal cord; recovery of upper limb function following brachial plexus injury

Table 3.11 Stem Cell Transplantation

Bone marrow stem cells	Animal study reports	• Neuronal and glial differentiation and neurologic recovery following bone marrow stem cell implants into SCI site
	Advantages	• Ease of obtaining autologous tissue
		• "Homing instinct" of marrow cells
		• Administer intravascularly or intrathecally
	Park et al study	• Improvements in ASIA grades in patients receiving marrow stem cell transplants within 7 to 14 days of injury
		• Patients also received granulocyte-macrophage colony-stimulating factor (GM-CSF)
Peripheral blood stem cells	Janson et al study	• Intrathecal administration to ALS patients
		• Few details of study found
Umbilical cord stem cells	China study	• Homologous umbilical cord stem cell transplants in chronic SCI patients
		• Performed intravenously, intrathecally, or directly into spinal cord
		• Reportedly showed benefits in some published trials; no definite proof
Fetal porcine stem cell xenotransplantation		• Diacrin Company performed trial, injecting pig stem sells directly into human spinal cord; no publication of results
Human embryonic stem cells		• At least one study in United States with no reports yet; one planned trial of particular interest involves differentiation in vitro of human embryonic cell line to an oligodendrocytic phenotype with functional competence for myelination, which could be very beneficial in SCI patients where demyelination is extensive

stem cells in experimental SCI that have shown some benefit.[53,54]

Transplantation of Olfactory Ensheathing Glia and Olfactory Bulb (Table 3.12)

Transplantation of OEG is currently being performed in patients with SCI in several countries, including China, Portugal, Russia, and Australia, and is based on many favorable reports in experimental models.[55,56] The strategy is attractive because of the ease with which autologous tissue can be obtained for transplantation in patients with SCI. Huang et al[57] in China has had the largest experience with this technique, and in 2003, they reported the results in 171 patients, mostly in the chronic phase, in a case series report. They transplanted OEGs or olfactory bulb tissue from human fetuses into the spinal cord at open surgery. Unfortunately, there was no blinding of examiners and no randomization, and neurologic improvement was reported after follow-up of only 8 weeks. Recently, Huang reported that he has performed transplantation of autologous OEG cells into the spinal cord in more than 300 SCI patients (personal communication). Guest et al[58] reported rapid recovery of one of Huang's cases but could not determine the exact mechanism. As noted above, Dobkin et al[21] criticized this trial on the basis of poor trial design, and they recorded complications, including meningitis. These authors also recorded the absence of neurologic improvement in all seven patients who had objective neurologic assessment before and after

Table 3.12 Olfactory Ensheathing Glia and Olfactory Bulb Transplantation

Advantages	• Autologous tissue obtained easily for use in SCI patients
	• Has shown benefits in experimental models
Huang et al[57] studies	• Use of human fetal olfactory ensheathing glia (OEG) or olfactory bulb transplanted into spinal cord at open surgery
	• Guest et al[58] reported rapid recovery of one case
	• Dobkin et al[21] criticized trial design and recorded subsequent cases of serious complications, including meningitis
	• More trials in progress; incomplete reporting of results and poor trial design

Table 3.13 Schwann Cell Transplantation

Miami Project	Has studied Schwann cell strategy for years in experimental animals
Zhu study	Injection of Schwann cells from peripheral nerves into spinal cord of SCI patients showed improvements in ASIA and sensory scores
Feng study	Injection of Schwann cells from sural nerve into spinal cord of SCI patients showed some recovery

transplantation of the OEG cells. Other investigators in China have also been performing this treatment (personal communication), and a similar large trial of OEG transplantation is in progress in Lisbon, Portugal, by Lima et al,[59] who reported the results in seven ASIA grade A patients, all of whom improved in a pilot study that was not a randomized control trial.[59] An Australian phase 1 trial of OEG transplants in three patients was reported in 2005,[60] and a larger trial is being planned for Australia and New Zealand.

Schwann Cell Transplantation (Table 3.13)

The Schwann cell strategy has been pursued in experimental SCI for several decades by many investigators, especially those at the Miami Project. Based on animal studies with human Schwann cells transplanted into the spinal cord of rats with demyelination,[61] there have been plans to transplant Schwann cells into the spinal cord of patients with conditions such as multiple sclerosis, but no clinical reports have been published in peer-reviewed journals. Recently, Zhu and colleagues in China injected human fetal Schwann cells harvested from peripheral nerves into the spinal cord of 47 patients with SCI and found improvement in ASIA motor and sensory scores (personal communication). Feng and colleagues in Tianjin, China, injected autologous Schwann cells from sural nerve into the spinal cord of nine SCI patients with apparent recovery in some (personal communication). There is no indication that the examiners were independent or blinded in these apparently phase 1 trials.

Fetal Porcine Stem Cell Xenotransplantation

In the United States, the Diacrin Company trial of fetal stem cells injected directly into the spinal cord involved 10 patients with SCI in two centers, St. Louis and Albany, New York (personal communication), but no report has appeared in the literature.

Human Embryonic Stem Cells

There are a large number of promising preclinical trials of various human embryonic stem cells, some of which have been differentiated toward a neural phenotype.[62,63] Some of the initial experimental paradigms in this field were not relevant to humans, such as mouse embryonic stem cells transplanted into rats with SCI.[64] However, there has been at least one phase 1 study of human embryonic stem cells in SCI patients in the United States (personal communication), but no published report has appeared. One of the most interesting has been a human embryonic cell line differentiated in vitro to favor an oligodendrocytic phenotype with functional competence for myelination in rats.[65–67] There is extensive demyelination associated with human SCI, and thus this strategy is very attractive. It is being prepared for a phase 1 trial in SCI (personal communication).

Immunomodulation (Table 3.14)

Some of the strategies already discussed, such as transplantation of autologous macrophages, may have an immunomodulation basis, but there have been other specific

Table 3.14 Other Strategies

Immunomodulation	• Alter immune response in spinal cord to enhance regeneration
	• Done via vaccination or depletion of circulating macrophages by liposome-encapsulated clodronate
	• Both cell-mediated and antibody-mediated immune responses can help in axonal regeneration
Fusion molecules (polyethylene glycol)	• Evidence that polyethylene glycol can repair neuronal membranes in vitro via "fusion"
	• Clinical trial being considered
Cyclic AMP	• Injected directly as dibutyryl cAMP or inhibition of cAMP hydrolysis by a phosphodiesterase IV inhibitor (rolipram); can enhance axonal regeneration following SCI
Rho antagonist	• Inactivation of Rho via Rho kinase inhibition can promote axonal regeneration after experimental SCI
	• Cethrin, a Rho inhibitor applied extradurally at time of surgery; phase 1 trial in patients has been completed with promising results

Table 3.15 Bioengineering in Neuroprotection and Regeneration

Examples	• Axonal guidance channels
	• Subarachnoid drug delivery systems
Advantages	• Opportunity to counteract secondary injury
	• Provides scaffolds to replace lost tissue and enhance regrowth of axons
	• Synaptic plasticity
	• Inhibition of astrocytosis
	• Structural and chemical versatility
Clinical trials	None yet

attempts at altering the immune response in the spinal cord designed to enhance regeneration by vaccination[68] or by depletion of circulating macrophages by measures such as liposome-encapsulated clodronate.[69] As discussed below, myelin contains molecules that inhibit regeneration of axons, and neutralizing the activity of these inhibitors can enhance axon regeneration. Thus, there are complex CNS–immune system interactions after SCI, and both cell-mediated and antibody-mediated immune responses can help in promoting axonal regeneration. The above efforts to develop an effective vaccine or cytokine treatment for experimental SCI have not yet been examined in human SCI.

Polyethylene Glycol Application

There is evidence that polyethylene glycol can repair neuronal membranes in vitro by "fusion," and there has been support for this concept in experimental SCI models.[70,71] A clinical trial is being considered (personal communication).

Scaffolds, Matrices, and Other Bioengineering Strategies (Table 3.15)

Bioengineering has been of major importance for exploring new methods of spinal cord repair, and our group has recently reviewed the field, including our experiences with some of these strategies, such as axonal guidance channels and subarachnoid drug delivery systems.[72] As stated above, the pathophysiology of SCI is multifactorial and multiphasic; therefore, it is likely that effective treatments will require combinations of neuroprotection and regeneration strategies. Bioengineering offers opportunities to counteract secondary injury, provide scaffolds to replace lost tissue, and enhance axonal regrowth, synaptic plasticity, and inhibition of astrocytosis.[73] Biomaterials have major advantages for spinal cord repair because of their structural and chemical versatility. For example, bioengineering technology can facilitate cellular treatment strategies, including Schwann cells,[74] olfactory ensheathing glia, or neural stem cells for repair of the injured spinal cord. Currently, the emphasis in our laboratory is on the use of naturally occurring agents, such as chitosan, and to make them biodegradable. To date, none of these strategies has been applied to humans for spinal cord regeneration.

Anti-Nogo-A Inhibition and Nogo-66-Receptor Inhibition (Table 3.16)

It is now known that there are several myelin-based proteins that are powerful inhibitors of neurite outgrowth in vitro and axonal regeneration in vivo. The most extensively studied of these inhibitors is known as Nogo-A, and it has been cloned and characterized by Schwab and colleagues in Zurich. Nogo-A is a protein present in oligodendroglial myelin and is one of at least three myelin-based inhibitors of central axonal regeneration identified in the CNS. Schwab and colleagues have prepared an antibody to Nogo-A, and this anti–Nogo-A antibody counteracts the Nogo-A inhibitory protein in vitro and in vivo in several experimental models of SCI in various species, including

Table 3.16 Myelin-Based Protein Inhibitors

Function of myelin-based proteins	• Serve as powerful inhibitors of neurite outgrowth in vitro and axonal regeneration in vivo
Examples	• Nogo-A, Nogo-66 receptor
Anti–Nogo-A antibody	• Counteracts Nogo-A inhibitory protein in vitro and in vivo in rodent and primate studies; phase 1 trial in humans is under way

Table 3.17 Reducing Glial Scar Formation

Glial scar	• Contains extracellular matrix (ECM) molecules, including chondroitin sulfate proteoglycans (CSPGs), which are inhibitors of axonal growth in vitro
Chondroitinase ABC	• Administered intrathecally
	• Counteracts inhibitory proteoglycans of ECM
Reports	• Several reports from experimental SCI studies show effectiveness
	• Some reports show enzyme may even enhance collateral axonal sprouting in central nervous system (CNS) remote from injury
Clinical trials	• Likely will be subjected to clinical trials in humans with SCI

rodents and monkeys.[75,76] A "humanized" form of the anti–Nogo-A antibody is currently being administered intrathecally to patients with SCI in a phase 1 trial in Germany and Switzerland in the centers of the European Consortium (see below; personal communication).

Other recently described efforts in animal studies to overcome inhibitory factors include antibodies or inhibitors of the Nogo-66 receptor protein.[77,78] These agents might be more effective than anti–Nogo-A antibody, which may neutralize only Nogo and not the other myelin-based inhibitors.

Chondroitinase ABC (Table 3.17)

At sites of CNS injury, a glial scar develops, containing extracellular matrix (ECM) molecules, including chondroitin sulfate proteoglycans (CSPGs). CSPGs are inhibitory to axon growth in vitro, and regenerating axons stop at CSPG-rich regions in vivo. Chondroitinase ABC has been administered intrathecally to counteract these inhibitory proteoglycans in the ECM in experimental SCI.[79,80] Recently, several other reports have appeared showing the effectiveness of this enzyme on recovery from experimental SCI, including combination strategies with scaffolds and various cellular transplants.[81–86] Also, it is interesting that this enzyme may enhance collateral axonal sprouting in the CNS remote from the injury site, which may confer additional benefits.[87] It is highly likely that this agent will be subjected to clinical trials in humans with SCI.

Cyclic Adenosine Monophosphate

It was first reported in 1991 that cyclic adenosine monophosphate (cAMP) enhances neurite outgrowth in vitro,[88,89] and recently it has been shown that this agent can enhance axonal regeneration after experimental SCI.[90–92] It can be injected directly as dibutyryl cAMP, or cAMP levels can be increased by inhibition of cAMP hydrolysis by the phosphodiesterase IV inhibitor rolipram. This strategy has also been used in combination therapy with neurotrophic factors and with cellular transplants.[92] Clinical trials are likely to appear.

Rho Antagonist

McKerracher and colleagues[93,94] showed that inactivation of Rho by Rho kinase inhibition can promote axonal regeneration after experimental SCI. Cethrin is a Rho inhibitor and is now undergoing a multicenter phase 1 trial. The agent is applied extradurally at surgery following surgical treatment for decompression or fusion within 14 days of SCI in ASIA grade A cervical or thoracic patients. It is uncertain whether this type of downstream intracellular inactivation of the inhibitory pathways is more effective than inhibition at the axonal membrane as afforded by anti–Nogo-A.

Electrical Stimulation with Direct Current Fields (Table 3.18)

It has been well established that electrical stimulation with direct current (DC) fields enhances the growth and alters the direction of neurite outgrowth in vitro.[95–97] Many studies of this modality were performed in experimental SCI by Borgens et al[98] in a variety of animal models of SCI and with several different forms of electrical stimulation. For many years this strategy was actively pursued in my laboratory but was ultimately abandoned because the therapeutic index was so unfavorable.[99,100] A phase 1 trial of pulsed oscillating current in 10 patients was reported by Shapiro et al[101] in cervical and thoracic ASIA grade A cases. Stimulation began within 18 days of injury with surgically implanted electrodes, and some patients showed neurologic improvement. Pulsed electrical stimulation of the spinal cord after SCI in humans has also been performed by Xu and Liu in Beijing, China, on more than 100 patients (personal communication).

Table 3.18 Technology and Rehabilitation in Regeneration Enhancement

Electrical stimulation with direct current fields	• Enhances growth and alters direction of neurite outgrowth in vitro
	• Many trials done
	• Has unfavorable therapeutic index
Functional electrical stimulation (FES)	• Stimulation of muscles to augment intact neurologic input or serve as the sole stimuli to produce movements
	• Remains questionable whether it plays a role in neurologic recovery
	• Treatments require much labor and are expensive
Gravity-assisted ambulation and automated locomotor training	• Gravity-assisted ambulation (body weight support) embodies treadmill training
	• Can improve walking, especially in incomplete SCIs
	• Great need for randomized prospective controlled trial but effectiveness is proven
Electrical stimulation with alternating currents	• Some evidence that this can assist in motor recovery; unproven value
	• Unknown relation to neurologic recovery
Rehabilitation and exercise strategies	• Exercise enhances recovery via regeneration (e.g., treadmill training)
	• Does so through elaboration of neurotrophic factors
	• Also provides muscle strength and joint mobility

Rehabilitation-Exercise Strategies Enhance Regeneration (Table 3.18)

It has been shown that certain physical rehabilitation measures can enhance neurologic recovery by enhancing regeneration, and it is likely that these measures should begin immediately after SCI to derive the maximum benefit. It is now known that physical exercise enhances regeneration of the CNS through the elaboration of neurotrophic factors. Cotman's group[102–104] has been at the forefront in defining the physiologic basis of exercise through the elaboration from the CNS of neurotrophic factors such as BDNF. In experimental SCI, the effect of exercise on neurologic function has been firmly established.[105,106] Thus, physiotherapy and occupational therapy in patients with SCI not only enhance muscle strength and preserve joint mobility, they also increase neurotrophic factors capable of promoting axonal regeneration. These findings have prompted clinical SCI trials to include early, vigorous, and consistent rehabilitation practices to maximize neurologic recovery. Also, investigators must ensure that defined rehabilitation programs are applied equally across treatment and control groups. In experimental SCI, these goals of enhanced and consistent physical activity are extremely difficult to achieve, but excellent studies have been done in experimental SCI, showing that measures such as treadmill training likely enhance regeneration.[107,108]

Functional Electrical Stimulation and "Patterned Neural Activity"

Functional electrical stimulation (FES) is accomplished through stimulation of the muscles to augment any intact neurologic input or to provide the sole stimuli to produce muscle contraction to perform a patterned, sequential function, such as walking or peddling a bicycle. The current question being examined is whether patterned neural activity such as provided by FES can play a role in improving neurologic recovery. Also, it is important to examine the mechanism of this modality in experimental models. It is unknown whether recovery is based on axonal regeneration. This treatment modality was applied to Christopher Reeve in a much publicized report purporting to show that his neurologic recovery was attributable to the treatment.[109] These treatments are labor intensive and involve large expenditures for equipment, training, and personnel, and thus, they impact significantly on clinical trials. Phase 1 trials of this modality have been reported.[110] There is a need for intensive examination of this strategy in experimental SCI.

Gravity-Assisted Ambulation and Automated Locomotor Training

This new modality of treatment of SCI patients has been termed gravity-assisted ambulation or body weight support and generally embodies treadmill training.[111] It has been shown that this method of rehabilitation can improve walking after SCI, especially in patients with incomplete injuries.[5] A multicenter trial to evaluate this modality has shown that walking is improved in ASIA grade C and D patients.[6] Further study by a randomized prospective controlled trial is essential for the same reasons noted above for FES. The precise mechanism for the improvements is not known, but one study with transcranial magnetic stimulation in patients with chronic SCI provided evidence that treadmill training increased locomotor function through an increase in function of the corticospinal tract.[112] A multicenter randomized trial commenced in 2003 and has not yet been reported.[113] It is conceivable that there is increased axonal sprouting or regeneration, even in chronic cases. Thus, there is a great need for further clinical and experimental studies of this modality.

Electrical Stimulation of the Spinal Cord by Alternating Current

There is a long history of the use of various forms of alternating current for stimulation of the spinal cord in experimental SCI to improve function,[114] and there is some evidence that electrical stimulation can assist motor recovery in patients. There is one report of improvement in walking in an ASIA grade C patient with an implanted extradural spinal cord stimulator.[115] It is unknown whether the functional improvement is related to neurologic recovery.

■ Conclusion

A large number of strategies have been proven to enhance regenerative processes in experimental in vitro and in vivo studies related to regeneration of the spinal cord. Many of these involve elaboration or administration of growth factors, and many involve stimulation of the body's endogenous regenerative mechanisms. Transplantation of various cells, especially a large variety of stem cells, has shown impressive effects on the pathologic picture. For example, it is possible to produce enough new tissue to completely fill the major cavities left behind after severe SCI. However, functional restoration of complex activities such as grasping and locomotion continue to elude investigators at both the experimental and clinical levels. In clinical SCI, a large number of trials of strategies to enhance regeneration are in progress in many countries, and several hundred SCI patients have been treated with cellular transplantation techniques. Most of the trials have been phase 1 with no controls, no independent examiners, and no reports in peer-reviewed literature or other sources in the public domain. Lack of rigorous attention to trial design and lack of detailed reporting make scientific evaluation impossible. Further, well-designed trials are necessary based on sound experimental SCI study of these strategies in clinically relevant experimental models.

References

1. Tator CH. Review of treatment trials in human spinal cord injury: issues, difficulties, and recommendations. Neurosurgery 2006;59: 957–982, discussion 982–957

2. Hurlbert RJ. The role of steroids in acute spinal cord injury: an evidence-based analysis. Spine 2001;26(suppl):S39–S46

3. De Girolami U, Frosch MP, Tator CH. Diseases of the spinal cord and vertebral column. In: Graham DI, Lantos P, eds. Greenfield's Neuropathology. 7th ed. Regional Neuropathology, vol 1. London: Arnold, 2002:1063–1101

4. Tator CH. Update on the pathophysiology and pathology of acute spinal cord injury. Brain Pathol 1995;5:407–413

5. Ladouceur M, Barbeau H. Functional electrical stimulation-assisted walking for persons with incomplete spinal injuries: longitudinal changes in maximal overground walking speed. Scand J Rehabil Med 2000;32:28–36

6. Wirz M, Zemon DH, Rupp R, et al. Effectiveness of automated locomotor training in patients with chronic incomplete spinal cord injury: a multicenter trial. Arch Phys Med Rehabil 2005;86:672–680

7. Fehlings MG, Sekhon LH, Tator C. The role and timing of decompression in acute spinal cord injury: what do we know? What should we do? Spine 2001;26(suppl):S101–S110

8. Kulbatski I, Mothe AJ, Nomura H, Tator CH. Endogenous and exogenous CNS derived stem/progenitor cell approaches for neurotrauma. Curr Drug Targets 2005;6:111–126

9. Lu J, Ashwell K. Olfactory ensheathing cells: their potential use for repairing the injured spinal cord. Spine 2002;27:887–892

10. Coumans JV, Lin TT, Dai HN, et al. Axonal regeneration and functional recovery after complete spinal cord transection in rats by delayed treatment with transplants and neurotrophins. J Neurosci 2001;21:9334–9344

11. Okano H, Ogawa Y, Nakamura M, Kaneko S, Iwanami A, Toyama Y. Transplantation of neural stem cells into the spinal cord after injury. Semin Cell Dev Biol 2003;14:191–198

12. Clifton GL, Donovan WH, Dimitrijevic MM, et al. Omental transposition in chronic spinal cord injury. Spinal Cord 1996;34: 193–203

13. Reier PJ. Cellular transplantation strategies for spinal cord injury and translational neurobiology. NeuroRx 2004;1:424–451

14. Sagen J. Cellular therapies for spinal cord injury: what will the FDA need to approve moving from the laboratory to the human? J Rehabil Res Dev 2003;40(suppl 1):71–79

15. Schwab ME, Bartholdi D. Degeneration and regeneration of axons in the lesioned spinal cord. Physiol Rev 1996;76:319–370

16. Fehlings MG, Perrin RG. The role and timing of early decompression for cervical spinal cord injury: update with a review of recent clinical evidence. Injury 2005;36(suppl 2):B13–B26

17. Tsai EC, Tator CH. Neuroprotection and regeneration strategies for spinal cord repair. Curr Pharm Des 2005;11:1211–1222

18. McDonald JW. Repairing the damaged spinal cord: from stem cells to activity-based restoration therapies. Clin Neurosurg 2004;51:207–227

19. Cesaro P. The design of clinical trials for cell transplantation into the central nervous system. NeuroRx 2004;1:492–499

20. Hofstetter CP, Holmstrom NA, Lilja JA, et al. Allodynia limits the usefulness of intraspinal neural stem cell grafts; directed differentiation improves outcome. Nat Neurosci 2005;8:346–353

21. Dobkin BH, Curt A, Guest J. Cellular transplants in China: observational study from the largest human experiment in chronic spinal cord injury. Neurorehabil Neural Repair 2006;20:5–13

22. Bareyre FM, Schwab ME. Inflammation, degeneration and regeneration in the injured spinal cord: insights from DNA microarrays. Trends Neurosci 2003;26:555–563

23. Ramer LM, Ramer MS, Steeves JD. Setting the stage for functional repair of spinal cord injuries: a cast of thousands. Spinal Cord 2005;43:134–161

24. Namiki J, Kojima A, Tator CH. Effect of brain-derived neurotrophic factor, nerve growth factor, and neurotrophin-3 on functional recovery and regeneration after spinal cord injury in adult rats. J Neurotrauma 2000;17:1219–1231

25. Cheng H, Liao KK, Liao SF, Chuang TY, Shih YH. Spinal cord repair with acidic fibroblast growth factor as a treatment for a patient with chronic paraplegia. Spine 2004;29:E284–E288

26. Penn RD, Kroin JS, York MM, Cedarbaum JM. Intrathecal ciliary neurotrophic factor delivery for treatment of amyotrophic lateral sclerosis (phase I trial). Neurosurgery 1997;40:94–99 discussion 99–100

27. Kalra S, Genge A, Arnold DL. A prospective, randomized, placebo-controlled evaluation of corticoneuronal response to intrathecal BDNF therapy in ALS using magnetic resonance spectroscopy: feasibility and results. Amyotroph Lateral Scler Other Motor Neuron Disord 2003;4:22–26

28. Reynolds BA, Weiss S. Clonal and population analyses demonstrate that an EGF-responsive mammalian embryonic CNS precursor is a stem cell. Dev Biol 1996;175:1–13

29. Kulbatski I, Mothe AJ, Keating A, Hakamata Y, Kobayashi E, Tator CH. Oligodendrocytes and radial glia derived from adult rat spinal cord progenitors: morphological and immunocytochemical characterization. J Histochem Cytochem 2007;55:209–22

30. Tator CH. Pathophysiology and pathology of spinal cord injury. In: Wilkins RH, Rengachary SS, eds. Neurosurgery. vol 2. New York: McGraw-Hill; 1996:2847–2859

31. Kolb B, Morshead C, Gonzalez C, et al. Growth factor-stimulated generation of new cortical tissue and functional recovery after stroke damage to the motor cortex of rats. J Cereb Blood Flow Metab 2007;27:983–997

32. Geisler FH, Dorsey FC, Coleman WP. Recovery of motor function after spinal-cord injury: a randomized, placebo-controlled trial with GM-1 ganglioside. N Engl J Med 1991;324:1829–1838

33. Geisler FH, Coleman WP, Grieco G, Poonian D. Measurements and recovery patterns in a multicenter study of acute spinal cord injury. Spine 2001;26(suppl):S68–S86

34. Geisler FH, Coleman WP, Grieco G, Poonian D. The Sygen multicenter acute spinal cord injury study. Spine 2001;26(suppl):S87–98

35. Reier PJ, Houle JD, Jakeman L, Winialski D, Tessler A. Transplantation of fetal spinal cord tissue into acute and chronic hemisection and contusion lesions of the adult rat spinal cord. Prog Brain Res 1988;78:173–179

36. Iwashita Y, Kawaguchi S, Murata M. Restoration of function by replacement of spinal cord segments in the rat. Nature 1994;367:167–170

37. Falci S, Holtz A, Akesson E, et al. Obliteration of a posttraumatic spinal cord cyst with solid human embryonic spinal cord grafts: first clinical attempt. J Neurotrauma 1997;14:875–884

38. Wirth ED III, Reier PJ, Fessler RG, et al. Feasibility and safety of neural tissue transplantation in patients with syringomyelia. J Neurotrauma 2001;18:911–929

39. Schwartz M, Lazarov-Spiegler O, Rapalino O, Agranov I, Velan G, Hadani M. Potential repair of rat spinal cord injuries using stimulated homologous macrophages. Neurosurgery 1999;44:1041–1045, discussion 1045–1046

40. Knoller N, Auerbach G, Fulga V, et al. Clinical experience using incubated autologous macrophages as a treatment for complete spinal cord injury: phase I study results. J Neurosurg Spine 2005;3:173–181

41. Schwartz M, Yoles E. Macrophages and dendritic cells treatment of spinal cord injury: from the bench to the clinic. Acta Neurochir Suppl 2005;93:147–150

42. Richardson PM, McGuinness UM, Aguayo AJ. Axons from CNS neurons regenerate into PNS grafts. Nature 1980;284:264–265

43. Cheng H, Cao Y, Olson L. Spinal cord repair in adult paraplegic rats: partial restoration of hind limb function. Science 1996;273:510–513

44. Barros TE, Oliveira R, Barros EMK, et al. The use of peripheral nerve bridges to spinal cord injury. J Spinal Cord Med 2003;26:S33

45. Brunelli GA. Direct neurotization of muscles by presynaptic motoneurons. J Reconstr Microsurg 2001;17:631–636

46. von Wild KR, Brunelli GA. Restoration of locomotion in paraplegics with aid of autologous bypass grafts for direct neurotisation of muscles by upper motor neurons—the future: surgery of the spinal cord? Acta Neurochir Suppl 2003;87:107–112

47. Tadie M, Liu S, Robert R, et al. Partial return of motor function in paralyzed legs after surgical bypass of the lesion site by nerve autografts three years after spinal cord injury. J Neurotrauma 2002;19:909–916

48. Carlstedt T, Anand P, Hallin R, Misra PV, Noren G, Seferlis T. Spinal nerve root repair and reimplantation of avulsed ventral roots into the spinal cord after brachial plexus injury. J Neurosurg 2000;93(suppl):237–247

49. Chopp M, Zhang XH, Li Y, et al. Spinal cord injury in rat: treatment with bone marrow stromal cell transplantation. Neuroreport 2000;11:3001–3005

50. Hofstetter CP, Schwarz EJ, Hess D, et al. Marrow stromal cells form guiding strands in the injured spinal cord and promote recovery. Proc Natl Acad Sci U S A 2002;99:2199–2204

51. Park HC, Shim YS, Ha Y, et al. Treatment of complete spinal cord injury patients by autologous bone marrow cell transplantation and administration of granulocyte-macrophage colony stimulating factor. Tissue Eng 2005;11:913–922

52. Janson CG, Ramesh TM, During MJ, Leone P, Heywood J. Human intrathecal transplantation of peripheral blood stem cells in amyotrophic lateral sclerosis. J Hematother Stem Cell Res 2001;10:913–915

53. Nishio Y, Koda M, Kamada T, et al. The use of hemopoietic stem cells derived from human umbilical cord blood to promote restoration of spinal cord tissue and recovery of hindlimb function in adult rats. J Neurosurg Spine 2006;5:424–433

54. Saporta S, Kim JJ, Willing AE, Fu ES, Davis CD, Sanberg PR. Human umbilical cord blood stem cells infusion in spinal cord injury: engraftment and beneficial influence on behavior. J Hematother Stem Cell Res 2003;12:271–278

55. Li Y, Field PM, Raisman G. Regeneration of adult rat corticospinal axons induced by transplanted olfactory ensheathing cells. J Neurosci 1998;18:10514–10524

56. Ramon-Cueto A, Plant GW, Avila J, Bunge MB. Long-distance axonal regeneration in the transected adult rat spinal cord is promoted by olfactory ensheathing glia transplants. J Neurosci 1998;18:3803–3815

57. Huang H, Chen L, Wang H, et al. Influence of patients' age on functional recovery after transplantation of olfactory ensheathing

cells into injured spinal cord injury. Chin Med J (Engl) 2003; 116:1488–1491

58. Guest J, Herrera LP, Qian T. Rapid recovery of segmental neurological function in a tetraplegic patient following transplantation of fetal olfactory bulb-derived cells. Spinal Cord 2006;44: 135–142

59. Lima C, Pratas-Vital J, Escada P, Hasse-Ferreira A, Capucho C, Peduzzi JD. Olfactory mucosa autografts in human spinal cord injury: a pilot clinical study. J Spinal Cord Med 2006;29:191–203 discussion 204–196

60. Feron F, Perry C, Cochrane J, et al. Autologous olfactory ensheathing cell transplantation in human spinal cord injury. Brain 2005; 128(pt 12):2951–2960

61. Kohama I, Lankford KL, Preiningerova J, White FA, Vollmer TL, Kocsis JD. Transplantation of cryopreserved adult human Schwann cells enhances axonal conduction in demyelinated spinal cord. J Neurosci 2001;21:944–950

62. Wu P, Tarasenko YI, Gu Y, Huang LY, Coggeshall RE, Yu Y. Region-specific generation of cholinergic neurons from fetal human neural stem cells grafted in adult rat. Nat Neurosci 2002;5:1271–1278

63. Tarasenko YI, Yu Y, Jordan PM, Bottenstein J, Wu P. Effect of growth factors on proliferation and phenotypic differentiation of human fetal neural stem cells. J Neurosci Res 2004;78:625–636

64. McDonald JW, Liu XZ, Qu Y, et al. Transplanted embryonic stem cells survive, differentiate and promote recovery in injured rat spinal cord. Nat Med 1999;5:1410–1412

65. Keirstead HS, Nistor G, Bernal G, et al. Human embryonic stem cell-derived oligodendrocyte progenitor cell transplants remyelinate and restore locomotion after spinal cord injury. J Neurosci 2005;25:4694–4705

66. Keirstead HS. Stem cells for the treatment of myelin loss. Trends Neurosci 2005;28:677–683

67. Totoiu MO, Keirstead HS. Spinal cord injury is accompanied by chronic progressive demyelination. J Comp Neurol 2005;486: 373–383

68. David S, Ousman SS. Recruiting the immune response to promote axon regeneration in the injured spinal cord. Neuroscientist 2002;8:33–41

69. Popovich PG, Guan Z, Wei P, Huitinga I, van Rooijen N, Stokes BT. Depletion of hematogenous macrophages promotes partial hindlimb recovery and neuroanatomical repair after experimental spinal cord injury. Exp Neurol 1999;158:351–365

70. Shi R, Borgens RB, Blight AR. Functional reconnection of severed mammalian spinal cord axons with polyethylene glycol. J Neurotrauma 1999;16:727–738

71. Borgens RB, Shi R. Immediate recovery from spinal cord injury through molecular repair of nerve membranes with polyethylene glycol. FASEB J 2000;14:27–35

72. Nomura H, Tator CH, Shoichet MS. Bioengineered strategies for spinal cord repair. J Neurotrauma 2006;23:496–507

73. Jimenez Hamann MC, Tator CH, Shoichet MS. Injectable intrathecal delivery system for localized administration of EGF and FGF-2 to the injured rat spinal cord. Exp Neurol 2005;194: 106–119

74. Chau CH, Shum DK, Li H, et al. Chondroitinase ABC enhances axonal regrowth through Schwann cell-seeded guidance channels after spinal cord injury. FASEB J 2004;18:194–196

75. Schwab ME. Experimental aspects of spinal cord regeneration. Curr Opin Neurol Neurosurg 1993;6:549–553

76. Schwab ME. Nogo and axon regeneration. Curr Opin Neurobiol 2004;14:118–124

77. Li S, Liu BP, Budel S, et al. Blockade of Nogo-66, myelin-associated glycoprotein, and oligodendrocyte myelin glycoprotein by soluble Nogo-66 receptor promotes axonal sprouting and recovery after spinal injury. J Neurosci 2004;24:10511–10520

78. Li S, Strittmatter SM. Delayed systemic Nogo-66 receptor antagonist promotes recovery from spinal cord injury. J Neurosci 2003;23:4219–4227

79. Yick LW, Wu W, So KF, Yip HK, Shum DK. Chondroitinase ABC promotes axonal regeneration of Clarke's neurons after spinal cord injury. Neuroreport 2000;11:1063–1067

80. Bradbury EJ, Moon LD, Popat RJ, et al. Chondroitinase ABC promotes functional recovery after spinal cord injury. Nature 2002;416:636–640

81. Huang WC, Kuo WC, Cherng JH, et al. Chondroitinase ABC promotes axonal re-growth and behavior recovery in spinal cord injury. Biochem Biophys Res Commun 2006;349:963–968

82. Houle JD, Tom VJ, Mayes D, Wagoner G, Phillips N, Silver J. Combining an autologous peripheral nervous system "bridge" and matrix modification by chondroitinase allows robust, functional regeneration beyond a hemisection lesion of the adult rat spinal cord. J Neurosci 2006;26:7405–7415

83. Massey JM, Hubscher CH, Wagoner MR, et al. Chondroitinase ABC digestion of the perineuronal net promotes functional collateral sprouting in the cuneate nucleus after cervical spinal cord injury. J Neurosci 2006;26:4406–4414

84. Ikegami T, Nakamura M, Yamane J, et al. Chondroitinase ABC combined with neural stem/progenitor cell transplantation enhances graft cell migration and outgrowth of growth-associated protein-43-positive fibers after rat spinal cord injury. Eur J Neurosci 2005;22:3036–3046

85. Caggiano AO, Zimber MP, Ganguly A, Blight AR, Gruskin EA. Chondroitinase ABCI improves locomotion and bladder function following contusion injury of the rat spinal cord. J Neurotrauma 2005;22:226–239

86. Fouad K, Schnell L, Bunge MB, Schwab ME, Liebscher T, Pearse DD. Combining Schwann cell bridges and olfactory-ensheathing glia grafts with chondroitinase promotes locomotor recovery after complete transection of the spinal cord. J Neurosci 2005;25:1169–1178

87. Barritt AW, Davies M, Marchand F, et al. Chondroitinase ABC promotes sprouting of intact and injured spinal systems after spinal cord injury. J Neurosci 2006;26:10856–10867

88. Ono K, Katayama N, Yamagata Y, Tokunaga A, Tsuda M. Morphology of neurites from N18TG2 cell induced by protein kinase inhibitor H-7 and by cAMP. Brain Res Bull 1991;26:605–612

89. Sanna PP, Bloom FE, Wilson MC. Dibutyryl-cAMP induces SNAP-25 translocation into the neurites in PC12. Brain Res Dev Brain Res 1991;59:104–108

90. Spencer T, Domeniconi M, Cao Z, Filbin MT. New roles for old proteins in adult CNS axonal regeneration. Curr Opin Neurobiol 2003;13:133–139

91. Pearse DD, Pereira FC, Marcillo AE, et al. cAMP and Schwann cells promote axonal growth and functional recovery after spinal cord injury. Nat Med 2004;10:610–616

92. Lu P, Yang H, Jones LL, Filbin MT, Tuszynski MH. Combinatorial therapy with neurotrophins and cAMP promotes axonal regeneration beyond sites of spinal cord injury. J Neurosci 2004;24:6402–6409

93. Lehmann M, Fournier A, Selles-Navarro I, et al. Inactivation of Rho signaling pathway promotes CNS axon regeneration. J Neurosci 1999;19:7537–7547

94. Dubreuil CI, Winton MJ, McKerracher L. Rho activation patterns after spinal cord injury and the role of activated Rho in apoptosis in the central nervous system. J Cell Biol 2003;162:233–243

95. Jaffe LF, Poo MM. Neurites grow faster towards the cathode than the anode in a steady field. J Exp Zool 1979;209:115–128

96. McCaig CD. Spinal neurite reabsorption and regrowth in vitro depend on the polarity of an applied electric field. Development 1987;100:31–41

97. Patel N, Poo MM. Orientation of neurite growth by extracellular electric fields. J Neurosci 1982;2:483–496

98. Borgens RB, Blight AR, McGinnis ME. Behavioral recovery induced by applied electric fields after spinal cord hemisection in guinea pig. Science 1987;238:366–369

99. Hurlbert RJ, Tator CH, Theriault E. Dose-response study of the pathological effects of chronically applied direct current stimulation on the normal rat spinal cord. J Neurosurg 1993;79: 905–916

100. Hurlbert RJ, Tator CH. Characterization of longitudinal field gradients from electrical stimulation in the normal and injured rodent spinal cord. Neurosurgery 1994;34:471–482 discussion 482–473

101. Shapiro S, Borgens R, Pascuzzi R, et al. Oscillating field stimulation for complete spinal cord injury in humans: a phase 1 trial. J Neurosurg Spine 2005;2:3–10

102. Cotman CW, Berchtold NC. Exercise: a behavioral intervention to enhance brain health and plasticity. Trends Neurosci 2002;25: 295–301

103. Cotman CW, Engesser-Cesar C. Exercise enhances and protects brain function. Exerc Sport Sci Rev 2002;30:75–79

104. Neeper SA, Gomez-Pinilla F, Choi J, Cotman C. Exercise and brain neurotrophins. Nature 1995;373:109

105. Gomez-Pinilla F, Ying Z, Opazo P, Roy RR, Edgerton VR. Differential regulation by exercise of BDNF and NT-3 in rat spinal cord and skeletal muscle. Eur J Neurosci 2001;13:1078–1084

106. Van Meeteren NL, Eggers R, Lankhorst AJ, Gispen WH, Hamers FP. Locomotor recovery after spinal cord contusion injury in rats is improved by spontaneous exercise. J Neurotrauma 2003;20: 1029–1037

107. Edgerton VR, Tillakaratne NJ, Bigbee AJ, de Leon RD, Roy RR. Plasticity of the spinal neural circuitry after injury. Annu Rev Neurosci 2004;27:145–167

108. Engesser-Cesar C, Anderson AJ, Basso DM, Edgerton VR, Cotman CW. Voluntary wheel running improves recovery from a moderate spinal cord injury. J Neurotrauma 2005;22:157–171

109. McDonald JW, Becker D, Sadowsky CL, Jane JA Sr, Conturo TE, Schultz LM. Late recovery following spinal cord injury: case report and review of the literature. J Neurosurg 2002; 97(suppl): 252–265

110. Thrasher TA, Flett HM, Popovic MR. Gait training regimen for incomplete spinal cord injury using functional electrical stimulation. Spinal Cord 2006;44:357–361

111. Dietz V, Colombo G. Recovery from spinal cord injury–underlying mechanisms and efficacy of rehabilitation. Acta Neurochir Suppl 2004;89:95–100

112. Thomas SL, Gorassini MA. Increases in corticospinal tract function by treadmill training after incomplete spinal cord injury. J Neurophysiol 2005;94:2844–2855

113. Dobkin BH, Apple D, Barbeau H, et al. Methods for a randomized trial of weight-supported treadmill training versus conventional training for walking during inpatient rehabilitation after incomplete traumatic spinal cord injury. Neurorehabil Neural Repair 2003;17:153–167

114. Wallace MC, Tator CH, Gentles WM. Effect of alternating current stimulation of the spinal cord on recovery from acute spinal cord injury in rats. Surg Neurol 1987;28:269–276

115. Herman R, He J, D'Luzansky S, Willis W, Dilli S. Spinal cord stimulation facilitates functional walking in a chronic, incomplete spinal cord injured. Spinal Cord 2002;40:65–68

4 Spinal Injury Classification Systems

F. C. Öner

Different classification systems have been used in traumatology to stratify and categorize injuries. Most surgeons consider them necessary tools to provide a conceptual framework for diagnosis and treatment. Furthermore, these schemes are used as systems for communication about the relative severity of the injuries and the result of different treatment options. However, these schemes have been gradually introduced into the field without a proper discussion of their meanings and consequences. Although indispensable in modern clinical practice and academic discussions, a thorough understanding of the types of classifications and what they mean together with an understanding of their strengths and weaknesses is necessary for proper use of these important tools. Especially the advancements in diagnostic imaging and our increasing capacity to help severely injured patients survive make this an urgent task.

A clinically relevant classification system not only should take into account the natural history of an injury pattern but also should predict outcome. Ideally, such a system should provide a universal language to describe spinal injuries and should guide clinical decision making. This system must be easy to remember and to use in clinical practice and should provide a platform for prospective research on spinal injuries. The system must be able to stratify injury severity and suggest the prognosis of a given injury.[1]

Classification of spinal injuries has been an exceptionally contentious subject (**Table 4.1**). Different schemes have been proposed, discussed, and criticized in an ongoing debate. Considering the complexity of the spine with its central role in the locomotor as well as the nervous system, it is no wonder that this discussion has at times been seen as intractable. The main difficulty lies in the fact that, unlike the fractures of long bones, the pattern of spine fractures may be progressive, evolving into an increasing deformity, and that the spine fractures represent complex injuries of a structure composed of parts with

Table 4.1 Classification Systems

Uses	• Stratify and categorize injuries
	• Conceptual framework for diagnosis and treatment
	• Used as system of communication about severity of injury and result of different treatments
Characteristics	• An account of the history of injury and prediction of outcomes
	• Provide universal language describing injuries
	• Guide decision making
	• Must be easy to remember
	• Provide platform for prospective research
	• Must be able to distinguish severity and suggest prognosis
Difficulties with spinal injury classification	• Spine fracture patterns may be progressive
	• Spine fractures are structural injuries with different injury susceptibilities and different healing potentials
	• Approach mechanical and neurologic injury separately
Requirement	• System must allow physician to assess three kinds of stability:
	1. Immediate mechanical
	2. Neurologic
	3. Long-term

different susceptibility to injury and different healing potentials. Adding to the confusion, injury to the mechanical integrity of the spinal column and the neurologic injury have been approached separately. *Stability* has been a key concept, but it is usually poorly defined, and the term is used inconsistently. The most reliable and mentally reproducible concept of stability was described in the 1970s by White and Panjabi:[2]

> Clinical instability is defined as a loss in the ability of the spine under physiologic loads to maintain relationships between vertebrae in such a way that there is neither damage nor subsequent irritation to the spinal cord or nerve roots. In addition there is no development of incapacitating deformity or pain due to structural changes.

This means that a useful classification system should enable the surgeon to make an educated guess about three kinds of stability:

- Immediate mechanical stability
- Neurologic stability
- Long-term stability

Classification of Neurologic Injury

Classification of the neurologic injury as a result of traumatic spinal conditions has been one of the fields where people can reach a consensus easily, but a lot of uncertainty remains due to the practical difficulties of conducting a thorough neurologic exam by trauma victims. In general, the neurologic syndromes associated with spinal cord or cauda equina are well defined, and a trained clinician can usually define the place and extent of pathology quite accurately as soon as a complete neurologic exam is possible (**Table 4.2**). In trauma patients, however, many factors, such as multiple injuries, and subdued consciousness levels as a result of brain injury, substance use, or emergency intubation, make it often impossible to carry out a reliable neurologic exam. It is generally accepted that a reliable neurologic status can be determined only after multiple neurologic exams within 48 to 72 hours

of the injury. The treating surgeons should always keep this uncertainty in mind during their decisions on treatment. There is a big difference in the prognosis between complete and incomplete spinal cord injuries, and it is advisable not to declare a patient a total paraplegic unless one is absolutely sure.

The Frankel classification was the first universally used system to categorize the patients with neurologic injury according to their remaining useful function for rehabilitation. As a result, this was a rather coarse classification. The American Spinal Injury Association (ASIA) has refined this scheme and developed a system to determine sensory and motor levels separately and finally to reach an ASIA impairment scale[3] (**Fig. 4.1**). Although the reproducibility of this scale has not been studied sufficiently, this scheme has found general acceptance and is recommended in every patient with spinal injury.

Classification of Fractures

All classification systems in traumatology are based on the assumption that the interaction between the chaotic forces causing the trauma and the human body would yield some recognizable, reproducible, and meaningful patterns of injury. Although the evidence for this basic assumption is frustratingly weak, practitioners generally accept that this approach has led to substantial improvement in trauma care and education. Many fracture classification schemes have been introduced for different anatomical areas of the spinal column. Traditionally two basic approaches to classification can be recognized: descriptive and mechanistic. Many of the schemes are a combination of these two basic approaches.

Anatomical Areas of the Spine

Although the basic anatomical plan of the spine is the same throughout the spinal column, very ancient and specific adaptations exist in the cranial and caudal extremities. Cranially, the occiput–C spine junction is formed by a special anatomical structure called the occipito-atlanto-axial complex. The most caudal section is formed by the fusion

Table 4.2 Neurologic Injury Classification

Neurologic syndromes	Usually well defined and can define place and extent of pathology accurately through neurologic exam
Trauma patients	• Reliable neurologic exam often not attainable due to extenuating circumstances of emergency
	• Accepted that reliable neurologic status can only be determined within 48 to 72 hours of injury
Frankel classification	• First universally accepted system categorizing neurologic injury
	• Classified according to remaining function useful for rehab
	• Refined by American Spinal Injury Association (ASIA); system now determines sensory and motor levels separately to reach an ASIA impairment scale

STANDARD NEUROLOGICAL CLASSIFICATION OF SPINAL CORD INJURY

Patient Name _____

Examiner Name _____ Date/Time of Exam_____

ASIA — AMERICAN SPINAL INJURY ASSOCIATION

ISCoS

MOTOR
KEY MUSCLES (scoring on reverse side)

R L
- C5 Elbow flexors
- C6 Wrist extensors
- C7 Elbow extensors
- C8 Finger flexors (distal phalanx of middle finger)
- T1 Finger abductors (little finger)

UPPER LIMB TOTAL
(MAXIMUM) ☐ (25) + ☐ (25) = ☐ (50)

Comments:

- L2 Hip flexors
- L3 Knee extensors
- L4 Ankle dorsiflexors
- L5 Long toe extensors
- S1 Ankle plantar flexors

Voluntary anal contraction (Yes/No)

LOWER LIMB TOTAL
(MAXIMUM) ☐ (25) + ☐ (25) = ☐ (50)

SENSORY
KEY SENSORY POINTS

LIGHT TOUCH / PIN PRICK
R L R L

0 = absent
1 = impaired
2 = normal
NT = not testable

C2, C3, C4, C5, C6, C7, C8, T1, T2, T3, T4, T5, T6, T7, T8, T9, T10, T11, T12, L1, L2, L3, L4, L5, S1, S2, S3, S4-5

Any anal sensation (Yes/No)

TOTALS { ☐ (56) + ☐ (56) } = ☐ (56) + ☐ (56)

PIN PRICK SCORE (max: 112)
LIGHT TOUCH SCORE (max: 112)

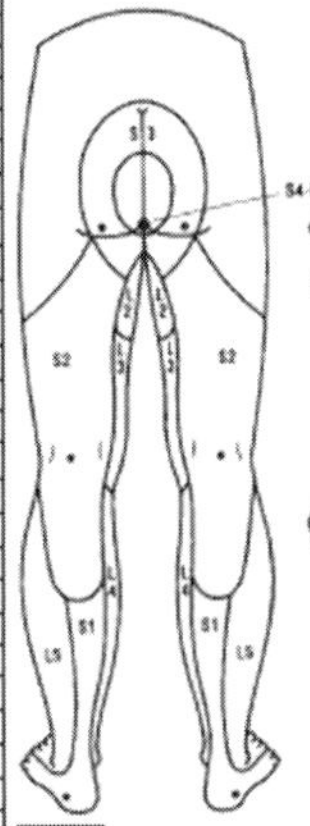

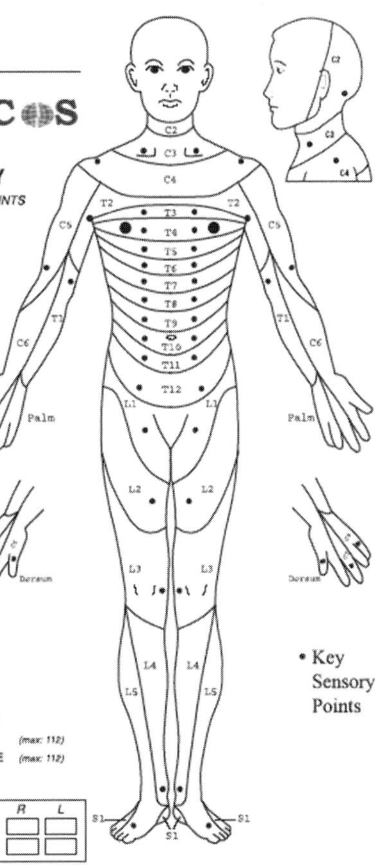

- Key Sensory Points

NEUROLOGICAL LEVEL
The most caudal segment with normal function

R L
SENSORY ☐ ☐
MOTOR ☐ ☐

COMPLETE OR INCOMPLETE? ☐
Incomplete = Any sensory or motor function in S4-S5

ASIA IMPAIRMENT SCALE ☐

ZONE OF PARTIAL PRESERVATION
Caudal extent of partially innervated segments

R L
SENSORY ☐ ☐
MOTOR ☐ ☐

This form may be copied freely but should not be altered without permission from the American Spinal Injury Association.

REV 03/06

MUSCLE GRADING

0 total paralysis

1 palpable or visible contraction

2 active movement, full range of motion, gravity eliminated

3 active movement, full range of motion, against gravity

4 active movement, full range of motion, against gravity and provides some resistance

5 active movement, full range of motion, against gravity and provides normal resistance

5* muscle able to exert, in examiner's judgement, sufficient resistance to be considered normal if identifiable inhibiting factors were not present

NT not testable. Patient unable to reliably exert effort or muscle unavailable for testing due to factors such as immobilization, pain on effort or contracture.

ASIA IMPAIRMENT SCALE

☐ A = **Complete:** No motor or sensory function is preserved in the sacral segments S4-S5.

☐ B = **Incomplete:** Sensory but not motor function is preserved below the neurological level and includes the sacral segments S4-S5.

☐ C = **Incomplete:** Motor function is preserved below the neurological level, and more than half of key muscles below the neurological level have a muscle grade less than 3.

☐ D = **Incomplete:** Motor function is preserved below the neurological level, and at least half of key muscles below the neurological level have a muscle grade of 3 or more.

☐ E = **Normal:** Motor and sensory function are normal.

CLINICAL SYNDROMES (OPTIONAL)

☐ Central Cord
☐ Brown-Sequard
☐ Anterior Cord
☐ Conus Medullaris
☐ Cauda Equina

STEPS IN CLASSIFICATION

The following order is recommended in determining the classification of individuals with SCI.

1. Determine sensory levels for right and left sides.

2. Determine motor levels for right and left sides.
   Note: in regions where there is no myotome to test, the motor level is presumed to be the same as the sensory level.

3. Determine the single neurological level.
   This is the lowest segment where motor and sensory function is normal on both sides, and is the most cephalad of the sensory and motor levels determined in steps 1 and 2.

4. Determine whether the injury is Complete or Incomplete (sacral sparing).
   If voluntary anal contraction = No AND all S4-5 sensory scores = 0 AND any anal sensation = No, then injury is COMPLETE. Otherwise injury is incomplete.

5. Determine ASIA Impairment Scale (AIS) Grade:

   Is injury **Complete?** If YES, AIS=A Record ZPP
   (For ZPP record lowest dermatome or myotome on each side with some (non-zero score) preservation)

   NO ↓

   Is injury motor **incomplete?** If NO, AIS=B
   (Yes=voluntary anal contraction OR motor function more than three levels below the motor level on a given side.)

   YES ↓

   Are **at least** half of the key muscles below the (single) neurological level graded 3 or better?

   NO ↓ → AIS=C   YES ↓ → AIS=D

   If sensation and motor function is normal in all segments, AIS=E
   Note: AIS E is used in follow up testing when an individual with a documented SCI has recovered normal function. If at initial testing no deficits are found, the individual is neurologically intact; the ASIA Impairment Scale does not apply.

Fig. 4.1 Classification of neurologic injury according to the American Spinal Injury Association.

Table 4.3 Vertebral Regions Reacting Differently to Trauma Due to Structure

Occipito-atlanto-axial junction	C0-C2
Subaxial spine	C3-C6
Cervicothoracic junction	C7-T3
Thoracic spine	T4–T9
Thoracolumbar junction	T10-L2
Lumbar spine	L3-L5
Sacrum	

of the last five or six spinal segments into the sacrum, which is also a part of the pelvic ring. Besides these special forms in the extremities, the vertebrae of the cervical, thoracic, and lumbar spine show variations in the different parts of the basic plan and react differently to traumatic forces. Usually these regions are treated separately (**Table 4.3**).

Conventionally, separate systems have been used for the upper cervical, subaxial, thoracic, and lumbar and sacral fractures.

Upper Cervical Injuries and Fractures

The first two vertebrae have evolved into a radically different body plan to form a special structure, allowing the junction of the cranium with the cervical spine (**Table 4.4**). This special occipitocervical junction containing the occipital condyle–atlas and atlas–axis connection is capable of extreme rotation, especially between C1 and C2. This is achieved by the fusion of the central section of the body of C1 to C2 as the odontoid process, and the conversion of the rest of the intervertebral disk space into a special kind of a facet joint, allowing an orientation parallel to the base of the skull. This atlantoaxial complex is joined to the skull through occipital condyles and strong ligaments (**Fig. 4.2**). Although injuries are usually classified under condyle fractures, atlas fractures, and axis fractures, one should not forget that this is a strongly integrated complex, and injury to one part has consequences for the whole complex. The classification systems used for this complex are descriptive and not validated.

Occipitocervical Dislocations

These dislocations are uncommon injuries probably because of their fatal outcomes. Thanks to advanced trauma life support (ATLS), however, more patients survive these injuries and are diagnosed. They are more common in children because of their relatively bigger head size. In autopsy studies, they represent more than 10% of cervical injuries. A descriptive classification has been suggested, but its value is questionable because of the infrequency of reported cases. According to this classification, type I represents anterior, type II vertical, and type III posterior displacements. Also, a type IIA injury has been described where the vertical displacement takes place between C1 and C2.[4]

Occipital Condyle Fractures

The most commonly used classification is that of Anderson and Montesano from 1988, based on the description of only six cases (**Fig. 4.3; Table 4.5**). A type I fracture is a comminuted impaction fracture resulting from axial loading, whereas type II is a condylar fracture with extension into the base of the skull. Type III is an avulsion-type fracture at the insertion of the alar ligament. Accordingly, Anderson and Montesano suggested that only the type III would be considered unstable. Tuli et al proposed in 1997 a new system of classification, because of the difficulty in predicting stability simply by the displacement of the occipital condylar fracture without confirmation by other means, such as

Table 4.4 Upper Cervical Fractures and Occipitocervical Dislocations

Structure	• Contains occipital condyle–atlas and atlas–axis connection capable of extreme rotation
Occipitocervical dislocation	• Uncommon due to high fidelity rate
	• More common in children
	• Represent 10% of cervical injuries
	• Classification:
	1. Type I: anterior dislocation
	2. Type II: vertical dislocation
	3. Type IIA: vertical between C1 and C2
	4. Type III: posterior dislocation

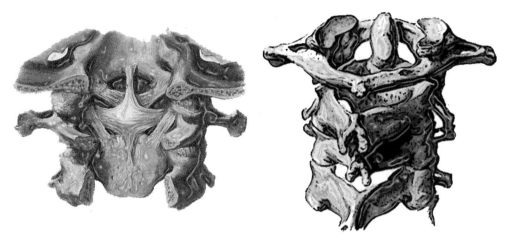

Fig. 4.2 The occipitocervical junction is formed by a special adaptation of the first two vertebrae and a strong network of ligaments.

magnetic resonance imaging (MRI), to establish whether there was a ligament injury. In this system, type I fractures are undisplaced and stable, and type II fractures are divided into subtypes A and B. Type IIA is a displaced fracture of the occipital condyle with stability at the occiput–C1-C2 levels. In type IIB fractures, there is instability at the occiput–C1-C2 levels as demonstrated by radiography.[5]

Atlas (C1) Fractures

This is a relatively common injury constituting approximately 10% of cervical injuries (**Table 4.6**). In almost half of the cases they occur in combination with C2 fractures. Three common types are observed: posterior arch fractures, lateral mass fractures, and burst (Jefferson) fractures (**Fig. 4.4**). Theoretically, the integrity of the

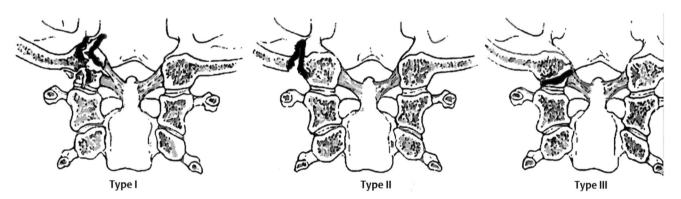

Type I Type II Type III

Fig. 4.3 Three basic types of condyle fractures.

Table 4.5 Occipital Condyle Fractures

Anderson and Montesano classification	• Type I: comminuted impaction fracture resulting from axial loading
	• Type II: condylar fracture with extension into base of skull
	• Type III: avulsion-type fracture at insertion of alar ligament; only one considered "unstable"
Tuli et al classification	• Type I: fracture undisplaced and stable
	• Type IIA: displaced fracture of occipital condyle with stability of the occiput–C1-C2 levels
	• Type IIB: instability at the occiput–C1-C2 levels demonstrated via radiography

transverse ligament is crucial in the stability of the atlantoaxial complex.

Axis (C2) Fractures

Due to its special anatomy, the axis is exceptionally vulnerable at two points: the odontoid process and the isthmus. The odontoid process (dens) is the only vertebral body type (cancellous) structure in the spine, which must resist forces other than compression. This explains the high incidence of these fractures in the osteoporotic spine. Because the C1-C2 connection lacks a real facet joint, the C2 body is connected to the facet of C3 through an elongated pedicle-isthmus. The motion planes of the proximal and distal joints of C2 also make a sharp angle and have a considerable offset between them. The motion plane of C1-C2 joint is ventral, whereas the C2-C3 joint is dorsal to the spinal canal. This connection is further

Table 4.6 Fractures of Atlas and Axis

Atlas (C1)	• Relatively common; approximately. 10% of cervical injuries
	• Approximately 50% associated with C2 fractures
	• Three common types:
	1. Posterior arch fractures
	2. Lateral mass fractures
	3. Burst (Jefferson) fractures
	• Integrity of transverse ligament crucial to stability
Axis (C2)	• Anatomically vulnerable at two points:
	1. Odontoid process (dens): common fractures in osteoporotic spine
	2. Isthmus: common spondylolisthesis of C2 (hangman's fracture)
Odontoid fracture	• 8 to 18% of cervical fractures
	• Neurologic injury occurring in 10 to 20% of cases
	• Two peaks of incidence:
	1. Childhood injury: hyperflexion
	2. Elderly injury: hyperextension
	• Anderson and D'Alonzo classification system used:
	Type I: tip of dens; uncommon
	Type II: fracture at dens–axis junction; most common, with high rate of nonunion
	Type III: fracture through body of axis
Hangman's fracture	• Traumatic spondylolisthesis of axis
	• Effendi classification used (modified by Levine and Edwards):
	Type 1: fracture through isthmus posterior to body; vertical fracture line
	Type 1A: "atypical hangman's fracture"; fracture lines of left and right isthmus not parallel
	Type 2: significant angulation and more than 3 mm of translation; vertical fracture lines; caused by combination of hyperextension and axial loading, causing type 1 fracture, followed by flexion force
	Type 2A: uncommon; little or no translation but significant angulation; oblique fracture line, from anterior-inferior to posterior-superior; caused by flexion-distraction forces
	Type 3: multiple configurations:
	Type 1 fracture with bilateral dislocation of C2-C3 facet joints
	Unilateral facet dislocation and contralateral isthmus fracture

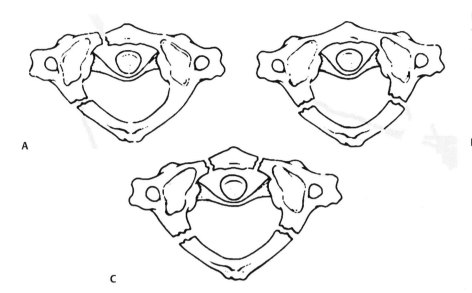

Fig. 4.4 The most common patterns of C1 fractures. **(A)** Lateral mass. **(B)** Posterior arch. **(C)** Burst (Jefferson).

weakened by the vertebral artery penetrating the axis just at the base of the pedicles. This explains the common occurrence of the traumatic spondylolisthesis of the C2, which is also (erroneously) called the hangman's fracture.

Odontoid (Dens) Fractures

These fractures constitute 8 to 18% of the cervical fractures, with neurologic injuries occurring in 10 to 20% of the cases. There are two peaks of incidence with distinctive patterns: one in childhood injuries usually as a result of hyperflexion, and one in the elderly with hyperextension forces.[6] The descriptive-anatomical classification of Anderson and D'Alonzo is the most commonly used system (**Fig. 4.5**):

- *Type I:* fractures at the tip of the dens. Although uncommon, they may be the result of an avulsion fracture of the alar ligaments as part of an occipitocervical dissociation.
- *Type II:* fractures occurring at the junction of the dens with the body of axis. These are the most common fractures and have a high rate of nonunion, especially if there is displacement or treatment delay.
- *Type III:* fractures through the body of axis.

Traumatic Spondylolisthesis of the Axis (Hangman's Fracture)

The most commonly used scheme is the Effendi classification modified by Levine and Edwards[7] (**Fig. 4.6**). This scheme is based on the morphology, presumed mechanism of injury, and the measured amount of angulation and translation between C2 and C3:

- *Type 1:* the fracture is through the isthmus just posterior to the body, and the fracture line is predominantly vertical.

- *Type 1A:* also called "atypical hangman's fracture." The fracture lines of the left and right isthmus are not parallel; therefore, they may not be easily visible on radiograms.

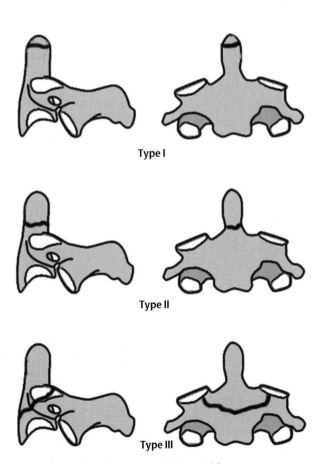

Type I

Type II

Type III

Fig. 4.5 The three basic types of odontoid fractures.

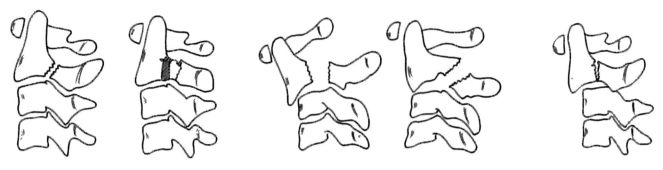

Fig. 4.6 Observed patterns of traumatic spondylolisthesis (hangman's fracture) of C2.

- *Type 2:* these injuries show significant angulation and more than 3 mm of translation. The fracture lines are similar to type 1 and are predominantly vertical. It is generally believed that this type is caused by a combination of hyperextension and axial loading, leading to a type 1 injury followed by a flexion force. This flexion force in the presence of type 1 fracture causes the disruption of the disk where the anterior longitudinal ligament is stripped off together with a crushed anterosuperior corner of the C3 end plate.
  - *Type 2A:* an uncommon but potentially confusing injury type. There is little or no translation but a significant angulation. The direction of the fracture line is oblique, running from anterior-inferior to posterior-superior. This injury is a result of flexion-distraction forces. The isthmus fails in tension as a result of hyperflexion forces, causing a rupture of the disk from posterior to anterior. There is no crushing of the C3 end plate, and the anterior longitudinal ligament (ALL) is intact.
- *Type 3:* may occur in several configurations. The most common form is a type 1 fracture in combination with bilateral dislocation of C2-C3 facet joints. Another potential pattern is a unilateral facet dislocation and contralateral isthmus fracture. The mechanism is unclear. It has been suggested that these result from a

flexion injury causing the facet dislocation followed by a hyperextension force causing the fracture. The neural arch in this type of injury has become a free-floating fragment with disruption of the posterior ligamentary complex (PLC) between C2 and C3 as well as the bony connection to the body of the axis.

Subaxial Cervical Injuries

Due to the relatively big size of the human head and frequent human activities leading to acceleration-deceleration forces, these are common injuries varying from minor sprains (whiplash) to major fracture dislocations (**Table 4.7**).[8] The anatomical adaptations in the C-spine allowing the highest degree of motion of the whole spinal column also predisposes it to highly unstable injury patterns. Cervical spine injuries are responsible for more than 55% of traumatic spinal cord injuries. Many of the concepts developed for the classification of thoracolumbar injuries have also been applied with modifications to the cervical spine.[9] For a discussion of these concepts, see Thoracic and Lumbar Spine Fractures (next subsection). The most commonly used system in the C-spine is the mechanistic classification proposed by Ferguson and Allen.[10] In this scheme the injuries are grouped into

Table 4.7 Subaxial Cervical Injuries

Injury type	• Vary from minor sprain ("whiplash") to fracture dislocations
	• Anatomically predisposed highly unstable injury patterns
Characteristics	• Common
	• Approximately 55% of traumatic spinal cord injuries
Allen and Ferguson classification	• Six phylogenies (according to inferred mode of failure):
	1. Flexion-compression
	2. Vertical compression
	3. Flexion-distraction
	4. Extension-compression
	5. Extension-distraction
	6. Lateral flexion

six phylogenies according to the inferred mode of failure of the C-spine:

1. Flexion-compression
2. Vertical compression
3. Flexion-distraction
4. Extension-compression
5. Extension-distraction
6. Lateral flexion

Within each phylogeny there is a series of stages based on the severity of anatomical disruption. This system is a highly complex combination of mechanistic classification at the phylogeny level and anatomical-descriptive categorization at the subphylogeny level. Because of its complexity, this scheme has not been used extensively in clinical practice, and no studies have been conducted on the validity and reproducibility of this scheme. More recent classification proposals are discussed later (see The Concept of Injury Severity Scores).

Thoracic and Lumbar Spine Fractures

There has been a great deal of controversy about the classification of fractures of the thoracolumbar spine since the first attempts by Böhler in 1929[1] (**Table 4.8**).

Table 4.8 Thoracic and Lumbar Spine Fractures

Böhler classification	• Based on five injury types:
	1. Compression fractures
	2. Flexion-distraction injuries
	3. Extension fractures
	4. Shear fractures
	5. Torsion injuries
Watson-Jones and Nicoll classification	• Developed this scheme further by introducing concept of "instability" and the crucial role of ligamentous structures:
	1. Wedge compression fractures
	2. Comminuted fractures
	3. Fracture dislocations
Holdsworth classification	• Abstracts the vertebral stability with an architectonic concept of two columns:
	1. Anterior column: vertebral body, intervertebral disks, and anterior and posterior ligaments
	2. Posterior column: facet joints, laminae, and posterior ligaments
	• First to describe burst fracture as separate entity
Kelly and Whitesides classification	• Further developed Holdsworth system:
	1. Anterior column: vertebral bodies
	2. Posterior column: neural arches
Roy-Camille classification	• Emphasized role of "segment moyen" (middle segment)
Louis classification	• Introduced three-column architecture:
	1. Anterior: vertebral bodies and disks
	2 & 3. Posterior: facet joints, articular process, and isthmus
	• Three columns connected by tree arches:
	1. Neural arch: two posteriors
	2. Two pedicles: posterior with anterior
	• Quantified instability: (instability = score of 2 or more)
	1. Each column = 1.0 point
	2. Arches = 0.5 point
	3. Other elements = 0.25 point

Böhler's descriptive scheme based on radiographic images identified five injury types:

1. Compression fractures
2. Flexion-distraction injuries
3. Extension fractures
4. Shear fractures
5. Torsion injuries

Watson-Jones and Nicoll further popularized and developed this descriptive scheme. Watson-Jones was the first who introduced the concept of *instability* and recognized the importance of ligamentary injuries for the mechanical stability of the spinal column. Based on three predominant injury categories—wedge compression fractures, comminuted fractures, and fracture-dislocations—he tried to define instability patterns so that the classification can be used as a predictive tool and a guide for treatment. Holdsworth tried to capture the problem of stability in a columnar spine concept in the 1960s. He tried to abstract the vertebral stability with an architectonic concept of two columns: (1) anterior column, consisting of the vertebral body, the intervertebral disks, and the anterior and posterior ligaments; and (2) posterior column, consisting of the facet joints, laminae, and posterior ligaments. This abstraction has been influential not only in the thoracolumbar but also in the cervical spine pathologies ever since (**Fig. 4.7**). Holdsworth was also the first author to describe the burst fracture as a separate entity. The columnar spine concept of Holdsworth was further developed by Kelly and Whitesides, with the anterior column represented by the vertebral bodies and the posterior column by the neural arches. Roy-Camille in the

1970s emphasized in that context the role of what he called the "segment moyen" (middle segment) formed by the posterior part of the disk, anulus fibrosus, and posterior longitudinal ligament, together with the pedicles and the facet joints. Louis tried to elaborate the spinal columns concept with the introduction of a three-column architecture of the spine. One column is the anterior, composed of the vertebral bodies and the disks; the other two columns are posterior, consisting of the facet joints, articular processes, and isthmus. These three columns are connected by three arches: the neural arch connecting the two posterior columns and the two pedicles connecting the posterior columns with the anterior column. Louis tried to quantify instability with this structure. Each column counts as 1, the arches as $\frac{1}{2}$, and the other elements as $\frac{1}{4}$. Instability is defined by a total score of 2 or more. Louis believed that this basic structure was maintained along the vertical column system, consisting of two columns at C1-C2 and three columns from C2 to the sacrum.

Introduction of computed tomography (CT) during the second half of the 1970s for spinal fractures provided new insight into the fine structure of these injuries (**Table 4.9**). The possibility of imaging the spine in transverse sections drew attention to the comminution of the fractures and canal encroachment, which would not even have been suspected with traditional radiograms. These CT findings had a large impact on the thinking about a new classification system, based on the more accurate description of the extent and place of injury. Some authors showed in extensive studies the indispensability of CT for an exact description of the injuries. Efforts in this direction in the early 1980s culminated in the three-column concept of Denis.[9]

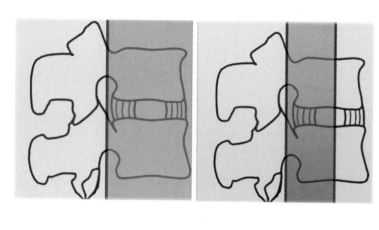
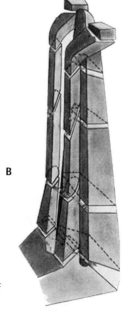

Fig. 4.7 Different columns of the spinal column. **(A)** The two columns of Holdsworth. **(B)** The three columns of Denis. **(C)** Columns of Louis.

Table 4.9 Thoracic and Lumbar Spine Fracture Classification Following Introduction of Computed Tomography (CT) Imaging

Denis classification	• Three-column conceptual model following introduction of CT imaging
	• Emphasized Roy-Camille's "middle column" (posterior half of vertebral body)
	1. Anterior: anterior longitudinal ligament to midvertebral body
	2. Middle: midvertebral body to posterior longitudinal ligament
	3. Posterior: all structures posterior to posterior longitudinal ligament
	• Classified fracture into four types:
	1. Compression fractures
	2. Burst fractures
	3. Seat-belt injuries
	4. Fracture dislocations
	• Introduced concept of three degrees of instability:
	First degree: mechanical instability with risk of progressive kyphosis
	Second degree: neurologic instability
	Third degree: both mechanical and neurologic instability
	• System has come under some criticism
McCormack classification	• Load-sharing classification, designed to help predict problem of failure of posterior fixation:
	A = comminution of vertebral body
	B = apposition of fragments
	C = deformity correction
	• Those with screw fracture had 7 or more points

Denis proposed a different three-column system derived from the Roy-Camille concept by emphasizing the middle column (posterior half of the vertebral body), stating that involvement of this column was paramount to accurately depicting instability in certain injury patterns. The anterior column included the ALL to the midvertebral body. The middle column included the midvertebral body to the posterior longitudinal ligament (PLL), and the posterior column included all structures posterior to the PLL. According to this concept, Denis classified fractures into four types (**Fig. 4.8**):

1. *Compression fractures:* failure under compression of the anterior column; the middle column is intact
2. *Burst fractures:* failure of the anterior and middle columns under axial loads
3. *Seat-belt injuries:* failure of both the posterior and middle columns under tension forces generated by flexion and distraction
4. *Fracture-dislocations:* failure of all columns under compression, tension, rotation, or shear

Denis also introduced the concept of different degrees of instability:

1. *Instability of the first degree* is a mechanical instability with risk of progressive kyphosis.
2. *Instability of the second degree* is a neurologic instability.
3. *Instability of the third degree* is both a mechanical and a neurologic instability. Fracture-dislocations and unstable burst fractures are in this category.

Although this classification was a refinement in the understanding of the nature of these injuries and was widely used for thoracolumbar as well as subaxial cervical fractures, it was amenable to many simplifications and led to some confusion that still exists. As usual, this scheme was also introduced without a proper analysis of reproducibility or the predictive power. Although Denis emphasized that his columns are formed by osseous and nonosseous structures, no attempt has been made to further the diagnosis of nonosseous injuries. The three-column concept was reduced to what is visible with transverse CT images. It has been

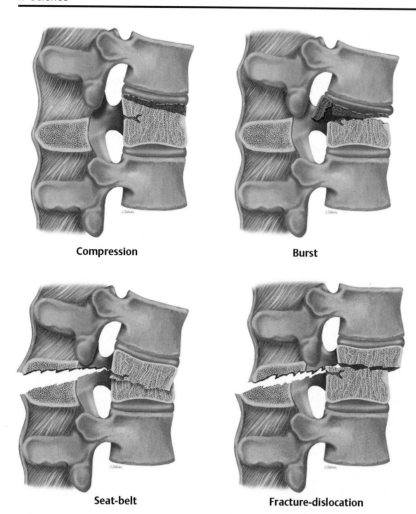

Compression

Burst

Seat-belt

Fracture-dislocation

Fig. 4.8 The four basic fracture types according to Denis.

simplified and reduced to a simple rule of thumb, which states that any injury to two of the three columns, as seen on CT (e.g., bony injury), makes the spine unstable. Further, an intact middle column has been seen as a guarantee of stability, although Denis mentioned some of these lesions as first-degree unstable. Also, the differentiation among first-, second-, and third-degree instability has been lost, leading to a vague, poorly defined, and alarming instability concept, which has remained dominant during the past two decades.

Despite its widespread acceptance, there has been criticism of the three-column concept of Denis and attempts to modify it from the beginning. Ferguson and Allen[10] in 1984 called the columns a "poor semantic choice" because these tissues do not anatomically or biomechanically resemble a column. They stated, "The term, although appealing for its verbal ring, is anatomically and biomechanically incorrect." They suggested a mechanistic classification instead, according to a presumed mechanism of injury deduced from the patterns of tissue failure. The vertebral body in this system is divided into two regions dissimilar to the Denis column system, with the anterior and posterior demarcation being drawn at the junction of the anterior two thirds and posterior one third of the vertebral body.

Dissatisfaction with these vague concepts led to attempts to define some specific questions disturbing the practitioners. One of the most remarkable attempts was the load-sharing classification proposed by McCormack et al[11] in 1994. This scheme is a specific elaboration of the Denis system with a specific problem in mind. The authors were disturbed by the high rate of failure of posterior fixation in their patients with some type of fractures and searched for factors predictive of this failure. Their conclusion was that the degree of comminution of the vertebral body together with the apposition of fragments and the degree of deformity correction were factors predictive of the failure of posterior fixation. The authors developed a rating system:

A: *comminution of the vertebral body:* little (1 point), more (2 points), gross (3 points)
B: *apposition of fragments:* minimal (1 point), spread (2 points), wide (3 points)
C: *deformity correction:* little (1 point), more (2 points), most (3 points)

McCormack et al observed that, in their series of 28 patients, all 10 patients with a screw fracture had a

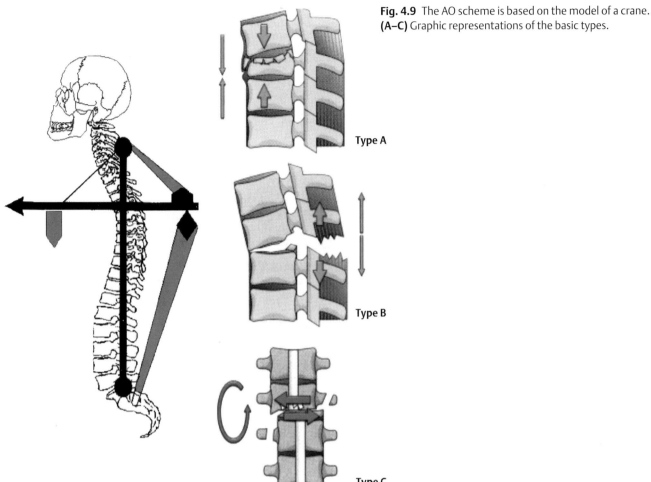

Fig. 4.9 The AO scheme is based on the model of a crane. **(A–C)** Graphic representations of the basic types.

Type A

Type B

Type C

sum of 7 or more points, and no patient with a sum of 6 or less points had a screw fracture.

The classification scheme of the AO group introduced in the early 1990s was a culmination of efforts of many practitioners during a 10-year period.[12] This scheme is primarily based on the pathomorphologic characteristics of the injuries and is based on the mechanical model of a crane (**Fig. 4.9**). Three main categories with a common injury pattern, the types, are formed (**Fig. 4.10**):

- Type A: vertebral body compression
- *Type B:* anterior and posterior element injury with distraction
- *Type C:* anterior and posterior element injury with rotation or translation

The AO group abandoned the three-column concept and went back to the two-column concept of Holdsworth, that is, an anterior column consisting of the vertebral body and the disk and a posterior osseous-ligamentary complex functioning as a tension band. The AO group also depended on the mechanistic classification of Ferguson and Allen for identification of common denominators of the types: type A injuries represent compression forces,

type B tensile forces, and type C axial torque or shear forces. Biomechanical studies showed a good relation between this type of categorization of the scheme and the resulting mechanical instability in a cadaveric fracture model. For further subclassification, the AO group used the common

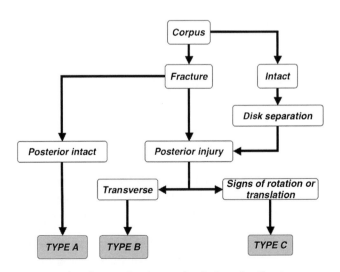

Fig. 4.10 Flow diagram for the type level of AO classification.

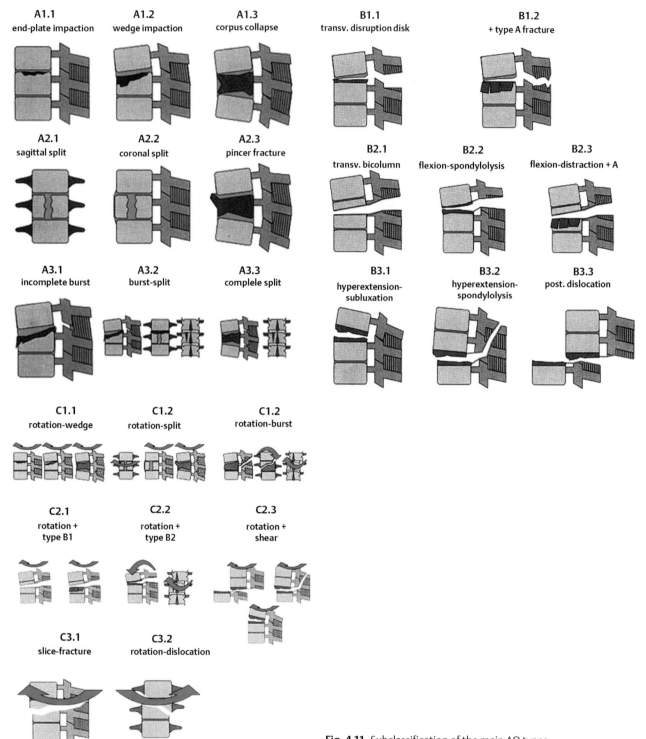

A1.1
end-plate impaction

A1.2
wedge impaction

A1.3
corpus collapse

B1.1
transv. disruption disk

B1.2
+ type A fracture

A2.1
sagittal split

A2.2
coronal split

A2.3
pincer fracture

B2.1
transv. bicolumn

B2.2
flexion-spondylolysis

B2.3
flexion-distraction + A

A3.1
incomplete burst

A3.2
burst-split

A3.3
complele split

B3.1
hyperextension-
subluxation

B3.2
hyperextension-
spondylolysis

B3.3
post. dislocation

C1.1
rotation-wedge

C1.2
rotation-split

C1.2
rotation-burst

C2.1
rotation +
type B1

C2.2
rotation +
type B2

C2.3
rotation +
shear

C3.1
slice-fracture

C3.2
rotation-dislocation

Fig. 4.11 Subclassification of the main AO types.

AO 3–3–3 grid (**Fig. 4.11**). Subclassification of the type B and C injuries essentially follows the subclassification of type A injuries (**Table 4.10**):

- Type A injuries: caused mainly by axial compression, resulting in predominantly an injury to the anterior elements (vertebral body and disk). There is no or insignificant injury to the tension band function of the posterior column. The subtypes of type A are as follows:
  - A1: impaction fractures. The deformation of the vertebral body is due to compression (plastic deformation) of the cancellous bone rather than fragmentation.
    - A1.1: end-plate impaction with minor wedging up to 5 degrees

Table 4.10 AO Group Classification of Spinal Injury

Type	Fracture	Class	Subclass
Type A	Vertebral body compression	A1: Impaction fractures	A1.1: end-plate impaction with minor wedging up to 5 degrees A1.2: wedge impaction with loss of anterior vertebral height resulting in angulation of more than 5 degrees A1.3: vertebral body collapse
		A2: Split fractures	A2.1: sagittal split fractures A2.2: coronal split fractures A2.3: pincer fracture
		A3: Burst fractures	A3.1: incomplete burst fracture A3.2: burst split fractures A3.3: complete burst fracture
Type B	Anterior and posterior element injury with distraction	B1: Posterior disruption predominantly ligamentary	B1.1: associated with transverse disruption of disk B1.2: associated with type A fracture of vertebral body
		B2: Posterior disruption predominantly osseous	B2.1: transverse bicolumn fracture B2.2: posterior disruption predominantly osseous with transverse disk disruption B2.3: posterior disruption predominantly osseous associated type A vertebral body fracture
Type B	Anterior and posterior element injury with distraction	B3: Anterior disruption through the disk	B3.1: hyperextension-subluxation B3.2: hyperextension-spondylolysis B3.3: posterior dislocation
Type C	Anterior and posterior element injury with rotation or translation	C1: Type A with rotation	C1.1: rotation and wedge fracture C1.2: rotation and split fracture C1.3: rotation and burst fracture
		C2: Type B with rotation	C2.1: rotation and type B1 C2.2: rotation and type B2 C2.3: rotation and type B3
		C3: Rotational shear injuries	C3.1: slice fracture C3.2: rotation and dislocation

- A1.2: wedge impaction with loss of anterior vertebral height resulting in an angulation of more than 5 degrees
- A1.3: vertebral body collapse; symmetrical loss of vertebral body such as observed in osteoporotic spines without significant extrusion of fragments
- A2: split fractures. The vertebral body is split in the coronal or sagittal plane with dislocation of fragments and filling of the defect with disk material.
  - A2.1: Sagittal split fractures
  - A2.2: Coronal split fractures
  - A2.3: Pincer fracture, in which the central part of the body is crushed and filled with disk material
- A3: burst fractures, with fragments of posterior wall extruding in the canal
  - A3.1: incomplete burst fractures; burst of the upper or lower half of the body

- A3.2: burst-split fracture; burst of one half of the vertebra and split of the rest
- A3.3: complete burst fracture; entire body is burst
- Type B injuries: the main criterion is a transverse disruption of one or both spinal columns leading to failure of the tension band. The subtypes of type B are as follows:
- B1: posterior disruption predominantly ligamentary
  - B1.1: associated with transverse disruption of the disk
  - B1.2: associated with type A fracture of the vertebral body
- B2: posterior disruption predominantly osseous
  - B2.1: transverse bicolumn fracture
  - B2.2: posterior disruption predominantly osseous with transverse disruption of the disk
  - B2.3: posterior disruption predominantly osseous associated with type A fracture of the vertebral body

- B3: anterior disruption through the disk
  - B3.1: hyperextension-subluxation
  - B3.2: hyperextension-spondylolysis
  - B3.3: posterior dislocation
- Type C injuries: anterior and posterior element injuries with rotation or translation. The subtypes of type C are as follows:
  - C1: type A with rotation
    - C1.1: rotation + wedge fracture
    - C1.2: rotation + split fracture
    - C1.3: rotation + burst fracture
  - C2: type B with rotation
    - C2.1: rotation + type B1
    - C2.2: rotation + type B2
    - C2.3: rotation + type B3
  - C3: rotational shear injuries
    - C3.1: slice fracture
    - C3.2: rotation-dislocation

This classification represents a taxonomic beauty in that each and every injury can be fitted to a certain category in ever-expanding detail. But one should not forget that the dream of a taxonomist might be the nightmare of a practitioner. Although conceptually sound, the apparent complexity frightened many practitioners and obstructed the diffusion of the basic ideas behind this sophisticated scheme.

Sacrum Fractures

The sacrum is the keystone in the junction between the pelvic ring and the spine. Its fractures have consequences for the stability of the pelvic ring as well as the spinal column and may cause injury to the sacral roots or the sacral plexus (**Table 4.11**). They are usually seen as part of the pelvic injuries and are classified according to the stability of the pelvic ring. Their consequences for the stability of the spinal column received little attention. There is no universally accepted unifying concept for their classification.

Table 4.11 Fractures of Sacrum

Implications	Junction between pelvic ring and spine: stability of both, as well as sacral plexus, is a concern in fractures
Denis classification	• Three zones:
	1. Lateral to neural foramina
	2. Through the neural foramina
	3. Central canal

Denis classified them into three zones: (1) lateral to the neural foramina, (2) through the neural foramina, and (3) in the central canal. For the sagittal deformity caused by fractures through zone 3, the classification of Roy-Camille has generally been accepted (**Fig. 4.12**). These are all descriptive schemes, and their usefulness has not been studied systematically.

■ Problems with Classification Systems

Any classification system is based on a presumption about an underlying common characteristic of the subsets of a domain. A fracture classification system is based on the presumption that the interaction of various forces with the parts of a living organism involved create some basic observable patterns. The main difficulty of all fracture classification schemes lies in the innumerable variables involved in a traumatic lesion. The classification has to presuppose an all-or-none result of some of these interactions. A classification scheme tries to compress the available information into reproducible categories without loss of information content, which means it is an algorithmic compression process (**Table 4.12**). It is then inevitable that two kinds of problems arise with categorization schemes:

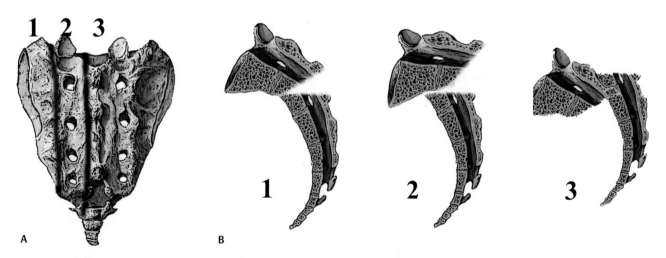

Fig. 4.12 (A) Three zones of sacrum (Denis) and **(B)** the classification of zone 3 fractures according to Roy-Camille.

Table 4.12 Problems with Classification Systems

• Main difficulty	• Innumerable variables involved in a traumatic lesion
• Problems arising in algorithmic compression process	• Loss of information content in favor of simplicity, thus higher reproducibility
	• Loss of simplicity and reproducibility in favor of higher fidelity to information content
• Commonalities	• All systems based on pattern recognition
	• Neutral construct or model of complex phenomenon providing information on injury severity and consequences, thus providing a reasonable estimation of outcomes of different treatments

either there is a loss of information content in favor of simplicity and thus higher reproducibility, or there is a loss of simplicity and reproducibility in favor of higher fidelity to the information content. Changes in the information content, for example as a result of novel technology, may have different effects on these two different strategies.[1]

All classification systems are actually based on pattern recognition. A classification of different injury patterns only makes sense if it helps us predict the final outcome better than a simple chance distribution. Recognition of some patterns of injury does not necessarily lead to a better understanding of the prognosis. Only if the observed patterns are shown to be related to certain outcome parameters can we speak of their prognostic significance. A classification scheme is actually a mental construct or a model of a complex phenomenon that is supposed to inform us about the severity of the injury and the possible consequences. This information should finally provide us with a reasonable estimation of the outcome of different treatment modalities. Simple recognition of a pattern may not be meaningful at all if we cannot develop it into a tool of prediction. Such a system should enable us to develop a hypothesis about the outcomes of certain kinds of intervention, which consequently can be tested in the real world. None of the schemes discussed has developed a treatment algorithm that can adequately be tested in the treatment of patients.

Influence of Diagnostic Modality

Although all authors emphasize the importance of soft tissue injuries and included them in the classification schemes, there were usually no conventional clinical or radiologic means to detect them **(Table 4.13)**. Although flexion-extension radiograms have been commonly used to verify ligamentary injury in the cervical spine, their use has been limited to conscious patients without neurologic involvement with suspected soft tissue injury at the subaxial cervical spine. The introduction of MRI offered the possibility of directly imaging all structures involved. Some early studies showed ligamentary involvement, which would be unsuspected on radiograms and CT scans. Cadaver studies in the 1990s showed excellent correlation between MRI findings and anatomical sections. These studies established MRI as a highly accurate modality for determining injury patterns and described the MRI features of different structures involved. In their 1996 review article about the role of imaging in the diagnosis and management of thoracolumbar fractures, Saifuddin et al[13] concluded that any future classification of thoracolumbar injuries should include MRI findings, allowing assessment of the discoligamentary element of the injury as well as of the bony element.

Oner et al[14] have categorized the MRI findings of thoracolumbar spine fractures in a prospective study of

Table 4.13 Influence of Diagnostic Modality

• Flexion-extension radiograms	• Limited use to conscious individual with no neurologic involvement with suspected soft tissue injury at subaxial cervical spine
• MRI	• Offers direct imaging of all structures
	• Shows ligamentary involvement, not detected on radiograms and CT scans (confirmed by Oner et al[14] study)
	• Highly accurate modality for determining injury patterns
	• Shows high incidence of ligament injuries in cervical fractures, whereas in conventional methods these injuries went undetected (e.g., 30% of cases missed posterior ligament complex injuries)
• Fate of intervertebral disk	• Degenerative disease and trauma-related injury now distinguished
• Shortcomings	• MRI detects vast amount of injuries but provides no simple answers to the creation of meaningful classification schemes

100 cases. Categorizing all possibly relevant structures (ALL, PLL, PLC, end plate, disk, and corpus), they found a wide variation of injury patterns in most cases unsuspected on conventional radiograms and CTs. The clinical relevance of these findings is not in every case evident. Fifty-three of these patients were prospectively followed up, and some interesting correlations with the final clinical and radiologic results were reported.[15] An unfavorable outcome in the conservative group was related to the progression of kyphosis, which in most cases was predictable with the use of trauma MRI findings concerning the end-plate comminution and vertebral body involvement. In the operatively treated group, recurrence of the kyphotic deformity was predictable by the lesion of the posterior longitudinal ligamentary complex together with end-plate comminution and vertebral body involvement as seen on trauma MRI. Some MRI studies have also shown a high incidence of ligament injuries in the cervical spine fractures. Since the advent of the AO classification and the following MRI studies, there has been more attention to the injuries of the posterior ligamentary complex injuries. It was shown in some series that at least in 30% of the cases, PLC injuries went undetected with conventional methods. Lee et al[16] compared MRI with perioperative findings of PLC injuries and found that fat-suppressed T2-weighted sagittal sequence of MRI was a highly sensitive, specific, and accurate method of evaluating posterior ligament complex injury.

Another point, which was insufficiently addressed in the existing schemes, was the fate of the intervertebral disk. Changes in the disk space were frequently observed, especially in thoracolumbar fractures, and were incriminated for progressive or recurrent kyphosis. Although it was assumed that this represented a process similar to the degenerative disk disease, it was shown that in the majority of the cases, the disks did not resemble degenerative disk disease patterns. Based on an MRI study of 63 patients minimally 18 months after trauma, a classification scheme of the post-traumatic disk types was developed.[17] The majority of the disks seemed to show predominantly morphologic changes with no change in signal intensity. Some disk types were associated with progressive kyphosis in the conservatively treated patients. In the operatively treated patients, recurrent kyphosis seemed to have resulted from the creeping of the disk in the central depression of the bony end plate rather than from disk degeneration.

Although these studies established MRI as a highly sensitive imaging modality capable of detecting all kinds of injury to a fractured spine, they did not provide answers to some of the essential problems of creating meaningful classification schemes.

Problems of Reproducibility

One of the main purposes of classification systems is to create a common language between the investigators of the field. This requires an acceptable degree of interobserver agreement on the main distinctions of a scheme. Also, each investigator or clinician should be able to reproduce the same classification in different occasions; that is, the scheme should also have reasonable interobserver repeatability. Both interobserver agreement and reproducibility have been problematic with fracture classification systems in general.

All of the conventional classification systems have been introduced without a proper study of their reproducibility. Studies later performed by independent groups raised serious concerns about the reproducibility issues.

Blauth et al[18] conducted a multicenter study to assess the interobserver reliability of the AO classification system using the radiographs of 14 fractures of the lumbar spine. The radiographs and CT scans were reviewed in 22 hospitals that were experienced in treating spinal trauma. The mean interobserver agreement for all 14 cases was found to be 67% (41–91%), when only the three main types (A, B, C) were used. The corresponding kappa value, however, of the interobserver reliability showed a coefficient of .33 (range, .30 to .35), indicating fair reliability. The reliability decreased by increasing the categories. Oner et al[19] studied the reproducibility of the Denis and AO schemes of thoracolumbar fractures using radiograms, CT, and MRI in 53 patients. Five observers of varying professions and experience were involved. They found that the main distinction of the AO system on the primary type level (A/non-A) was fairly reproducible with CT (kappa .34). With MRI this reached only moderate levels (kappa .42). The same was true for type (A, B, C) distinction. Subclassification of type A (groups) yielded higher kappa values corresponding to substantial agreement, which dropped with A subgroups. Intraobserver kappa values between CT and MRI readings were A/non-A .45, for Type .41, for A group .76, and for A subgroup .47.

The agreement was in general better with the Denis classification (CT type kappa .60; CT whole classification .45; MRI type .52; MRI whole classification .39), but the variance was higher due to difficulties of finding proper categories for some injury patterns.

Wood et al[20] repeated this study in 31 cases assessed by 19 experienced spine surgeons and got similar results both for the AO and the Denis classifications.

Thus, the AO scheme seems to focus on fidelity to the information content by providing categories for all kinds of possible injury patterns. This leads inevitably to an increase in the complexity of the scheme but also provides means for classification in accordance with increasing information content following novel technology. But, although the AO scheme recognizes the difference in injuries with or without transverse plane soft tissue involvement, the means to make this distinction reliably were not sufficiently explored. The classification presupposes that the posterior ligamentary complex is either injured or not, although the authors recognize that transient forms do exist.

However mechanically sound this distinction may be, in reality one observes varying degrees of involvement of the posterior ligamentary complex. It is not clear which MRI findings are indicative of *mechanically significant* failure of the tension band system.

The Denis classification, for its time, was based on the novel technology of transverse CT images and represents a strategy of simplification. Refinement of the imaging technology in the form of CT with multiplanar reconstruction (CT-MPR) and MRI proved that much of the information from these new modalities is difficult to integrate into this scheme. Much of the ligamentary involvement of the posterior column cannot be accounted for in the scheme. As a result, injury patterns either with or without posterior ligamentary complex involvement are grouped together into categories based on the patterns of bony involvement, or injury patterns with posterior ligamentary complex involvement are assigned to higher categories constituting an overestimation of the severity. In the study of Oner et al, the more experienced observer more often assigned these injuries to higher categories, leading to marked variance in the results. This type of confusion may have contributed in the past to the widely different results of different treatment strategies reported in the literature.

■ The Concept of Injury Severity Scores

Although classification attempts have been going on for all kinds of traumatic injuries to the spinal column since the introduction of radiograms, critical assessment of these schemes was lacking until the last decade. Classifications of traumatic injuries have been developed as pattern recognition systems without a proper discussion on the question of whether these observed patterns are reproducible or meaningful. Parallel developments in the diagnostic imaging and surgical treatment of these injuries have urged the surgeons to critically assess these practices to reach scientifically sound methods to improve the care of these patients with a high personal, economic, and social burden. An international group of surgeons came together for this purpose in the Spine Trauma Study Group. After reviewing the available information, this group reached the following conclusions (**Table 4.14**).

The various classification systems proposed overlap in their basic description of injury (anatomical, mechanistic). Only a few attempts were seen to develop treatment recommendations based on presumed injury severity. No classification system has been universally adopted because

Table 4.14 Injury Severity Scores

Spine Trauma Study Group	Components of a good classification system:
	• Based on observed morphology of injury
	• Comprehensive
	• Characterize injury by mechanical, neurologic, and long-term stability
	• Reproducible
	• Allow development of testable hypothesis based on treatment recommendations
	• Remain evolvable (room for refinement)
Injury Severity Score: Thoracolumbar Injury Classification and Severity Score (TLICS)	1. Pattern or morphology: comparable to type level of AO system
	• Compression = 1 point
	• Burst = 2 points
	• Rotation/translation = 3 points
	• Distraction = 4 points
	2. Posterior ligamentary complex integrity: working as a tension band
	• Intact = 0 point
	• Suspected/intermediate = 2 points
	• Disrupted = 3 points
	3. Neurologic involvement: one of the most crucial parameters in clinical decision making
	• Intact = 0 point

(Continued on page 64)

Table 4.14 *(Continued)* **Injury Severity Scores**

	• Nerve root = 2 points
	• Cord/conus
	○ Complete (ASIA A) = 2 points
	○ Incomplete (ASIA B-D) = 3 points
	• Cauda equina = 3 points
Injury Severity Score: Subaxial Cervical Spine Injury Classification System (SLIC)	1. Pattern or morphology
	• Compression = 1 point
	• Burst = 2 points
	• Distraction (e.g., facet perch, hyperextension) = 3 points
	• Rotation/translation (e.g., facet dislocation, unstable teardrop, or advanced staged flexion compression injury) = 4 points
	2. Discoligamentous complex
	• Suspected/intermediate = 1 point
	• Disrupted = 2 points
	4. Neurologic involvement: one of the most crucial parameters in clinical decision making
	• Nerve root = 1 point
	• Cord
	○ Complete (ASIA A) = 2 points
	○ Incomplete (ASIA B-D) = 3 points
	○ Continuous cord compression in setting of neuro deficit = +1
Score interpretation	Sum of scores yields severity score:
	• ≤ 3 points = nonoperative
	• ≥ 5 points = operative
	• 4 points = nonoperative or operative

of particular shortcomings that weaken their ability to guide general treatment and offer prognostication for future functionality.

The Spine Trauma Study Group decided that a good classification scheme should meet the following criteria:

1. It should be based on the observed morphology of injury.
2. It should be comprehensive, meaning that all types of injury can be included and classified based on the severity of the injury.
3. It should characterize the injury in terms of mechanical, neurologic, and long-term stability.
4. It should be reasonably reproducible.
5. It should allow the development of testable hypotheses based on treatment recommendations.
6. It should be evolvable, meaning that the results of clinical studies based on the treatment recommendations

can be integrated into the scheme, allowing a continuous refinement process.

The Spine Trauma Study Group's work resulted in the development of the Injury Severity Score first for the thoracic and lumbar fractures (TLISS), which was later expanded to the Thoracolumbar Injury Classification and Severity Score (TLICS).[21]

Thoracolumbar Injury Classification and Severity Score

In this scheme three separate factors are critical for the determination of the injury severity:

• Pattern or morphology
• Integrity of the posterior ligamentary complex
• Neurologic involvement

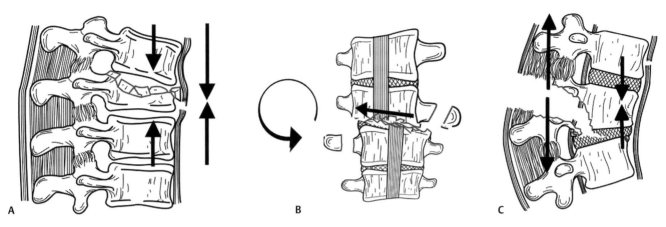

Fig. 4.13 The three main fracture patterns according to the Thoracic and Lumbar Injury Classification and Severity Score (TLICS). **(A)** Compression. **(B)** Rotation/translation. **(C)** Distraction.

Pattern or Morphology

This is basically the same as the type level of the AO classification. Three main injury types are recognized: compression, distraction, and rotation/translation (**Fig. 4.13**).

Integrity of the Posterior Ligamentary Complex

The importance of the PLC working as a tension band is an independent prognostic factor that has been shown in different studies. It was also thought to be important to dissociate the injury to the PLC from the injury pattern because this seemed to be a main problem in the reproducibility of the AO classification, as frank fracture-dislocations have to be grouped together with compression-type fractures with associated PLC injury.

Neurologic Involvement

As neurologic involvement is usually seen as one of the most crucial parameters in the clinical decision process, it should be included in the severity score. The ASIA impairment scale is used here (ASIA classes A to E).

The basic idea is to assign points for the different severity indices for each of the above three factors and finally to reach a combined injury severity score. Treatment recommendations can then be based on this combined score. A panel of experienced spine trauma surgeons decided on these factors and their relative weights. This provides the opportunity to use this semiquantitative system to design multicenter studies and accordingly change the relative weights based on the data. In this way the scheme can evolve on the basis of new investigations. Besides these three basic items, some clinical modifiers, such as polytrauma, age, osteoporosis, degree of deformity, and ankylotic spine, can be used in the same way, and research can be initiated to determine the relative importance of these factors in the clinical decision and prognosis.

A comprehensive Injury Severity Score (**Table 4.15**) is calculated from the injury characteristics to assist in determining treatment. Each of the subgroups in the three main injury categories has a numerical value associated with it. As the injury is sequentially classified into these subgroups, the values are added across the three main injury categories to provide a comprehensive severity score. One to 4 points (1 indicates least severe; 4 indicates most severe/urgent) are assigned to reflect the degree of injury severity and the potential impact on mechanical or neurologic stability. In the presence of multiple contiguous or noncontiguous injuries, only the most severely

Table 4.15 Comprehensive Injury Severity Score

• Pattern or morphology:	
○ Compression	1 point
■ Burst	2 points
○ Rotation/translation	3 points
○ Distraction	4 points
• Posterior ligamentary complex	
○ Intact	0 point
○ Suspected/indeterminate	2 points
○ Disrupted	3 points
• Neurology	
○ Intact	0 point
○ Nerve root	2 points
○ Cord/conus	
■ Complete (ASIA A)	2 points
■ Incomplete (ASIA B-D)	3 points
○ Cauda equina	3 points

involved level is scored. The sum of these scores yields a final Injury Severity Score. Eventually points can be added or subtracted using the clinical modifiers. This final score can be used for a treatment proposal. Fractures with 3 points or less are considered nonoperative cases. Fractures with scores of 5 and higher are considered for operative treatment. Cases with 4 points can be treated operatively or nonoperatively.

Studies done by the Spine Trauma Study Group showed an acceptable reproducibility of this scheme, especially in the final treatment decision point.[22] This system is expected to assist surgeons involved in the treatment of spinal trauma patients. Furthermore, it will stimulate further research and can be used as an instrument for education.

Subaxial Cervical Spine Injury Classification System

Adaptation of this same idea for the subaxial cervical spine has yielded the *Subaxial* Cervical Spine Injury Classification System (SLIC).[23]

Comparable to the TLICS, the most important factors are defined as follows: (1) injury morphology, as determined by the pattern of spinal column disruption on available imaging studies; (2) integrity of the discoligamentous complex, represented by both anterior and posterior ligamentous

structures as well as the intervertebral disk; and (3) neurologic status of the patient. These three injury characteristics are recognized as largely independent predictors of clinical outcome. Within each of the three categories, subgroups were identified and graded from least to most severe and are assigned points according to the severity. This is a promising idea in that the thoracolumbar and subaxial cervical injuries can be approached in a unified manner.

■ Conclusion

Classification systems have helped us to progress in the understanding and treatment of spinal injuries. However, we should not forget the inherent uncertainties and possible flaws in our conceptions. Spinal fractures are less frequent than other injuries, and no one center is able to answer the questions on the prognosis and the proper treatment of these patients. Therefore, it is essential that data be collected from many centers to facilitate developing scientifically valid conclusions. Some kind of abstraction of all these various patients and experiences is necessary if we want to improve our understanding of these injuries. The Spinal Injury Severity Score approach seems to be the most promising project at this moment, and its use should be encouraged.

References

1. Oner FC. Thoracolumbar spine fractures: diagnostic and prognostic parameters [academic thesis]. Utrecht: University of Utrecht, 1999 (http://www.library.uu.nl/digiarchief/dip/diss/1885237/inhoud.htm)
2. White AA, Panjabi MM. Clinical Biomechanics of Spine. Philadelphia: Lippincott; 1978
3. http://www.asia-spinalinjury.org
4. Mark NH. Guidelines for management of acute cervical spine injuries. Neurosurgery 2002;50:1
5. Alcelik I, Manik KS, Sian PS, et al. Occipital condylar fractures: review of the literature and case report. J Bone Joint Surg Br 2006;88:665–669
6. Maak TG, Grauer JN. The contemporary treatment of odontoid injuries. Spine 2006;31(suppl):S53–S60
7. Levine AM. Traumatic spondylolisthesis of the axis, "hangman's fracture." In: The Cervical Spine Research Society Editorial Committee. The Cervical Spine. 3rd ed. Philadelphia: Lippincott-Raven; 1998:429–448
8. Kwon BK, Vaccaro AR, Grauer JN, et al. Subaxial cervical spine trauma. J Am Acad Orthop Surg 2006;14:78–89
9. Denis F. The three-column spine and its significance in the classification of acute thoracolumbar spinal injuries. Spine 1983;8:817–831
10. Ferguson RL, Allen BL. A mechanistic classification of thoracolumbar spine fractures. Clin Orthop Relat Res 1984;189:77–88
11. McCormack T, Karaikovic E, Gaines RW. The load-sharing classification of spine fractures. Spine 1994;19:1741–1744
12. Magerl F, Aebi M, Gertzbein SD, et al. A comprehensive classification of thoracic and lumbar injuries. Eur Spine J 1994;3:184–201

13. Saifuddin A, Noordeen H, Taylor BA, et al. The role of imaging in the diagnosis and management of thoracolumbar burst fractures: current concepts and a review of the literature. Skeletal Radiol 1996;25:603–613
14. Oner FC, van Gils AP, Dhert WJ, et al. MRI findings of thoracolumbar spine fractures: a categorisation based on MRI examinations of 100 fractures. Skeletal Radiol 1999;28:433–443
15. Oner FC, van Gils APG, Faber JAJ, et al. Some complications of common treatment schemes of thoracolumbar spine fractures can be predicted with magnetic resonance imaging. Prospective study of 53 patients with 71 fractures. Spine 2002;27:629–636
16. Lee HM, Kim HS, Kim DJ, et al. Reliability of magnetic resonance imaging in detecting posterior ligament complex injury in thoracolumbar spinal fractures. Spine 2000;25:2079–2084
17. Oner FC, van der Rijt RR, Ramos LM, et al. Changes in the disc space after fractures of the thoracolumbar spine. J Bone Joint Surg Br 1998;80:833–839
18. Blauth M, Bastian L, Knop C, et al. [Inter-observer reliability in the classification of thoraco-lumbar spinal injuries.] Orthopade 1999;28:662–681
19. Oner FC, Ramos LMP, Simmermacher RKJ, et al. Classification of thoracic and lumbar spine fractures: problems of reproducibility. A study of 53 patients using CT and MRI. Eur Spine J 2002;11:235–245
20. Wood KB, Khanna G, Vaccaro AR, Arnold PM, Harris MB, Mehbod AA. Assessment of two thoracolumbar fracture classification systems as used by multiple surgeons. J Bone Joint Surg Am 2005;87:1423–1429

21. Vaccaro AR, Lehman RA Jr, Hurlbert RJ, et al. A new classification of thoracolumbar injuries: the importance of injury morphology, the integrity of the posterior ligamentous complex, and neurologic status. Spine 2005;30:2325–2333

22. Vaccaro AR, Baron EM, Sanfilippo J, et al. Reliability of a novel classification system for thoracolumbar injuries: the Thoracolumbar Injury Severity Score. Spine 2006;31(suppl): S62–S69

23. Vaccaro AR, Hulbert JR, Fisher C, et al. The Sub-axial Cervical Spine Injury Classification System (SLIC): a novel approach to recognize the importance of morphology, neurology and integrity of the disco-ligamentous complex. Spine 2007;32: 2365–2374

5 Imaging Spinal Cord Injuries

Paul D. Campbell Jr. and John A. Carrino

In the setting of trauma, imaging of the spine is often of paramount importance. There are 30,000 traumatic spinal injuries each year in the United States.[1] The majority of injuries sustained to the spine are a result of motor vehicle accidents. Most patients who have sustained acute injuries to the spine present with pain, and appropriate radiologic examinations are obtained, which are tailored to help make specific diagnoses. The preliminary evaluation often consists of radiographs, but with the widespread availability, increased speed,[2,3] and improved sensitivity of computed tomography (CT),[4-10] it has become increasingly the initial evaluation of choice. However, radiographs and CT, although quite sensitive in the diagnosis of bony injury, are less sensitive in the detection of soft tissue and spinal cord injury. The pattern of spinal cord injury without radiographic abnormality (SCIWORA) is often encountered and introduces the need for further advanced imaging techniques, such as magnetic resonance imaging (MRI), which are better suited for such evaluation (**Table 5.1**). Furthermore, the determination of neurologic deficit is often difficult when a patient presents with altered mental status, further complicating the clinical picture. The clinician must integrate the clinical history, mechanism of injury, and physical examination to appropriately tailor diagnostic radiologic evaluations to quickly and effectively obtain diagnoses so that appropriate patient management can be initiated.

Spinal cord injury can be divided into the segment of the spine that is injured—cervical, thoracic, or lumbar. Injuries within these portions of the spine can be further subdivided based on the mechanism of injury. This chapter discusses the most common types of injury in these classifications and their radiologic manifestations.

■ Cervical Spine

Normal Anatomy and Imaging Modalities

Radiographs

In the initial evaluation of trauma, a standard three-view radiographic series of the cervical spine is often obtained (**Table 5.2**). This series includes anteroposterior (AP), lateral, and odontoid views. Of these views, the lateral is usually the most helpful. A normal lateral view of the cervical spine is illustrated in **Fig. 5.1**. There are many important landmarks to recognize on the lateral view, and distortion or absence of any of these is often a clue to the presence of cervical injury. There are five important lines to recognize in the evaluation of the lateral radiograph. The first is the anterior prevertebral soft tissue line. This line is usually curvilinear, with an expected convexity at or about the level of C4-C5 near the origin of the esophagus. The second and third lines, the anterior and posterior vertebral lines, correspond to lines linking the anterior and posterior cortices of continuous vertebral bodies and are curvilinear in a fashion that mimics the usual slight lordosis of the cervical spine. The fourth line is the spinolaminar line, which is also curvilinear and corresponds to the location where the paired laminae meet at the base of the spinous process. The final line, the spinous process line, is another curvilinear line that corresponds to the posterior border of the respective spinous processes.

There are additional structures that should be evaluated in the approach to the lateral cervical spine radiograph. The axis ring is the circular structure that projects over the C2 vertebral body. The junction of the C2 vertebral body and pedicle forms the anterior arc of the axis ring.

Table 5.1 Imaging Modalities

Radiography	Preliminary Evaluation
CT	• Faster, increased sensitivity, widespread availability
	• More commonly used now for initial evaluation
	• More sensitive for osseous than soft tissue abnormalities, can result in spinal cord injury without radiographic abnormality (SCIWORA)
MRI	• Better suited for comprehensive evaluation; sensitive to bone, soft tissue, and spinal cord

Table 5.2 Cervical Spine Imaging

Radiographs	Initial evaluation: three-view series is done:	
	1. Lateral	• Five important lines to recognize:
		1. Anterior prevertebral soft tissue line
		2. Anterior vertebral line
		3. Posterior vertebral line
		4. Spinolaminar line
		5. Spinous process line
		• Additional structures:
		1. Axis ring
		2. Intervertebral disk spaces; heights should be equal
		3. Cervical facet joints
		4. Interspinous distance
		5. Prevertebral soft tissue; no wider than 7 mm anterior to C2
		6. Atlantoaxial interval (ADI); no more than 2.5 mm
		7. Cervicothoracic junction (C7-T1)
	2. Anteroposterior (AP)	Visualization from C3; cervicothoracic junction
		• Lateral margin of articular masses should be smooth
		• Spinous processes should align linearly
	3. Odontoid	Visualization of atlantoaxial and atlantooccipital joints
		• Lateral C1 should align with adjacent lateral C2
CT	• Increased sensitivity over radiographs to evaluate bone	
	• Better imaging of soft tissue adjacent to spine	
	• Has become the evaluation of choice for osseous abnormality	
MRI	• Capacity to detect subtle spinal cord and ligamentous injury	
	• Useful in instances of	
	1. Posttraumatic myelopathy/radiculopathy	
	2. Symptoms unexplained via other radiographic images	
	3. Impaired neurologic exam	

The junction of the odontoid process and the C2 vertebral body forms the superior arc. The posterior arc corresponds to the posterior cortex of the C2 vertebral body, and the projection of the C2 transverse process forms the inferior apex. Disruption of any portion of the ring is secondary to disruption of the structure that forms that part of the ring and is indicative of an abnormality.

Many other structures should be evaluated on the lateral radiograph. The respective intervertebral disk spaces should be visualized, and their heights should be essentially equal to one another. If there are one or more disk spaces that are decreased in height, this can be secondary to acute or chronic disk disease. On the lateral view, the cervical facet joints are well visualized and should parallel one another. Another space that should be evaluated is the interspinous distance, which is the distance between continuous spinous processes. If one or more of these spaces is abnormally widened with respect to the others, it is often an indicator of cervical spine injury. The prevertebral soft tissues should be thoroughly evaluated. The soft tissues anterior to the upper cervical spine (C4 and above) should be no wider than 7 mm anterior to C2,[11] but may be greater inferiorly, with the increased distance anterior to the lower cervical spine due to the interposed esophagus. Another important distance to evaluate is the atlantoaxial interval (ADI), which is the distance between the posterior cortex of the anterior C1 arch and the anterior cortex of the odontoid process. This distance should be no greater than 2.5 mm.[11] The cervicothoracic (C7-T1) junction is the final landmark that must be evaluated on

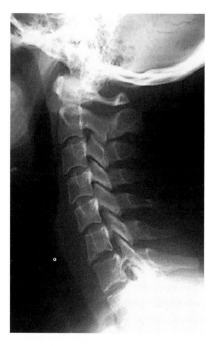

Fig. 5.1 Normal lateral cervical spine radiograph. Note the normal alignment of the anterior prevertebral soft tissue line, anterior and posterior vertebral body lines, spinolaminar line, and spinous process line.

the lateral radiograph. If the superior end plate of T1 is not visualized, a swimmer's view is performed. The swimmer's view is obtained by positioning the patient with one arm fully abducted over the head and the opposite shoulder slightly depressed in an attempt to visualize the complete cervical spine down to the level of the superior T1 end plate. However, positioning for this view can exacerbate instability in an injured spine, so if there is high clinical suspicion of injury, a CT should be performed instead.

The second view in the cervical spine series is the AP view. The AP view helps evaluate portions of the cervical spine that are not adequately evaluated on the lateral examination. Typically, the AP view permits visualization of the cervical spine from C3 to the cervicothoracic junction. The lateral margins of the articular masses should be smooth. The spinous processes should align in a linear fashion, except when normal variant bifid spinous processes are present, in which alignment is often distorted. On the AP view, the uncovertebral joints are well visualized, and subtle fractures as well as degenerative changes can be visualized.

The final view in the cervical spine series is the odontoid view. The odontoid view permits appropriate visualization of the atlantoaxial and atlanto-occipital joints. The lateral borders of C1 should align with the adjacent lateral margins of C2. The morphology of the odontoid process is visualized well with this view, and odontoid fractures can be detected. The odontoid view is often altered by rotation or head tilt, which narrows the atlantoaxial and

atlanto-occipital spaces that occur on the side opposite the head movement.

There are special considerations in the imaging of children primarily because children often exhibit radiographic manifestations of increased ligamentous laxity. The prevertebral soft tissues in children often appear increased in size due to poor positioning caused by ligamentous laxity. Imaging the cervical spine of the child at inspiration with the neck in flexion can prevent the so-called pseudomass in the prevertebral soft tissues. Another radiographic manifestation of ligamentous laxity in children is an increased ADI (up to 5 mm), secondary to laxity of the transverse atlantal ligament. A final manifestation of ligamentous laxity in children is physiologic pseudosubluxation of C2-C3 and C3-C4, manifested by up to 2 mm of subluxation of one vertebral body on another.

Computed Tomography

Computed tomography can identify essentially every bony landmark that is evaluated on the standard radiographic examination (**Table 5.2**). It has a significantly increased sensitivity over radiographs in the evaluation of bony injury. Furthermore, it has the advantage of better visualization of soft tissue structures adjacent to the spine. For these reasons, in addition to its speed and widespread availability, CT has become the evaluation of choice in the setting of spinal trauma in many institutions. The proliferation of multidetector CT with three-dimensional (3D) reconstruction capability has revolutionized imaging of spinal injury and has further increased the ability to quickly detect sequelae of spinal injury from the craniooccipital to cervicothoracic junctions.

Magnetic Resonance Imaging

Magnetic resonance imaging is particularly helpful in the evaluation of injury to the spinal cord. Although not indicated as the primary evaluation in the setting of spinal trauma, MRI can be a useful adjunct particularly when a patient experiences posttraumatic myelopathy/radiculopathy, when there are symptoms that cannot be explained by other radiographic studies, or when the patient has an impaired sensorium or difficult neurologic examination (**Table 5.2**). MRI has the capacity to detect even subtle injury to the spinal cord, which is a strength that radiographs and CT lack. MRI also is useful in the detection of ligamentous injury.[12]

Mechanisms of Injury

There are multiple types of cervical spine injury, which are best classified by the mechanism of injury. The mechanism of injury is described by the vector of the force that causes it. Most patients with cervical spine trauma have more than one injury.[13]

Table 5.3 Hyperflexion Injuries

Injury	Cause	Injury Characteristics	Imaging
Hyperflexion sprain (anterior subluxation)	"Whiplash"	• Injury to posterior ligamentary complex (PLC)	• Radiography: abrupt focal kyphosis at injury level
		• Posterior anulus fibrosus may also be disrupted	• MRI: adjunct modality; increased T2 signal in PLC injury
		• 50% show delayed instability	
Bilateral interfacetal dislocation (BID)	Disruption of anterior longitudinal ligament, posterior longitudinal ligament, intervertebral disk, and PLC	• Unstable with high risk of cord injury	• Radiography: 50% anterior subluxation of vertebral body in complete dislocation; bilateral perched facets in partial facet joint displacement
		• Bilateral locked facets	
		• Generally within low cervical spine	• CT: detects subtle fractures; "inverted hamburger sign"
Simple wedge compression	Compressive forces affecting anterosuperior end plate of vertebral body	• Anterior longitudinal ligament and disk intact	• Radiography: loss of vertebral height; impacted superior end plate; angulated anterior cortical margin of vertebral body
		• Deformity of anterosuperior end plate of affected vertebrae	
Clay shoveler's fracture	• Forced flexion of head and upper cervical spine	• Avulsion fracture of C6, C7, or T1 spinous process	
	• Downward traction on spinous processes by muscular attachments to scapulae while arms perform forceful lifting	• Stable due to intact PLC	
		• Mimicked by unfused apophysis	
Flexion teardrop fracture	Severe flexion with disruption of all ligaments and their stability	• Unstable; worst cervical spine injury compatible with life	• Radiography: visualize kyphosis, "teardrop" fragment, retropulsed bone, and significant prevertebral soft tissue swelling
		• Comminution of anterior vertebral body, "teardrop" fragment displaced	
		• Posterior vertebral body retropulses into spinal cord, resulting in injury to the spinal cord, with many patients presenting with acute anterior cord syndrome	

Hyperflexion Injuries (Table 5.3)

There are several types of hyperflexion injuries, in which there is compression of the anterior column and distraction of the posterior elements of the spine.

Hyperflexion Sprain (Anterior Subluxation)

Hyperflexion sprain injuries are most often caused by "whiplash" injury, usually from abrupt deceleration in a vehicle traveling less than 30 miles per hour. This mechanism often occurs when a stopped car is rear-ended. The hallmark of hyperflexion sprain is injury to the posterior ligament complex. The posterior anulus fibrosus and intervertebral disk are sometimes also disrupted, with presumptive injury to the facet capsule as well. Initially, hyperflexion sprain injuries are stable, but up to 50% of them can exhibit delayed instability.

Radiographically, hyperflexion sprain injuries often manifest by an abrupt focal kyphosis at the level of injury. Posteriorly, the interspinous and interlaminar spaces are widened. The facets become partially uncovered due to the increased kyphosis and probable loss of facet capsule integrity. There is also increased distance between the anterior cortex of the displaced vertebral body and the superior facets. In addition, the intervertebral disk space is widened posteriorly and narrowed anteriorly. MRI can be used as an adjunct modality and demonstrates increased T2 signal within the posterior ligamentary complex (PLC), signifying injury.

Bilateral Interfacetal Dislocation

In the second form of hyperflexion injury, bilateral interfacetal dislocation (BID), there is disruption of the anterior longitudinal ligament, posterior longitudinal ligament, intervertebral disk, and PLC. The inferior articular masses of the affected facet joint pass superiorly and anteriorly to the subjacent facet and are located within the neural foramina. BID is an unstable injury and is associated with a high risk of spinal cord damage. This injury is commonly referred to as "bilateral locked facets," although this is a misnomer because the facets are not in fact locked together but are instead unstable due to the extensive ligamentous injury present. BID usually occurs within the lower cervical spine.

Radiographically, if dislocation is complete, BID exhibits at least 50% anterior subluxation of the affected vertebral body on the subjacent vertebrae (**Fig. 5.2**). If the facet joints are partially displaced, *bilateral perched facets* result, in which the superior vertebral facets are subluxed superiorly and anteriorly on the subjacent facets but are not completely dislocated. When incomplete, overall anterior subluxation is less than 50%. In both complete and partial displacement of the facets, there are often small impaction fracture fragments present that are not clinically significant. CT easily demonstrates facet dislocation as well as other, more subtle fractures that are more difficult to see on the plain radiograph. On CT, facet joint articulations resemble the cross section of a hamburger bun. With facet dislocation, the hamburger bun is inverted, corresponding to the so-called inverted hamburger sign.

Simple Wedge Compression

Wedge compression fractures are usually found within the middle to lower cervical spine, with compressive forces from hyperflexion affecting the anterosuperior end plate of the vertebral body. The anterior longitudinal ligament and intervertebral disk are intact. There is a deformity of the anterosuperior end plate of the affected vertebrae along with buckling of the anterior cortex. This fracture is stable unless the PLC is injured and fails to heal, in which case there is delayed instability.

Radiographically, there is loss of vertebral body height and impaction of the superior end plate of the vertebral body. The impacted superior end plate usually demonstrates increased density. The anterior cortical margin of the vertebral body is angulated. If there is injury to the PLC, there is widening of the interspinous and interlaminar distances (as seen in hyperflexion sprain and BID).

Clay Shoveler's Fracture

The clay shoveler's fracture is an acute avulsion fracture of the C6, C7, or T1 spinous process (**Fig. 5.3**). This fracture

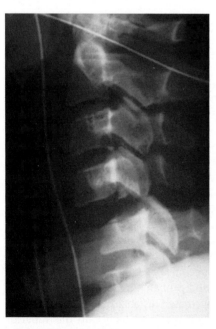

Fig. 5.2 Bilateral interfacetal dislocation. The facet joints of C4 are dislocated anteriorly with respect to C5.

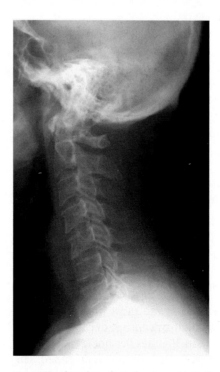

Fig. 5.3 Clay shoveler's fracture. Note the fracture through the spinous process of C7.

is caused by forced flexion of the head and upper cervical spine, resulting in opposing action of the supraspinous and interspinous ligaments. An alternative mechanism for this injury is downward traction on the spinous processes by muscular attachments to the scapulae while the arms perform forceful lifting. The injury with a clay shoveler's fracture is stable, as the posterior ligamentous structures are intact. The clay shoveler's fracture is mimicked by unfused apophyses, which typically have smoother, well-corticated margins.

Flexion Teardrop Fracture

The flexion teardrop fracture is an unstable fracture and is the most devastating cervical spine injury compatible with life. This injury is caused by severe flexion with resultant disruption of all ligaments and their associated stability. The anterior vertebral body is comminuted, with a triangular fragment, or "teardrop," anteroinferiorly. The posterior portion of the vertebral body retropulses into the spinal canal, causing injury to the spinal cord. Patients clinically present with acute anterior cord syndrome, characterized by complete paralysis, hypesthesia and hypalgesia to the level of injury, and preservation of dorsal column function.

On the lateral radiograph, kyphosis is demonstrated along with anterior compression and vertebral body fracture. The "teardrop" fragment is displaced from the anterior and inferior aspect of the vertebral body (**Fig. 5.4**). Retropulsed bone from the fractured vertebral body is present within the spinal canal, and there is increased interlaminar and interspinous distance consistent with posterior ligamentous injury. Significant prevertebral soft tissue swelling usually accompanies the fracture.

Hyperflexion Injuries with Rotation (Table 5.4)

Unilateral Interfacetal Dislocation

With unilateral interfacetal dislocation (UID), the mechanism of injury is similar to that of BID, except that the flexion force is accompanied by a rotational component. The dislocation occurs on the side opposite the direction of the rotation. The anterior longitudinal ligament, intervertebral disk, and posterior longitudinal ligaments are

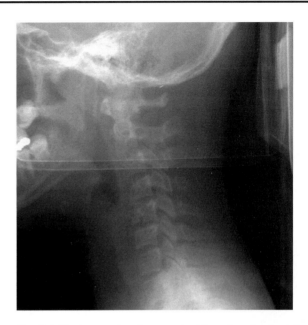

Fig. 5.4 Flexion teardrop fracture. In this patient, kyphosis is centered at C5 where there is a compression deformity and fracture of the anteroinferior vertebral body end plate.

intact, but there is disruption of the PLC and articular joint capsule. In up to 70% of cases, there are impaction fractures involving the tip of either articular mass. These injuries are most common at C5-C6 and C6-C7. The injury is stable unless the fracture isolates the articular process. Because UID is usually a stable injury, the term *unilateral locked facet* is appropriate, unless the articular mass or contralateral facet is injured. CT is required when UID is present because it can detect subtle fractures and injuries that deem the injury unstable.[14]

In UID, the lateral radiograph demonstrates the classic "bow-tie" sign, which is due to the lack of superimposition of the articular masses at the level of injury (**Fig. 5.5**). The degree of anterior subluxation is greater than 3 mm but less than one half of the width of the vertebral body. Due to injury to the PLC, there is increase in the interlaminar and interspinous distances. On the AP view, rotation of the spinous processes at and above the level of involvement in the direction of the injury is observed.

Table 5.4 Hyperflexion Injury with Rotation

Injury	Cause	Injury Characteristics	Imaging
Unilateral interfacetal dislocation (UID)	Mechanism similar to bilateral interfacetal dislocation (BID) except accompanied by rotation	• Most common at C5-C6 and C6-C7	• Radiography: classic "bow-tie" sign
		• Dislocation on opposite side of rotation	• CT: required to detect subtle fractures
		• Disruption of posterior ligamentary complex and articular joint capsule	
		• 70% with impaction fracture	
		• Unilateral locked facet when stable	

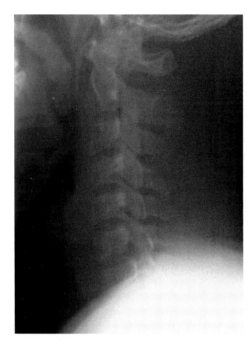

Fig. 5.5 Unilateral interfacetal dislocation. The "bow-tie" sign is present, as there is lack of superimposition of the articular masses at the level of injury.

Vertical Compression Injuries (Table 5.5)

With vertebral compression (axial load) injuries, a force is delivered to the top of the skull that is transmitted through the occipital condyles to the cervical spine at the instant that the spine is straight. Two types of axial load injuries are commonly encountered.

Jefferson Fracture

In the Jefferson fracture, the ring of C1 is fractured in its anterior and posterior components. The Jefferson fracture

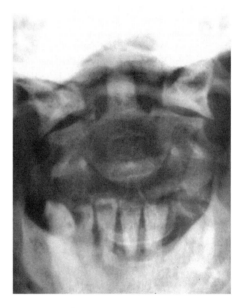

Fig. 5.6 Jefferson fracture. Note the step-off between the lateral borders of the C1 arch relative to C2.

was initially described as a four-part fracture, but two- and three-part fractures also occur. The fractures can be unilateral or bilateral. Fracture fragments are displaced laterally. Up to one half of patients have associated C2 fractures.[15] The odontoid view usually shows displacement of the lateral borders of C1 off the C2 superior articular facets (**Fig. 5.6**). If displaced more than 7 mm, there is disruption of the transverse ligament.[16] However, displacement of less than 7 mm does not exclude injury to the transverse ligament. Lateral radiographs often demonstrate fractures of the C1 arch as well as prevertebral soft tissue swelling. If the ADI is greater than 4 mm, injury to the transverse ligament is more likely. CT easily identifies a Jefferson fracture, which is an unstable injury when associated with

Table 5.5 Vertical Compression (Axial Load) Injuries

Injury	Cause	Injury Characteristics	Imaging
Jefferson fracture	Force to top of skull, transmitted through occipital condyles to cervical spine	• Stability dependent on status of transverse ligament	• Radiography: displacement of lateral C1 borders off C2
		• Ring of C1 fractured anteriorly and posteriorly	• Superior articular facet in odontoid view
		• Uni- or bilateral fractures	• CT: easily identifiable
		• 50% associated with C2 fracture	
Burst fracture	Nucleus pulposus protrudes into vertebral body, causing vertebral body rupture	• Common at C3-C7 levels, usually involving cord injury	• Radiography: vertical fracture line best seen on anteroposterior view
		• Stable, as ligamentous structures intact	• CT: evaluates fracture fragments
			• MRI: evaluates cord, disk, and ligaments

injury to the transverse ligament, but stable when the ligament is intact. A developmental variant that mimics the Jefferson fracture is incomplete fusion of the posterior C1 arch. This is a solitary defect in the cortex of C1, whereas and Jefferson fractures involve two or more fracture foci.

Burst Fracture

The burst fracture is analogous to the Jefferson fracture within the lower cervical spine, usually occurring at the C3–C7 levels. In theory, a vertical compression force causes the nucleus pulposus to protrude into the vertebral body through the inferior end plate, leading to "burst" or rupture of the vertebral body. There is usually injury to the spinal canal. The anterior longitudinal ligament, intervertebral disk, and PLC are intact. The burst fracture is a stable injury. The AP view best characterizes a burst fracture, and the vertical fracture lines are readily seen on that view. CT is used to further characterize the extent of injury and evaluate fracture fragments. MRI is also used as an adjunct to evaluate the spinal cord, intervertebral disk, and ligamentous attachments.

Hyperextension Injuries (Table 5.6)

Hangman's Fracture

The hangman's fracture is a bilateral fracture of the C2 arch and is also referred to as *traumatic spondylolisthesis of the axis*. The hangman's fracture is the most common

Table 5.6 Hyperextension Injuries

Injury	Cause	Injury Characteristics	Imaging
Hangman's fracture	Most common fracture in fatal motor vehicle accidents	• Bilateral fracture of C2 arch = traumatic spondylolisthesis of axis • Neurologic involvement rare • May involve transverse foramina	• Radiography: shows extent of anterior dislocation and involvement of transverse foramina
		• Effendi classification used: I: most common, little displacement, stable II: C2 body anteriorly displaced, C2-C3 disk disruption, facet joints intact III: rare, greater displacement of II, articular facet joints displaced	• CT: fracture lines visible
Hyperextension dislocation	Direct blow to forehead or "whiplash"	• Unstable with significant soft tissue injury and ligament disruption • Common in low cervical spine • Paralysis, acute central cervical cord syndrome	• Radiography: "normal" but with prevertebral soft tissue swelling and anterior widening of disk space • MRI: evaluates cord, tissues, and ligaments
Anterior arch avulsion of atlas	Hyperextension	• Site at middle or inferior anterior arch of C1 • At attachments of longus colli muscles or atlantoaxial ligaments • Stable, no neurologic deficits	• Radiography: prevertebral soft tissue swelling; fracture line seen in odontoid view
Posterior arch atlas fracture	Forceful hyperextension trapping posterior arch of C1 between occiput and spinous process of C2	• Bilateral fractures of posterior arches, posterior to articular masses • With significant prevertebral soft tissue swelling, Jefferson fracture considered • Unstable when associated with C2 fracture (50%)	• Radiography: appears on lateral radiograph

(Continued on page 76)

Table 5.6 *(Continued)* **Hyperextension Injuries**

Injury	Cause	Injury Characteristics	Imaging
Extension teardrop fracture	Acute avulsion fracture caused by attachments of anterior longitudinal ligament	• Vertical dimension greater than longitudinal dimension	• Radiography
		• Fragment originates from antero inferior vertebral body, most commonly at C2	
		• Common in elderly with osteopenia	
		• Unstable in neck extension, stable in flexion	
Laminar fracture	Compression between superior and inferior lamina in neck extension	• Stable	Best modalities are lateral radiograph and CT
		• Common in low cervical spine	

fracture in fatal motor vehicle accidents. Neurologic involvement is rare because even though these fractures can involve significant displacement, the spinal cord occupies only one third of the spinal canal at the C2 level, and there is room for "autodecompression." The Effendi classification divides hangman's fracture into three types.[17,18] Type I is the most common and is associated with minimal displacement (**Fig. 5.7**). These fractures are mechanically stable, and the anterior longitudinal ligament and C2-C3 disk are intact. Type I fractures are often difficult to detect on radiographs. The fracture is deemed type II when the C2 vertebral body is displaced anteriorly and the C2-C3 disk is disrupted (**Fig. 5.8**). With type II injury, facet joints are intact. Type II fractures are often associated with fractures of the anterosuperior C3 end plate. Type III fractures are rare but are associated with greater displacement than in a type II fracture as well as displacement of one or both of the articular facet joints. Neurologic involvement is more common in type II and most common with type III injuries. Fractures can also extend to involve the transverse foramina, resulting in injury to the vertebral arteries.

Radiographs as well as CT demonstrate the extent of anterior dislocation as well as the presence of transverse foramina involvement. With CT using multiplanar reconstruction, fracture lines are easily visible, which traverse from the superior-posterior aspect to the inferior-anterior aspect of C2. The bilateral fractures usually involve the pars interarticularis or the adjacent articular processes.

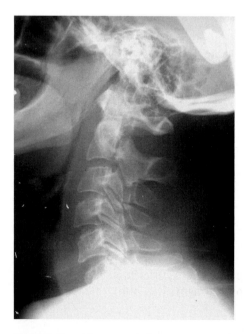

Fig. 5.7 Type I hangman's fracture seen in this patient without spondylolisthesis.

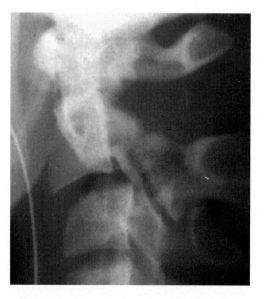

Fig. 5.8 Type II hangman's fracture with anterolisthesis of C2 on C3. There are often C3 fractures associated with this injury.

Hyperextension Dislocation

Hyperextension dislocation is a significant injury that affects soft tissues. It entails disruption of the anterior longitudinal ligament, posterior longitudinal ligament, and intervertebral disk. The hyperextension dislocation injury typically occurs in the lower cervical spine and can result from a direct blow to the forehead or "whiplash." The anterior component of the spinal cord is compressed by the posterior aspect of the vertebral body, and the posterior aspect of the spinal cord is compressed by the disrupted ligamentum flavum. When the force is removed, structures spontaneously reduce, leading to the classic clinical scenario of a patient with paralysis or acute central cervical cord syndrome and a normal cervical spine radiograph. The radiograph is not entirely normal, and associated findings usually include prevertebral soft tissue swelling as well as anterior widening of the disk space. In about 60% of cases, there is a small avulsion fracture from the anteroinferior end plate due to the dense Sharpey's fibers of the disk annulus.[19] Hyperextension dislocation is an unstable injury, and MRI is used to further characterize injury to the spinal cord, soft tissues, and associated ligamentous structures.

Anterior Arch Avulsion of the Atlas

The avulsion fracture of the anterior arch of C1 usually occurs in the middle or inferior portion of the arch and is secondary to the attachments of the longus colli muscles and atlantoaxial ligaments, which are stretched with hyperextension. The avulsion fracture of the anterior arch of the atlas is a stable fracture and does not have associated neurologic deficits. The radiograph demonstrates associated prevertebral soft tissue swelling. On the odontoid view, the fracture line extends past the lateral margin of the odontoid process. A condition that mimics this fracture is the presence of an accessory ossicle inferior to the anterior arch of C1. When this ossicle is present, the presence or absence of significant prevertebral soft tissue swelling helps one to decide if a fracture is present or not.

Posterior Arch of Atlas Fracture

The fracture of the posterior arch of C1 is another fracture that occurs by a hyperextension mechanism. With forceful hyperextension, the posterior arch of C1 becomes trapped between the occiput and the spinous process of C2. This fracture occurs through both sides of the posterior arch of the atlas, posterior to the articular masses, and is usually apparent on the lateral radiograph. If there is significant prevertebral soft tissue swelling, a Jefferson fracture should be considered instead of a fracture of the posterior arch of the atlas. The fracture of the posterior arch of C1 is a stable fracture unless it coexists with a fracture of C2, a situation that occurs about half of the time.[15]

Extension Teardrop Fracture

The extension teardrop fracture is an acute avulsion fracture caused by attachments of the anterior longitudinal ligament. The vertical dimension of the fragment is greater than or equal to its longitudinal dimension, separating it from the avulsion fracture seen with the hyperflexion dislocation injury. The fragment originates from the anteroinferior portion of the vertebral body, and there is associated prevertebral soft tissue swelling. This fracture most commonly occurs at C2 and is seen most often in elderly patients with osteopenia. The extension teardrop fracture is unstable with the neck held in extension but stable with the neck in flexion.

Laminar Fracture

The final injury related to hyperextension is the laminar fracture. The laminar fracture occurs due to compression between superior and inferior vertebral laminae when the neck is extended. The laminar fracture is a stable fracture most commonly occurring in the lower cervical spine, but fragments can extend into the spinal canal. The best imaging modalities to see this fracture are the lateral radiograph and CT.

Hyperextension Injuries with Rotation (Table 5.7)

This pattern of injury occurs with force applied to the forehead or upper face that is not central, causing rotation associated with hyperextension. There are two distinct patterns of injury with this mechanism.

Pillar Fracture

The pillar fracture is a fracture through the articular mass caused by impaction from the overlying superior articular mass. The fracture line is vertical and best seen on the AP view, pillar view, oblique view, or CT. The injuries are sometimes comminuted and extend to involve other structures in the posterior arch. If isolated to the articular mass, the injury is stable. However, there can be associated anterolisthesis and intervertebral disk injury. Patients typically present with radiculopathy and lateralizing neck and arm pain.

Pedicolaminar Fracture-Separation

The pedicolaminar fracture is an injury with a similar mechanism to that of the pillar fracture. In this injury, there are fractures through the ipsilateral pedicle and lamina, producing a free-floating lateral mass. The articular pillar fragment is often rotated, yielding the "horizontalized facet." If the injury produces only a free-floating lateral mass, then it is deemed a type I pedicolaminar fracture-separation. Anterolisthesis is often present, in which the injury is type II. A type II injury

Table 5.7 Hyperextension Injuries with Rotation

Injury	Cause	Injury Characteristics	Imaging
Pillar fracture	Fracture through articular mass caused by impaction from superior articular mass	• Vertical fracture line; may be comminuted • Stable if isolated to articular mass • Common patient presentation: radiculopathy, lateralizing neck and arm pain	• Radiography: AP, pillar, oblique • CT: also used

Pediculolaminar fracture	Similar to pillar fracture mechanism	• Fracture through ipsilateral pedicle and lamina, creating free-floating lateral mass
		
		• Classification:
		
		  I: only a free-floating lateral mass
		
		  II: anterolisthesis present
		
		  III: associated injury to disk
		
		  IV: involves contralateral UID (spine unstable)
			• Radiography
			
			• CT angiography: used if fracture extends to transverse foramina, thus injuring vertebral artery

with associated injury to the intervertebral disk is a type III injury. Type IV injury is present if the injury involves contralateral UID, in which case the spine is unstable. If the fracture extends into the transverse foramen, injury to the vertebral artery is also possible, and CT angiography is indicated.

Lateral Flexion Injury (Table 5.8)

There are a host of injuries that can occur secondary to accentuated lateral flexion. The mechanism is due to extreme lateral tilt in the coronal plane. The fractures are often associated with vertebral artery injury secondary to involvement of the transverse foramina. Injuries associated with lateral flexion include fractures of the occipital condyle, uncinate process, and transverse process. Lateral wedge compression deformities and eccentric atlas burst fractures can also occur. Odontoid fractures can also be caused by this mechanism and are further outlined below. Injuries sustained secondary to lateral flexion are best visualized on AP radiographs and CT.

Other Fractures/Injuries (Table 5.9)

Rotatory Atlantoaxial Fixation—Torticollis

Rotatory fixation of C1-C2 usually occurs secondary to mild trauma and can occur due to sleeping in an unusual position. Rotation and lateral tilt occur at the atlantoaxial joint, and when symptoms do not resolve within a few days, torticollis results. Imaging findings demonstrate incongruity of the articular surfaces of C1 and C2, best seen on the odontoid view. There is also asymmetry in the distance between the ring of C1 and the dens on the odontoid view. If the abnormality is secondary to trauma, there will be associated prevertebral soft tissue swelling. CT is used to further characterize it and demonstrates disruption of one or more of the facet joints, often including locking.

Odontoid Fractures

Over 10% of cervical spine injuries involve odontoid fractures. Of these, three quarters occur in children. Often, odontoid fractures are associated with Jefferson fractures or atlantoaxial dislocations. Radiographically, odontoid

Table 5.8 Lateral Flexion Injury

Injury	Cause	Injury Characteristics	Imaging
Host of injuries (fractures of occipital condyles, uncinate process, transverse process, lateral wedge compression, eccentric atlas burst fractures, odontoid fractures)	Extreme lateral tilt in coronal plane	Often involves transverse foramina, thus associated with vertebral artery injury	Best modalities are AP radiograph and CT

Table 5.9 Other Fractures/Injuries

Injury	Cause	Injury Characteristics	Imaging
Rotatory atlantoaxial fixation—torticollis	• Secondary to mild trauma; can occur when sleeping in unusual position • Torticollis results when symptoms not resolved within a few days	• Incongruity of C1 and C2 articular surfaces • Asymmetry in distance between ring of C1 and dens • Associated prevertebral soft tissue swelling (secondary to trauma)	• Radiography: odontoid view to visualize incongruity and asymmetry • CT: further visualize facet joint disruption

Odontoid fractures	Associated with Jefferson fractures and atlantoaxial dislocations	• > 10% of cervical spine injuries; ~75% of these are in children
		• May mimic mach line
		• Anderson and D'Alonzo classification:
		  I: rare; avulsion fracture at tip of dens from alar ligament
		  II: unstable; most common; base of dens; may heal in nonunion
		  III: unstable; through upper body of C2; involving facets
			• Radiography: II and III often visible in odontoid view
			• CT: definitive diagnosis and to exclude other bony injuries

Transverse atlantal ligament rupture	• Isolated tearing not involving dens • Trauma (blunt force to occiput) that involves trauma to dens	• Unstable; increase in ADI and anterior translation of skull and atlas • Associations: Jefferson fractures, systemic illnesses (inflammatory arthropathies or focal inflammatory disorders such as tuberculosis)	
Occipitoatlantal dissociation	Severe head trauma causing extensive ligamentous injury	• Often fatal, as there's often medullary transection • If incomplete, significant neurolgic and vascular compromise	• Radiography: shows increase of over 12 mm in basion-dental interval

fractures may be subtle; often, the only clue is the presence of prevertebral soft tissue swelling. The Anderson and D'Alonzo system is used to classify odontoid fractures. Type I odontoid fractures are rare and are small avulsion fractures off the tip of the dens caused by the alar ligament. Type II fractures occur at the base of the dens and are the most common (**Fig. 5.9**). They also have a great tendency to heal in a nonunion fashion.[20] Type III fractures are fractures through the upper part of the C2 vertebral body, usually involving the facets (**Fig. 5.10**).

Radiographically, type II and type III fractures are often visible on the odontoid view. Often, however, odontoid views are suboptimal, or not obtained due to patient condition, so other clues such as disruption of the axis ring must be observed. CT is definitive in the diagnosis of odontoid fractures. One must be aware of fracture mimics, such as the mach line when interpreting cervical spine radiographs. The mach line is a line through the dens that appears to represent a fracture but actually represents an

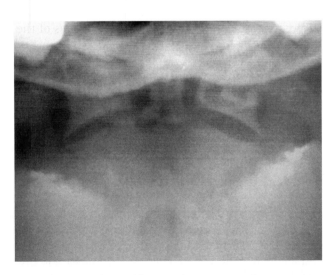

Fig. 5.9 Type II odontoid fracture demonstrating lucency representing fracture line through the base of the dens.

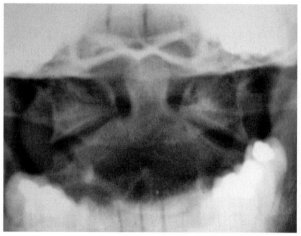
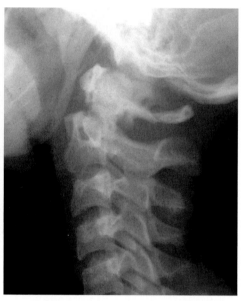

A

B

Fig. 5.10 Type III odontoid fracture. **(A)** Anteroposterior and **(B)** lateral views of a patient with a type III odontoid fracture, with extension of fracture to involve facets. There is posterior angulation of the superior dens, as seen on the lateral view.

interface and is caused by superimposition of the inferior cortex of the posterior arch of C1. The mach line can be differentiated from a fracture line by its extension beyond the lateral cortex of the dens.

Type II and type III fractures are unstable. If present, CT is performed to exclude the presence of other bony injuries. Neurologic compromise is more likely if there is displacement or angulation of the fracture fragment.

Transverse Atlantal Ligament Rupture

Isolated tearing of the transverse atlantal ligament can occur with or without trauma to the dens. If associated with trauma, there is usually a history of blunt force to the occiput. Radiographically, there is an increase in the ADI and anterior translation of the skull and atlas. Transverse atlantal ligament rupture is unstable and is associated with other injuries such as Jefferson fracture. There are systemic illnesses such as inflammatory arthropathies or focal inflammatory disorders such as tuberculosis that can weaken the transverse atlantal ligament and cause dislocation with only minor trauma.

Occipitoatlantal Dissociation

In severe head trauma, there can be extensive ligamentous injury that causes disruption of the craniovertebral articulation, or occipitoatlantal dissociation. Rotational and shearing forces cause injury to the alar and tectorial ligaments. This injury is often fatal, especially with complete dissociation, as there is often medullary transection. If incomplete, there is significant subluxation that is extremely unstable, and there is often significant neurologic and vascular compromise. Radiographically, there is an increase in the basion-dental interval (BDI) of greater than 12 mm.

■ Thoracolumbar Spine

Anatomy

The thoracolumbar spine consists of 17 vertebral bodies—12 thoracic and 5 lumbar. Within the thoracolumbar spine, there are three biomechanical regions (**Table 5.10**). The T1-T8 region is relatively rigid, anchored by the rib cage. From L3 to the sacrum, the spine is quite mobile and is prone to injury. It is the region from T9 to L2 that serves as a transition between immobile and mobile regions, and it is this trait that makes it the portion of the thoracolumbar spine most susceptible to traumatic injury. In addition to the mobility of the lower lumbar spine, it has other characteristic traits that explain its propensity to injury. There is a normal lordosis within the lumbar spine. For this reason, approximately 30% of the weight bearing of the lumbar spine is placed on the posterior elements. Furthermore, a flexion mechanism straightens the lumbar spine, and an extreme flexion can produce an axial-type loading injury.

Table 5.10 Three Biomechanical Regions of the Thoracolumbar Spine

T1-T8	Rigid, anchored by rib cage
T9-L2	Transition between immobile and mobile regions; the most susceptible to traumatic injury
L3-sacrum	Quite mobile; prone to injury due to its normal lordotic properties

Table 5.11 "Three-Column" Theory of Thoracolumbar Stability and Instability

Columns	Anterior column	Anterior longitudinal ligament, anterior vertebral body, anterior annulus
	Middle column	Posterior vertebral body, posterior annulus, posterior longitudinal ligament
	Posterior column	All three bony elements and posterior ligaments
Implications	Injury to any two of the three columns represents an unstable spine	

To fully understand how trauma affects the lumbar spine, it is important to appreciate the ligamentous structures that provide support and stability. Like the cervical spine, the vertebral bodies are stabilized by anterior and posterior longitudinal ligaments. In addition to these ligaments, the ligamentum flavum is present posterior to the central canal. Interspinous ligaments further stabilize the posterior structures.

It is also important to understand the anatomy of the spinal canal to appreciate the impact of trauma on the spinal cord and, subsequently, neurologic function. Within the thoracic spine, the central canal has a mean diameter of approximately 16×16 mm. This distance increases to 26×17 mm within the lumbar spine. The spinal cord terminates at the L1 level. For these reasons, less significant trauma can have a greater impact on the thoracic spine due to its smaller area and greater likelihood of injuring the spinal cord at any given level.

The neural foramina are the pathways in which the exiting nerve roots leave the spinal canal. The foramina are surrounded by many structures and are quite susceptible to injury. Trauma to the facet, pedicle, laminae, or transverse process can impinge upon the neural foramen and its exiting nerve root. Similarly, retropulsed bony fragments from the vertebral bodies and spondylolisthesis can have the same effect.

Stability and Instability

Thoracolumbar stability and instability are explained by the three-column theory, which states that the thoracolumbar spine is composed of three columns (**Table 5.11**). The anterior column consists of the anterior longitudinal ligament, the anterior portion of the vertebral body, and the anterior annulus. The middle column consists of the posterior portion of the vertebral body, posterior annulus, and posterior longitudinal ligament. The posterior column consists of all posterior bony elements and posterior ligaments. Injury to any two of the three columns produces an unstable spine. For instance, a common burst fracture injures the anterior and middle columns, with or without posterior column injury, and is deemed mechanically unstable. Similarly, an anterior wedge compression fracture with posterior ligamentous injury would also produce an unstable spine, even though the middle column remains intact. If only one column is injured, as in an anterior wedge compression fracture without posterior ligamentous injury, the spine remains stable.

Mechanisms of Injury (Table 5.12)

Most injuries to the thoracolumbar spine are secondary to motor vehicle accidents or falls. There are about 4000 traumatic thoracolumbar fractures diagnosed each year in the United States.[21] As in the cervical spine, there are a host of mechanisms that lead to predictable patterns of injury. Thorough knowledge of these patterns helps one to better appreciate and understand the pathogenesis of thoracolumbar injury as well as better interpret radiologic exams. Although standard radiographs are often used, CT has long been established as the superior imaging modality.[22,23]

Axial Load

An axial load injury is one in which force is applied to the thoracolumbar spine from a superior direction. The most common type of injury producing this mechanism is a fall from a significant height. In axial load injuries, the most common site of trauma is at the thoracolumbar junction. Almost half of all injuries have an additional injury at another level. A small fraction of these multiple-level injuries are noncontiguous, so if there is evidence for one focus of injury, imaging of the whole spine is necessary.

The axial load can also produce two types of fractures: compression and burst fractures. Compression fractures are seen radiographically as anterior wedge deformities. These fractures are stable, as there is only injury to the anterior column. A burst fracture is a comminuted fracture of the vertebral body caused by an axial load that is unstable secondary to disruption of the anterior and middle columns. The fracture causes bowing of the posterior portion of the vertebral body with retropulsion of bony fragments into the spinal canal. The retropulsed fragment is attached to the annulus and posterior longitudinal ligament and often rotates. Distraction usually helps reduce this injury. Radiographically, there is loss of vertebral body height on the lateral view and widening of the interpedicular distance on the AP view. Due to the wider spinal canal in the lower lumbar spine, the presence of retropulsed bone may not necessitate reduction. It is important to differentiate anterior wedge fractures from

Table 5.12 Mechanisms of Injury to Thoracolumbar Spine

Axial load	• Force applied from superior direction
	• Most common: fall from significant height
	• Most common site: thoracolumbar junction
	• Can produce two types of fractures:
	1. Compression (stable)
	2. Burst (unstable)
Flexion/compression	• Anterior wedge and burst fractures
	• Greater risk of posterior ligament disruption:
	1. > 50% loss of vertebral body height
	2. Widening of interspinous distance
	• MRI recommended to identify posterior ligament injury
Flexion/rotation	• Produce anterior wedge and burst fractures
	• Rotation also causes posterior element fractures and posterior ligament injury, especially in dislocations
	• Often at thoracolumbar junction
	• Often severe neurologic damage
Flexion/distraction	• Common seat belt injuries
	• Usually no neurologic damage
	• Produce Chance and Chance variant fractures:
	1. Chance: purely osseous
	2. Chance variant: osseous and ligamentous
Lateral flexion/compression	• Loss of lateral vertebral body height
	• Scoliotic deformities
	• Posterior elements often fractured
Shear injury	• Upper and lower body drawn in different directions
	• Severe ligamentous injury
	• Can produce spondylolisthesis
	• Neurologic impairment with fractures and dislocations
Extension	• Compression of posterior components, distraction of anterior components
	• Possible injury to anterior longitudinal ligament and anterior annulus, and fractures of posterior spine elements
Transverse process fractures	• Common, present at multiple levels
	• Often clue signifying more serious injury

burst fractures because one is a stable injury, whereas the other is an unstable injury (**Fig. 5.11**). CT is the best tool to help differentiate these two entities. MRI is a useful adjunct to look for ligamentous injury, especially of the PLC, or if there are significant neurologic symptoms present.

Flexion/Compression

With a flexion/compression mechanism, there are also anterior wedge and burst fractures. However, with this mechanism, there is greater risk for posterior ligamentous disruption. The degree of loss of vertebral body height should always be greater in the anterior aspect of the vertebral body. However, if the loss of height is greater than 50% of the height of either the vertebral body above or below the injury, a posterior ligament injury should be suspected. Another clue to the presence of posterior ligament injury is widening of the interspinous distance. It is important to recognize posterior ligamentous injury because if unrecognized, it can lead to progressive anterior

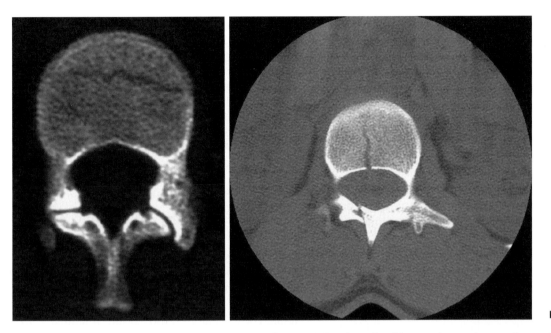

A   B

Fig. 5.11 Compression versus burst fracture. Compression fracture **(A)** with confined fracture line to the anterior portion of the vertebral body. Contrast this with a burst fracture **(B)** in which the fracture line extends through and involves the cortex of the posterior vertebral body.

collapse, compromise of middle column function, and delayed instability. Posterior ligamentous injury may be occult on radiography and CT, and in that case, MRI is recommended for further evaluation.

Flexion/Rotation

In a fashion similar to the flexion component of the flexion/compression mechanism, flexion injuries with the flexion/rotation phenomenon produce anterior wedge and burst fractures. However, the rotation component of this injury adds further instability and concordant posterior element fractures, as well as posterior ligamentous injury. These additional injuries can lead to dislocation. The flexion/rotation injury usually occurs at the thoracolumbar junction, and there is often severe neurologic compromise.

Flexion/Distraction

With the flexion/distraction injury, the axis of flexion is moved anteriorly, as seen in common seat belt injuries. When the flexion is applied, this results in large distractive forces, predominantly over the posterior elements. There is usually no neurologic compromise. The fractures produced by this mechanism are Chance fractures and Chance variant fractures.

Chance fractures are injuries that are purely osseous and are more common than Chance variants. Although Chance fractures are unstable, they have a good prognosis. Radiographically, with a Chance fracture there is a horizontal fracture line that extends entirely, through the vertebral body from its anterior to its posterior elements, as if the bone were being divided into two parts (**Fig. 5.12**).

There is usually greater distraction of the posterior portion of the fracture. Chance variants are injuries that are either a combination of bony and ligamentous injury or entirely ligamentous/disk related and have a greater risk of instability. Chance variants are not as prone to healing as well as the pure bony chance fracture.

Lateral Flexion/Compression

The mechanism of the lateral flexion/compression injury is similar to that of the flexion injury, except that the force is

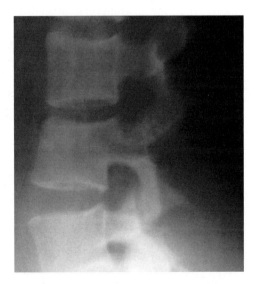

Fig. 5.12 Chance fracture. Note the horizontal fracture line extending through the extent of the vertebrae from its anterior to posterior elements as if it were being divided into two parts.

applied to a more parasagittal region rather than the central portion of the vertebral body. This asymmetric application of force produces fractures and loss of height of the lateral aspect of the vertebral body with scoliotic deformities. The posterior elements are often fractured as well. These fractures are synonymous with asymmetric burst fractures.

Shear Injury

A shear injury is one in which the upper and lower parts of the body are drawn in different directions, causing severe ligamentous damage. Shear injury can produce significant spondylolisthesis. Fractures and dislocations are quite common, often producing significant neurologic impairment.

Extension

Extension injuries produce effects that are the opposite of flexion injuries. There is distraction of anterior components and compression of posterior components. This causes possible injury to the anterior longitudinal ligament, anterior annulus, as well as fractures of the posterior elements of the vertebrae. Radiographically, this can be a subtle injury, with anterior disk widening being the only clue present. CT is more definitive to evaluate for fractures in this situation. MRI is useful to confirm disk disruption.

Transverse Process Fractures

Transverse process fractures are quite common and are often present at multiple levels. If only one transverse process fracture is present, it is usually due to avulsion from the adjacent paraspinal and psoas muscles. Transverse process fractures are often clues that signify more serious injury. A particular example of this is an L5 transverse process fracture, which usually coincides with a sacral injury due to its connection to the sacrum via the iliolumbar ligament. When the L5 transverse process is fractured, there is often injury to the adjacent ipsilateral L5 nerve root as well.

■ Spinal Cord Injury (Table 5.13)

Magnetic resonance imaging is indispensable in the evaluation of the soft tissue component of spinal cord injury. MRI has enabled the focus of spinal injury to shift from bony structures to the spinal cord itself.[24] It is much more sensitive in the detection of acute injury to the spinal cord than other anatomical imaging modalities such as CT. Thecal sac and spinal cord impingements are easily identified. Up to 40% of patients who present with acute spinal injury have evidence of disk herniation. Some studies report that patients with anterior cord syndrome have 100% incidence of disk herniation. Other sequelae of spinal injury such as epidural hematoma, spinal cord edema, spinal cord hematoma, ligamentous disruption, and vascular injury, as

Table 5.13 Spinal Cord Injury

MRI imaging	Indispensable in evaluation of soft tissue components of cord
Spinal injuries	• Thecal sac and cord impingements
	• Epidural hematoma
	• Spinal cord edema
	• Spinal cord hematoma
	• Ligamentous disruption
	• Vascular injury
	• Syringomyelia and myelomalacia

well as complications such as syringomyelia and myelomalacia, can be identified by MRI.

On MRI examination, often the first sign of injury to the spinal cord is manifestation of intramedullary swelling and edema. Edema/swelling can be seen with increased cord caliber on T1-weighted images and increased cord signal on T2-weighted images. The length/span of spinal cord edema is proportional to neurologic deficit and prognosis.[25] Intramedullary and extramedullary hemorrhage is often secondarily seen due to injury to the spinal cord, but it has a variable MR appearance that depends on the age of

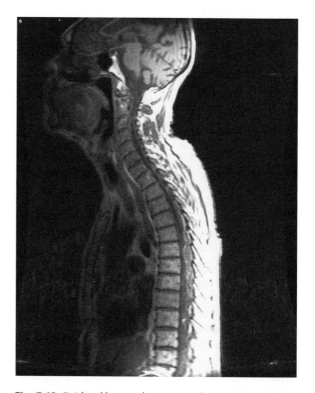

Fig. 5.13 Epidural hemorrhage secondary to trauma. Sagittal T1 image of the cervicothoracic spine demonstrating increased signal posterior to the thoracic cord representing acute epidural hemorrhage.

the blood that is present. Most commonly, acute/subacute hemorrhage on MR is characteristically intermediate to bright on T1-weighted images and dark on T2-weighted images (**Fig. 5.13**).

■ Conclusion

The spectrum of spinal injury is complex, and health care practitioners are challenged by its many different manifestations. However, along with the history and clinical examination, appropriate imaging modalities may be used that will optimally benefit the patient so that expedient diagnoses may be made and appropriate treatments may be employed. Radiographs and CT are most useful as the primary imaging modalities in the initial evaluation of spinal cord injury, with MRI serving as a useful adjunct. Many challenges still remain. Ultimately, the application of the many new and emerging technologies, along with coordination of care by physicians in all of the different subspecialties, will help facilitate optimal patient care.

References

1. Bagley LJ. Imaging of spinal trauma. Radiol Clin North Am 2006;44:1–12
2. Daffner RH. Cervical radiography for trauma patients: a time effective technique? AJR Am J Roentgenol 2000;175:1309–1311
3. Daffner RH. Helical CT of the cervical spine for trauma patients: a time study. AJR Am J Roentgenol 2001;177:677–679
4. Widder S, Doig C, Burrowes P, Larsen G, Hurlbert RJ, Kortbeek JB. Prospective evaluation of computed tomographic scanning for spinal clearance of obtunded trauma patients: preliminary results. J Trauma 2004;56:1179–1184
5. Blackmore CC, Ramsey SD, Mann FA, Koepsell TD. Cervical spine screening with CT in trauma patients: a cost effectiveness analysis. Radiology 1999;212:117–125
6. Grogan EL, Morris JA Jr, Dittus RS, et al. Cervical spine evaluation in urban trauma centers: lowering institutional costs and complications through helical CT scan. J Am Coll Surg 2005;200:160–165
7. Blackmore CC, Mann FA, Wilson AJ. Helical CT in the primary trauma evaluation of the cervical spine: an evidence based approach. Skeletal Radiol 2000;29:632–639
8. Brandt MM, Wahl WL, Yeom K, Kazerooni E, Wang SC. Computed tomographic scanning reduces cost and time of complete spine evaluation. J Trauma 2004;56:1022–1028
9. Nguyen GK, Clark R. Adequacy of plain radiography in the diagnosis if cervical spine injuries. Emerg Radiol 2005;11:158–161
10. Schenarts PJ, Diaz J, Kaiser C, Carillo Y, Eddy V, Morris JA Jr. Prospective comparison of admission computed tomographic scan and plain films of the upper cervical spine in trauma patients with altered mental status. J Trauma 2001;51:663–668
11. Berquist TH. Imaging of adult cervical spine trauma. Radiographics 1988;8:667–694
12. Lee HM, Kim HS, Kim DJ, Suk KS, Park JO, Kim NH. Reliability of magnetic resonance imaging in detecting posterior ligament complex injury in thoracolumbar spinal fractures. Spine 2000;25:2079–2084
13. Berquist TH. Imaging of Orthopedic Trauma and Surgery. Philadelphia: Saunders; 1986
14. Woodring JH, Goldstein SJ. Fractures of the articular processes of the cervical spine. AJR Am J Roentgenol 1982;139:341–344
15. Levine AM, Edwards CC. Treatment of injuries in the C1–C2 complex. Orthop Clin North Am 1986;17:31–44
16. Spence KF Jr, Decker S, Sell KW. Bursting atlantal fracture associated with rupture of the transverse ligament. J Bone Joint Surg Am 1970;52:543–549
17. McCall IW, Park WM, McSweeny T. The radiologic demonstration of acute lower cervical injury. Clin Radiol 1973;24:235–240
18. Mirvis SE, Young JWR, Lim C, Greenberg J. Hangman's fracture: radiologic assessment in 27 cases. Radiology 1987;163:713–717
19. Davis SJ, Teresi LM, Bradley WG, Ziemba MA, Bloze AE. Cervical spine hyperextension injuries: MR findings. Radiology 1991;180:245–251
20. Pathria MN, Petersilge CA. Spinal trauma. Radiol Clin North Am 1991;29:847–865
21. Van Goethem JW, Maes M, Ozsarlak O, Van den Hauwe L, Parizel PM. Imaging in spinal trauma. Eur Radiol 2005;15:582–590
22. McAfee PC, Yuan HA, Frederickson BE, Lubicky JP. The value of computed tomography in thoracolumbar fractures. J Bone Joint Surg Am 1983;65:461–473
23. Mann FA, Cohen WA, Linnau KF, Hallam DK, Blackmore CC. Evidence-based approach to using CT in spinal trauma. Eur J Radiol 2003;48:39–48
24. Demaerel P. Magnetic resonance imaging of spinal cord trauma: a pictorial essay. Neuroradiology 2006;48:223–232
25. Flanders AE, Spettell CM, Friedman DP, Marino RJ, Herbison GJ. The relationship between the functional abilities of patients with cervical spinal cord injury and the severity of damage revealed by MR imaging. AJNR Am J Neuroradiol 1999;20:926–934

6 Biomechanics of the Spine

Eve C. Tsai, Eric P. Roger, and Edward C. Benzel

The discipline of biomechanics embodies the application of the principles of physics to biologic systems. A basic understanding of the anatomy and of biomechanical principles facilitates a better understanding of spine injury and its effect on the normal function of the human vertebral column. Detailed anatomy is dealt with elsewhere in this text. This chapter defines some of the terms and principles used in clinical spinal biomechanics and illustrates how these biomechanical principles apply to spine injury in general. The biomechanical principles with respect to some of the most common and illustrative types of traumatic spine injury are discussed here.

■ Biomechanical Principles and Terms

A *scalar* is a quantity of magnitude and does not have a direction. When direction is given to a magnitude, it is then termed a *vector*. An action that changes the state of rest of the body to which it is applied can be defined as a *force*. Because force has no direction, it is a scalar. If a force has a direction, it is called a force vector or load vector. *Force* and *load* are used interchangeably in biomechanics.

When a force vector acts on a lever (moment arm), it causes a *bending moment*. When a bending moment is applied to a point in space, it causes *rotation,* or a tendency to rotate about an axis. This axis regarding the spine is termed the instantaneous axis of rotation (IAR). The moment arm *(M)* is equal to the force *(F)* multiplied by its perpendicular distance *(D)* from the IAR *(M = F × D)*. Therefore, the moment arm increases when the same force is applied farther away from the IAR.

The standard Cartesian coordinate system has been applied to the spine (**Fig. 6.1**). In this system, there are three axes: x, y, and z. Applied clinically, these axes can also be described by rostral-caudal, ventral-dorsal, and right-left. Rotational and translation movements can occur within these axes. Therefore, there are 12 potential movements about the IAR, as there are two translational movements (in each direction) along each of the three axes and two rotational movements (one in each direction) around each of the axes. With this coordinate system, all force vectors can be divided into their components and hence facilitate systematic study.

A deforming force vector results in strains. The deforming force vector can be translational or rotational. With a translational deforming force vector, there is a change in the length of the body. With a rotational deforming force

vector, there is a change in the angle of the body. *Strain* is the change in the body when a deforming force vector is applied to the body. A linear strain is the change in unit length, and a shear strain is the change in unit angle. When a deformation occurs in the direction of the force application, it is termed axial strain. When a deformation occurs transverse to the direction of the application of the force, it is termed transverse strain.

The application of a force vector or stress to the spine results in deformations or strains, as no solid is absolutely rigid. With respect to biologic systems, the stress/strain curve (**Fig. 6.2**) can be divided into different zones. Initially, when a force is applied to a biologic tissue in vivo, most solids (e.g., bones) subjected to the external force are buffered from the force by ligaments, disks, tendons, and other soft tissues. Therefore, the first zone that is passed is the neutral zone. Once the maximum strain capacity of the neutral zone is reached, the tissues are then deformed according to Hooke's law, where the size of the deformation is proportional to the deforming force and applies to small displacements. Once deformation ensues,

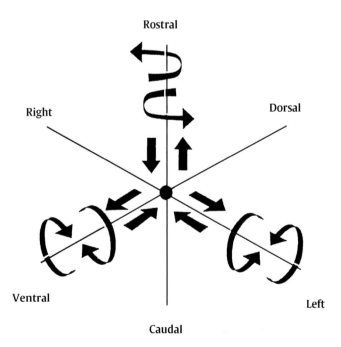

Fig. 6.1 The Cartesian coordinate system with the instantaneous axis of rotation as the center. Translation and rotation can occur in both of their respective directions about each axis. (From Benzel EC, ed. Biomechanics of Spine Stabilization. New York: Thieme; 2001:20, with permission.)

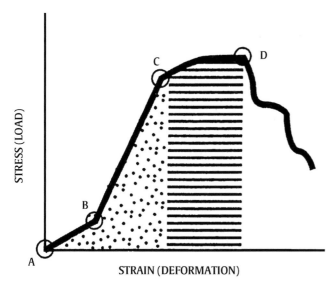

Fig. 6.2 A typical stress/strain curve for a biologic tissue, such as a ligament. Point A to point B is the neutral zone, and B to C is the elastic zone. When the elastic limit (yield point, C) is reached, permanent deformation can occur (permanent set). Point C to point D is the plastic zone, where a permanent set occurs. Past point D, failure occurs, and the load diminishes. Hashed plus dotted area represents strength, whereas the dotted area represents resilience. (From Benzel EC, ed. Biomechanics of Spine Stabilization. New York: Thieme; 2001:24, with permission.)

the stress/strain relationship enters the elastic zone. In the elastic zone, the tissue completely recovers when the strain is removed. The magnitude of the elastic zone is dependent on the elastic modulus of the tissue, and thus is obviously greater for ligaments than bone.

With further application of force, the elastic zone is exceeded, and the elastic limit (or yield point) is reached. At this point the relationship between stress (force) and strain (extent of deformation) is no longer linear. With even more application of force, the elastic limit is exceeded. The plastic zone is thus entered. In this zone, the tissue acquires a permanent set so that if the external forces are removed, the solid does not spring back to its undeformed configuration. With the continued further application of force, the tissue will fail, thus reaching the failure point. After damage has occurred, the segment is relatively lax, with an expanded neutral zone. This increase in the neutral zone defines, in part, segmental instability.

The ratio of stress to strain defines *stiffness* (**Fig. 6.2**). In the spine, the relationship between stress and strain is not always linear. Therefore, to determine the maximum stiffness or elastic modulus of a structure, the most linear portion of the stress/strain curve is often selected. *Flexibility* is the inverse of stiffness, or the ratio of the strain to an applied stress. *Range of motion* is a term that is frequently used in spine biomechanics. It describes the deformation, from one extreme to the other extreme, within the confines of the neutral and elastic zones of an intervertebral

joint. The area under the stress/strain curve defines the energy absorbed prior to failure and is a measure of strength. The area under the curve up to the yield point is a measure of an object's resilience.

The phenomenon of *coupling,* as it relates to the spine, is defined as a movement of the spine along or about an axis, which obligates another movement along or about another axis (of the Cartesian coordinate system). For example, when the cervical spine bends laterally, there exists an obligatory rotation of the spinous processes away from the concave side of the curve. This is due to the orientation of the facet joints and the presence of the uncovertebral joints (**Fig. 6.3**). In the lumbar spine, because of the different orientation of the lumbar facet joints (sagittal rather than coronal, as is the case in the cervical spine), the spinous processes rotate in the same direction as the concave side of the lateral bend.

■ Clinical Biomechanics and General Principles

The type of spine injury that occurs following trauma is influenced by the structural anatomy and the force vector(s) applied. Facet orientation, bony anatomy, associated ligaments, and supporting structures (e.g., the rib cage) generally affect the segmental motions that occur at the various spinal levels (**Fig. 6.4**). The anatomical effects can be illustrated by the example of the occipital-C1 facet. Because of the obliquity of the occipital-C1 facets and because the occipital condyles are medial to the superior articulating facets of C1, the ring of C1 is prone to injury from axial loading. The location of the dorsal arch of C1 can be injured with hyperextension and hyperflexion loading injuries. In general, flexion and extension are most prominent in the cervical and lumbar spine, and rotation is greatest in the atlantoaxial joint and to a lesser extent in the thoracic spine (**Fig. 6.5**).

In the cervical spine, pathologic stresses are increased by the substantial force vectors that are often applied during head trauma or with sudden deceleration of the torso. It has been reported that many upper cervical spine injuries result from trauma to the head.[1-6] As well, sudden deceleration of the torso, combined with restriction of movement of the cervical spine, can create a flexion-distraction mechanism of injury, which is a result of a torso deceleration-induced cervical spine-bending moment.

When a force vector is applied to the spine, the kinetic energy imparted is dissipated by the vertebrae and the surrounding spinal elements, which include the ligaments and calvarium. The kinetic energy imparted by the force vector dictates the magnitude of the injury; however, the relative strengths of the spine and the spinal elements influence the injury type. For example, when an axial load is applied to the cervical spine, a burst fracture of the atlas, a C2 burst-pedicle fracture, or

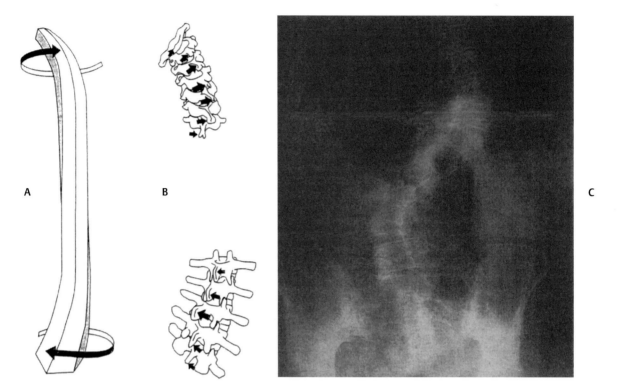

Fig. 6.3 An important manifestation of the coupling phenomenon is the relationship between lateral bending and rotation in the cervical and lumbar regions. This is depicted **(A)** diagrammatically and **(B)** anatomically. Note that the coupling phenomenon results in spinal rotation, in opposite directions, in these two regions. **(C)** A biconcave thoracic and lumbar curve, as depicted in an anteroposterior view, illustrates this phenomenon. Note that the lumbar spinous processes are rotated toward the concave side of the curve. (From Benzel EC, ed. Biomechanics of Spine Stabilization. New York: Thieme; 2001:28, with permission.)

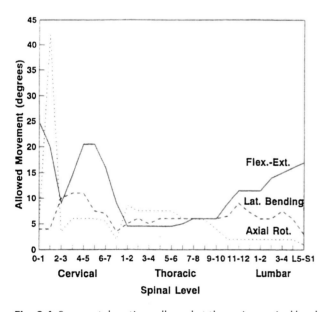

Fig. 6.4 Segmental motions allowed at the various spinal levels (combined flexion and extension, *solid line*; unilateral lateral bending, *dashed line*; and unilateral axial rotation, *dotted line*). (From Benzel EC, ed. Biomechanics of Spine Stabilization. New York: Thieme; 2001:4, with permission.)

a subaxial cervical spine burst fracture can result. The relative intrinsic strengths of the ring of C1, the body and pedicle of C2, and the subaxial cervical spine vertebral bodies affect the type of injury that follows a failure-producing force. More commonly, C1 or the subaxial spine is a relatively "weak link," so a C1 burst fracture or a subaxial spine fracture is common. Fractures of C2 or the calvarium and occipital condyles, however, can also occur.

■ Biomechanics and Specific Spine Injuries

This section addresses the principles of biomechanics with respect to some of the more common spine injuries, beginning with the occipital cervical complex and proceeding downward to the subaxial spine and sacrum. Because the anatomy of the subaxial spine, to the sacrum, is relatively similar, subaxial injuries are grouped together. Sacral injuries are discussed separately.

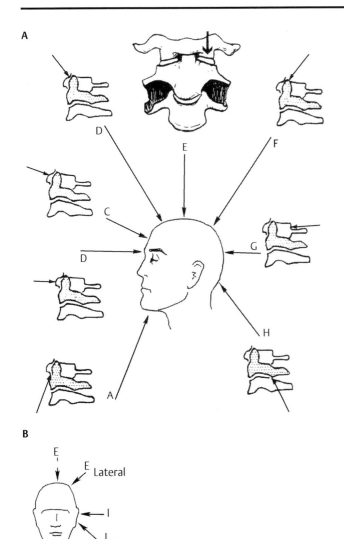

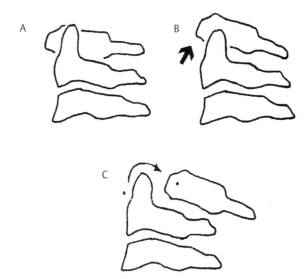

Fig. 6.6 The mechanism of injury of a dorsal C1-C2 dislocation. Note the requirement for at least some distraction (*heavy straight arrow*) to cause the ventral arch of C1 to slide over the dens (*curved arrow*). Dots portray original (pretraumatic) and posttraumatic ventral C1 arch location. (From Benzel EC, ed. Biomechanics of Spine Stabilization. New York: Thieme; 2001:64, with permission.)

Fig. 6.5 The mechanism of injury (orientation of injury force vector) partly dictates the type of injury incurred. **(A)** Sagittal plane injury. **(B)** Coronal plane injury.(From Benzel EC, ed. Biomechanics of Spine Stabilization. New York: Thieme; 2001:64, with permission.)

Occipital-Cervical Spine Injuries

Comprehension of the direction of the force vector that is applied to the occipital-cervical region aids in the understanding of the fracture patterns that occur. The common fracture patterns are discussed here, beginning with a rostral extension-oriented force vector and proceeding sequentially to other common, clinically relevant, orientations of force vectors, as illustrated in **Fig. 6.5**.

Superior-Dorsal-Oriented Force Vector

With a rostral-dorsal or rostral-extension-oriented force vector (**Fig. 6.5,** injury mechanism **A**), a judicial hangman's

fracture or, less commonly, a dorsal dislocation of C1 on C2 can occur. The judicial hangman's fracture (bilateral pars interarticularis fracture) of C2, with or without ventral subluxation, results from judicial hanging with the noose placed in the submental position. Other injury types, such as falls[7,8] and the use of a diagonal shoulder harness without an accompanying lap belt,[9] can cause this type of injury.

Rostral-dorsal-oriented force vectors can also cause dorsal C1-C2 dislocations.[10,11] In this situation, the force vector causes the ventral arch of C1 to sublux over the dens, resulting in locking the C1 ring behind the dens (**Fig. 6.6**).

Dorsal-Oriented Force Vector

A dorsal- or extension-oriented force vector applied to the head can cause the commonly occurring hangman's fracture or traumatic spondylolisthesis of the axis (**Fig. 6.5,** injury mechanism **B**) from bilateral C2 pars interarticularis fractures. Hangman's fractures have been classified by Effendi into three types[3] (**Fig. 6.7**). A dorsal-oriented force vector is associated with the Effendi type I fracture. The type I fracture is the most common and is an isolated hairline fracture of the pars interarticularis with less than 3 mm displacement between the dorsal dens and the dorsal body of C3.

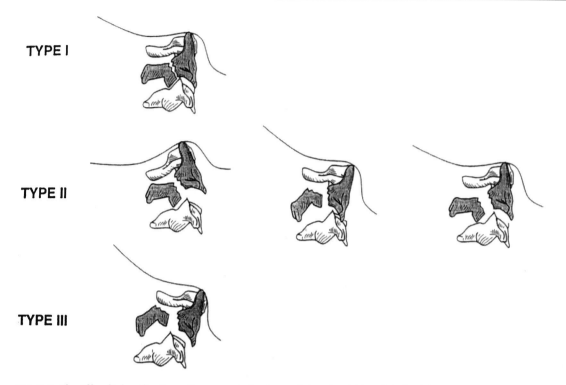

TYPE I

TYPE II

TYPE III

Fig. 6.7 The Effendi classification of hangman's fractures. A type I fracture is an isolated hairline fracture of the pars interarticularis with minimum displacement of the body of C2 on C3. A type II fracture involves the ventral displacement of the ventral fragment (C1 and C2 body) on C3. A type III fracture involves the ventral displacement as with type II fractures, but with the body of C2 resting in a flexed position. (From Benzel EC, ed. Biomechanics of Spine Stabilization. New York: Thieme; 2001:65, with permission.)

Dorsal with Axial Load Force Vector

When there exists a dorsal force vector, combined with a small axial load (**Fig. 6.5**, injury mechanism **C**), an Effendi type II fracture may occur. With the type II fracture, there is a greater than 3 mm displacement between the posterior dens and the posterior C3 body or angulation of C2 on C3, indicating potential disruption of the posterior longitudinal ligament and disk. The type II fracture also has a flexion force applied after the initial extension force. With the type III fractures, the facets of C2-C3 are bilaterally locked. These fractures are relatively rare and, unlike type I and type II fractures, involve a flexion compression mechanism.

Dorsal force vectors, combined with axial force vectors, can also cause other, more common fractures of C2. When the bony fault travels through the pedicle and the dorsal C2 vertebral body, it is termed a vertical coronally oriented C2 body fracture with C2-C3 subluxation (**Fig. 6.8**). When the dorsal force vector is applied to the high forehead region (**Fig. 6.5**, injury mechanism **D**), capital hyperextension forces, together with an axial load force, can be applied to the cervical spine. In this case, the fracture fault can pass through the ventral caudal aspect of the C2 body, resulting in a teardrop avulsion fracture, and through the ventral disk interspace between C2 and C3 and the dorsal C2 vertebral body (**Fig. 6.9**). This fracture is termed a dorsal C2 body fracture with C2-C3 subluxation and a ventral teardrop. Other variants include the isolated extension teardrop and hyperextension dislocation injuries (**Fig. 6.9**). The isolated extension teardrop fracture involves an avulsion injury of the ventral caudal aspect of the C2 vertebral body. If extension results in C2-C3 disk interspace disruption, a hyperextension dislocation injury results. Both of these variants are termed horizontal caudal C2 body fractures.

Axial Force Vectors

Axial loads applied to the cranial vertex (**Fig. 6.5**, injury mechanism **E**) can cause several injury types, depending on the relative strengths of the vertebral elements. Although occipital condyle fractures can also occur with axial loading, they are much less common than C1 fractures because the ring of C1 is relatively weak, compared with the occiput. Three types of occipital condyle fractures have been identified. Types I and II occur with axial loading. Type I fractures involve a medial disruption of the condyle and are rare, because the ring of C1 usually fails

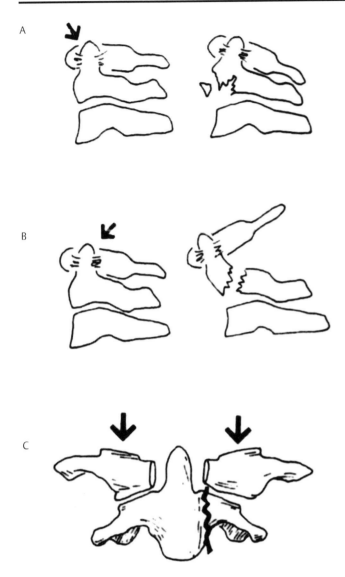

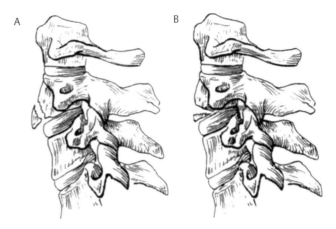

Fig. 6.9 The mechanism of injury of type I C2 body fracture variants. **(A)** Isolated extension teardrop fracture. **(B)** Hyperextension dislocation. (From Burke JT, Harris JH. Acute Injuries of the Axis Vertebra. Skeletal Radiol 1989;18:335–346, with permission.)

Fig. 6.8 Blows to the head cause an extension load **(A)** or a flexion load **(B)** to be applied to the odontoid process, unless a pure axial load is applied. If a pure axial load is applied, the lateral masses bear this load. A C2 fracture may result **(C)**. (From Benzel EC, ed. Biomechanics of Spine Stabilization. New York: Thieme; 2001:63, with permission.)

before the occipital condyle. With type II occipital condyle fractures, the fracture is usually an extension of a basal skull fracture. Type III occipital condyle fractures are more frequently associated with laterally directed force vectors and are discussed later in the chapter.

The most commonly occurring fracture in the upper cervical spine is the C1 burst fracture (Jefferson fracture) (**Fig. 6.10**). The oblique orientation of the occipital C1 facet joints results in a laterally directed force with axial compression that results in a fracture of the C1 ring.

This causes a C1 burst fracture (Jefferson fracture). Axial loads, with or without hyperextension, can result in C1 arch fractures, usually through the weakest point of the atlas. This is usually near the course of the vertebral artery. Axial loads with a component of hyperextension or hyperflexion moment application via ligamentous attachments to C1 may also result in C1 arch fractures.

To assess stability and the possible rupture of the transverse ligament of the atlas, the total lateral displacement of the C1 facet joints on C2 (summation of the total lateral displacement on both the right and left side) can be determined from an anteroposterior plain radiograph. A sum greater than 7 mm indicates that the fracture may be unstable (**Fig. 6.11**).[12] Although plain radiographs may be useful for screening, they may be misleading, and computed tomography (CT) and magnetic resonance imaging (MRI) may be more helpful regarding the assessment of the stability of an injury. Two types of transverse ligament injuries associated with C1 fractures have been identified. With type 1, the transverse ligament injury is ligamentous, whereas the type 2 injury is associated with an avulsion of the transverse ligament from its attachment to the bony ring of C1. With type 1 ligamentous injuries, surgery may be required to maintain stability, whereas with type 2 injuries, surgery may not be required, because stability can be achieved with fracture healing. It should be noted that the mechanism of injury is controversial.[13]

C2 body fractures may also occur if other structures, such as the occipital condyle, C1, or subaxial spine fractures do not occur first. With axial loads to the articular pillars of C2, comminuted sagittal fractures of the lateral aspect of the C2 body can occur. With this injury, the dorsal wall of the C2 vertebral body is thrust into the spinal canal.

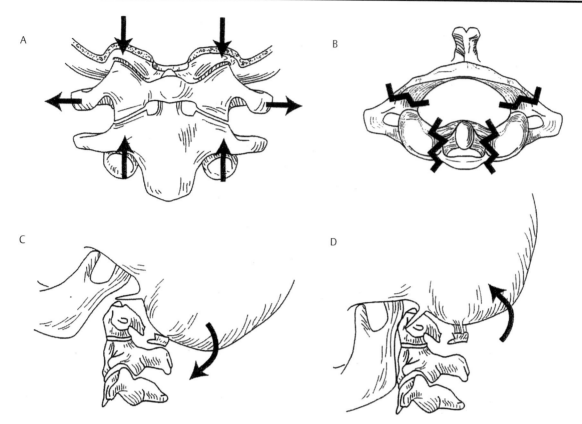

Fig. 6.10 (A) A coronal section of the C1-C2 articulations with surrounding elements. An axial load (*vertical arrows*) causes a laterally oriented resultant force vector (*horizontal arrows*) that, if substantial, causes **(B)** a bursting of the ring of C1 via fracture of the ring in four locations (Jefferson fracture). **(C)** Hyperextension of the calvarium can cause a fracture of the posterior arch of C1 by impingement on the dorsal arch of C1 via the occiput or the lamina of C2. **(D)** Hyperflexion can cause a similar injury via ligamentous attachments. The latter two injuries do not usually degrade spinal stability, as can the C1 burst fracture. (From Benzel EC, ed. Biomechanics of Spine Stabilization. New York: Thieme; 2001:62, with permission.)

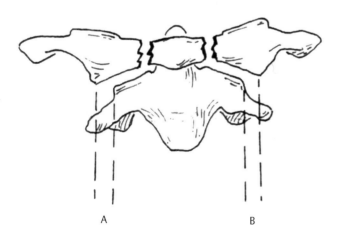

Fig. 6.11 A greater than 7 mm lateral displacement of the C1 facet on the C2 facet, adding the **(A)** right and **(B)** left displacements, implies disruption of the transverse ligament of the atlas and significant instability. (From Benzel EC, ed. Biomechanics of Spine Stabilization. New York: Thieme; 2001:66, with permission.)

Technically, this fracture can be considered a burst fracture via the Denis classification scheme.[14] These vertical sagittally oriented C2 burst-pedicle fractures are best seen with an anteroposterior view.

With purely axial loads, the compression is substantially borne by the facets. If an extension or flexion component, however, is added, a large portion of the load is borne by the odontoid process. In this case, the dens functions as a lever or moment arm by accepting the load and applying a bending moment. If a lateral component to the axial load is applied, the fracture may extend more laterally, passing through the foramina transversaria and along the pars interarticularis of C2 (**Fig. 6.12**).

Ventral Force Vectors

Ventrally applied force vectors with an axial component (**Fig. 6.5,** injury mechanism **F**) may result in a dorsal

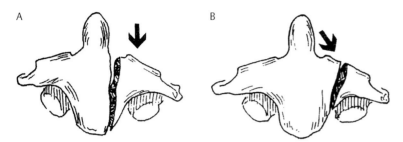

Fig. 6.12 The mechanism of injury of a vertical sagittally oriented C2 burst-pedicle fracture. **(A)** Note the absence of bony support immediately below the lateral mass of C2 (*shaded area*). **(B)** A more lateral orientation of the axial load (see **Fig. 6.5**) may result in a more laterally situated fracture. (From Benzel EC, ed. Biomechanics of Spine Stabilization. New York: Thieme; 2001:67, with permission.)

caudal C2 teardrop fracture with flexion and opening of the C2-C3 disk space. The orientation of the C2-C3 disk space is in line with the applied-force vector. This results in a C2-C3 subluxation. This vertical coronally oriented dorsal C2 body teardrop fracture with C2-C3 flexion-subluxation fracture may occasionally extend rostrally into the dens, or an isolated vertical dens fracture can occur. The latter fracture may be the result of the ventral foramen magnum impinging upon the dens as a result of the applied axial load.

A ventrally oriented force vector applied to the dorsal aspect of the head (**Fig. 6.5,** injury mechanism **G**) can result in true neck flexion and may injure C2 or the transverse ligament of the axis. Fractures of C2 include a horizontal fracture through the rostral portion of the body of C2.[5] This has been classified by Anderson and D'Alonzo[15] as a type III odontoid process fracture, although technically the fracture is located in the vertebral body of C2 and not the odontoid[16,17] (**Fig. 6.13C**). The complete classification of "odontoid" fractures is shown in **Fig. 6.13**.

In children, ventral force vectors do not commonly cause C2 fractures. Such vectors tend to cause fractures or, rather, failure through the synchondroses or ossification centers.

If the dens does not yield to a failure-producing force, the transverse ligament may rupture. The ligament, however, is usually stronger than C2, so transverse ligament rupture is less common. MRI may aid in the demonstration of the transverse ligament disruption.

Ventral Force Vector with Distraction

A ventral force vector with distraction (**Fig. 6.5,** injury mechanism **H**) is usually caused by deceleration over a fulcrum, such as over a shoulder harness. A flexion-distraction force is applied and can result in the application of a bending moment about the ventral caudal aspect of C2, with an accompanying opening of the disk interspace dorsally and the maintenance or exaggeration of disk height and the preservation of ventral soft tissue integrity. This fracture is termed a vertical coronally oriented dorsal C2 body fracture. It results from the application of flexion-distraction forces and has been termed an atypical hangman's fracture.[18] This atypical fracture can be caused by other mechanisms, including hyperextension with an axial load, hyperflexion with an axial load, and flexion-distraction (**Fig. 6.14**).

Laterally Directed Force Vectors

Laterally directed force vectors[19] (**Fig. 6.5,** injury mechanism **I**), with or without extension,[20] can cause type II odontoid or dens fractures. Lateral force vectors can also

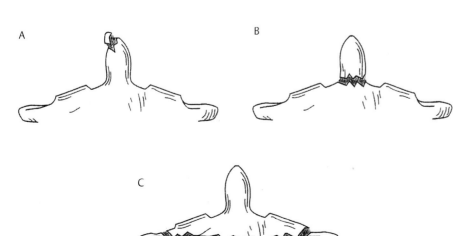

Fig. 6.13 The Anderson and D'Alonzo odontoid process fracture scheme. **(A)** A type I dens avulsion fracture. **(B)** A type II dens base fracture. **(C)** A type III horizontal upper C2 body fracture. (From Benzel EC, ed. Biomechanics of Spine Stabilization. New York: Thieme; 2001:68, with permission.)

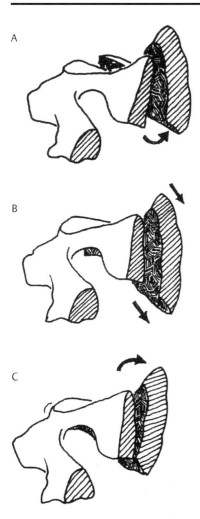

Fig. 6.14 Various mechanisms of injury of vertical coronally oriented C2 body fractures. **(A)** Hyperextension with varying degrees of axial loading (see **Fig. 6.5A,** injury mechanisms C and D), resulting in a bending moment (*arrow*). **(B)** Axial loading with some flexion (see **Fig. 6.5A,** injury mechanism F), resulting in a translational deformation (*arrows*). **(C)** Flexion-distraction (see **Fig. 6.5A,** injury mechanism H), resulting in a bending moment (*arrow*). (From Benzel EC, ed. Biomechanics of Spine Stabilization. New York: Thieme; 2001:69, with permission.)

result in type III occipital condyle fractures, in which an avulsion injury is caused by shearing forces that place tension on the occipital condyle via the alar and capsular ligaments.[17,21] Other injuries may also be associated, including open upper cervical injuries[22] and tectorial membrane injuries, particularly in children.[23]

Lateral Bending Rotation-Distraction Force

An applied lateral bending rotation-distraction force complex (**Fig. 6.5,** injury mechanism **J**) may result from lateral deceleration injuries. Atlanto-occipital dislocation has been attributed to the application of this force complex,

although hyperextension-distraction mechanisms have also been postulated.[1,24]

Torque

If a torque is applied about the long axis of the spine or dens, a rotatory injury may result.[25,26] The rotatory subluxation of C1 on C2 occurs because this region is the weakest link in the occiput-C1-C2 ligamentous complex. If the IAR is situated more laterally (e.g., through the facet joint), it may result in a contralateral unilateral rotatory subluxation (**Fig. 6.15**).

The biomechanical studies of Mouradian and colleagues[5] and Fielding and colleagues[27] have provided much of the evidence for the aforementioned statements. Their observations are summarized in **Fig. 6.16**.

Subaxial Spine

Whereas the considerable variation in anatomy of the upper cervical spine results in many complex patterns of injury, the anatomy of the subaxial spine is more consistent. As a result, the injury patterns are less varied. Therefore, they are examined as a group.

Like the occipital-cervical region, subaxial spine injury is also determined by force vectors. The magnitude of the force vector must be great enough to reach the failure point and cause injury. The magnitude can be influenced by the bending moment. The bending moment is the result of a force vector on a lever. When the same force is applied to a long lever compared with a short lever, the resulting force is greater in magnitude. Because the perpendicular distance of force application in relation to the IAR determines the length of the lever arm (moment arm), the bending moment can be significantly affected by the location of the point of force vector application in relation to the IAR.

The direction of the force vector affects the fracture pattern. For example, compressive forces that are applied ventral to the IAR often result in wedge compression fractures. Pure axial loading (i.e., in line with the IAR) results in a pure burst fracture. Distraction forces placed dorsal to the IAR result in a ligamentous or bony Chance fracture, whereas a compressive force in that same area (behind the IAR) results in hyperextension-shear injuries.

Axial Force Vectors Ventral to the Instantaneous Axis of Rotation: Ventral Wedge Compression Fractures

Ventral wedge compression fractures that are generated from an axial load placed ventral to the IAR create a ventrally oriented bending moment. In this situation, all elements of the spine that are located ventral to the IAR

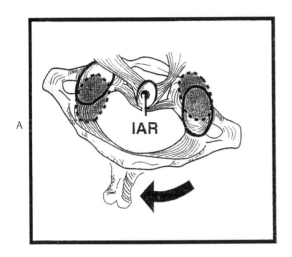

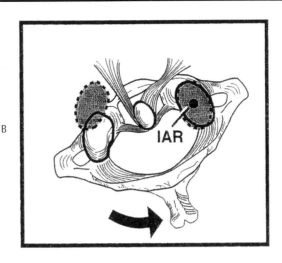

Fig. 6.15 C1-C2 rotatory subluxation. **(A)** If rotation occurs about the dens (e.g., the instantaneous axis of rotation (IAR) located in the region of the dens), bilateral facet dislocations may occur. **(B)** If the IAR is located more laterally, a unilateral and contralateral dislocation may occur. (From Benzel EC, ed. Biomechanics of Spine Stabilization. New York: Thieme; 2001:71, with permission.)

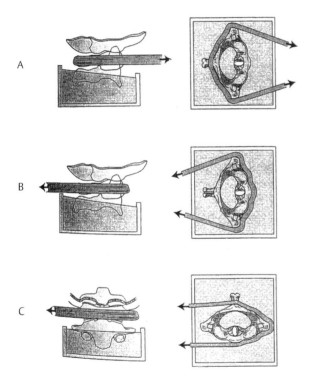

Fig. 6.16 Mouradian et al[5] and Fielding et al[27] produced fractures in the biomechanics laboratory in cadavers by applying forces (load) to the upper cervical spine. They applied loads to C1 in **(A)** ventral, **(B)** dorsal, and **(C)** lateral orientations with respect to C2 (which was fixed). **(A)** Ventral C1 loads resulted in either a C1 transverse ligament rupture or a dens fracture. Dorsal C2 loads failed to produce an injury. **(B)** C2 fracture in the epoxy failed first. **(C)** Lateral C2 loading produced a dense fracture (type II fracture of Anderson and D'Alonzo). (Adapted with permission from Fielding JW, Cochran GVB, Lawsing JF III, et al. Tears of the traverse ligament of the atlas: a clinical and biomechanical study. J Bone Joint Surg 1974;56A: 1683–1691; and Mouradian WH, Fietti VG Jr, Cochran GV, et al. Fractures of the odontoid: a laboratory and clinical study of mechanisms. Orthop Clin North Am 1978;9:985–1001.)

become closer together, and all the elements dorsal to the IAR become farther apart. Dorsal distraction is not significant because of the resistance of the dorsal ligamentous complex. At the ventral/dorsal plane of the IAR, the vertebral body height is unchanged. The bending moment causes an eccentric loading of the spine and concentrates the stresses ventrally. This increased stress concentration ventrally explains why failure is more likely when a bending moment is simultaneously applied with an axial load (**Fig. 6.17**). This contrasts with burst fractures (see below). Imaging demonstrates the flexion deformity where the ventral vertebral body height is less than the dorsal height.[1,28–31]

The thoracic spine, the thoracolumbar junction, and the cervical spine are all prone to these injuries. Although the natural kyphotic curve of the thoracic spine exposes it to an increased chance of a flexion component injury, the rib cage can be a significant source of stability to the upper and middle thoracic segments (**Fig. 6.18**). An increased chance of flexion injury also occurs at the thoracolumbar junction because of the kyphotic curvature of the thoracolumbar region of the spine, as well as its location between the relatively unyielding thoracic segment and rib cage rostrally and lumbar segment caudally. Although the middle to lower cervical spine has an intrinsic lordotic curvature, the occurrence of these fractures in the cervical spine is due to the flexibility of the cervical spine that often counterbalances the influences of the natural lordotic posture. When a flexed posture is assumed, the axial load is located ventral to the IAR, which predisposes the spine to a compression fracture. If the person has not assumed a flexion posture, the biomechanics of the natural lordotic posture will prevail, and a burst fracture may occur. The flexibility of the cervical spine and the often-assumed relatively flexed posture of these regions at the moment of impact are the factors that predispose the cervical spine

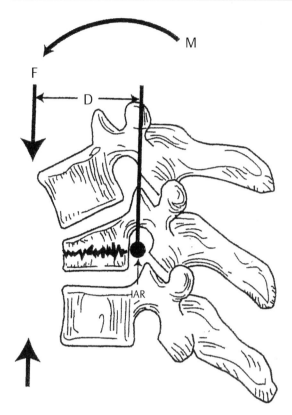

Fig. 6.17 A depiction of the injury force vector causing a ventral wedge compression fracture. *Abbreviations: F*, applied force vector; *D*, length of moment arm (from IAR to plane of *F*); *M*, bending moment. (From Benzel EC, ed. Biomechanics of Spine Stabilization. New York: Thieme; 2001:74, with permission.)

to ventral wedge compression fractures despite the natural lordotic posture.

Decreasing the flexion component eliminates or nearly eliminates the bending moment and therefore decreases

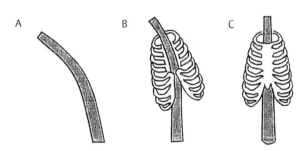

Fig. 6.18 An illustration of the stability provided to the spine by the rib cage. **(A)** The spine without a rib cage can bend excessively. **(B)** The addition of the rib cage moderately increases stability. **(C)** Sternal attachments are required for achievement of the full stabilization potential of the rib cage. Removal of the effects of either the sternum or the ribs causes a significant diminution of stability. (From Benzel EC, ed. Biomechanics of Spine Stabilization. New York: Thieme; 2001:39, with permission.)

the incidence of compression fractures. The flexion component is decreased with the intrinsic lordotic curves of the lower cervical region and the lumbar region. In addition, the massive size of the vertebral bodies of the lumbar spine makes them relatively unyielding. This decreases the likelihood of occurrence of a significant flexion component in a spinal fracture in this region. With no flexion, there is no bending moment applied, and an isolated axial load is applied to the middle to lower cervical and lumbar regions. The frequent assumption of a flexed, kyphotic cervical spine posture at the moment of impact (e.g., during "spear" tackling in American football) results in a greater incidence of wedge compression fractures in the cervical region than the lumbar region. When wedge compression fractures do occur in the lumbar spine, they tend to occur near the upper limits of the lumbar spine due to the lessening of the natural lordotic curvature observed as the lumbar spine ascends into the thoracolumbar junction. Bone or disk fragments can be retropulsed into the spinal canal when these fractures occur.

Axial Force Vector Alone: Burst Fractures

Because the vertebral body is the predominant axial load-bearing structure of the spine, pure axial loading with no bending moment or eccentric load outside of

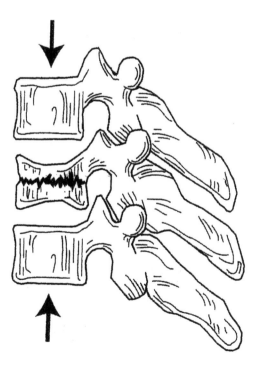

Fig. 6.19 The mechanism of injury of a burst fracture; true axial loading without a bending moment ($D = 0$). (From Benzel EC, ed. Biomechanics of Spine Stabilization. New York: Thieme; 2001:75, with permission.)

the IAR results in true or pure burst fractures of the vertebral body (**Fig. 6.19**). With burst fractures, a symmetric compression of the vertebral body results,[1,32–38] because there is no eccentric component to the force vector, and the moment arm length of the force vector (perpendicular distance from the force vector to the IAR) is zero. Due to the absence of an applied bending moment, eccentric loading, and the absence of stress concentration, greater or excessive forces may be required to generate a fracture. In fact, if the spine is preloaded along its axis (follower load), its resistance to angular deformation is increased.[39] If an eccentric load is present, an angular deformity results, as is the case with a ventral or lateral compression wedge fracture. Just as pressure on dough causes the dough to extrude, the symmetric compression of the vertebral body can cause extrusion of or retropulsion of bony fragments into the spinal canal, resulting in dural sac compression.[14,40] The extent of spinal canal compromise is associated with the loading rate.[38]

Because a pure axial load is required for burst fractures, they most frequently occur in the upper and middle cervical and lumbar regions. Burst fractures are common in the upper lumbar region because of the relatively limited flexibility of the lumbar spine, compared with the cervical spine, and the substantial lordotic posture present in the lower lumbar spine. The decreased incidence in the lower lumbar spine is also due to the spinal column's increased intrinsic compression-resisting ability secondary to the increased bony and muscle mass in this region.[35,41]

Although burst fractures compromise both the anterior and middle columns of the Denis classification scheme (see below) and hence are suggestive of instability, burst fractures of the middle or lower lumbar spine are often stable because of the preservation of the dorsal elements. If there is no neurologic impairment, nonoperative management is often sufficient.[42,43] In contrast, cervical burst fractures exposed to extension or further compression may worsen spinal canal compromise.[44]

Eccentric Axial Load Vector: Lateral Wedge Compression Fractures

Although wedge compression and burst fractures focus on sagittal plane deformations, coronal plane deformations can also occur. Anteroposterior radiographs demonstrate asymmetric loss of height of the vertebral body. These fractures are caused by an axial load placed eccentrically with respect to the IAR (**Fig. 6.20**). The mechanism of injury is secondary to the "buckling" of the spine that follows the application of an axial load, thus creating a lateral bending moment (**Fig. 6.21**). Although lateral wedge compression fractures can occur as isolated

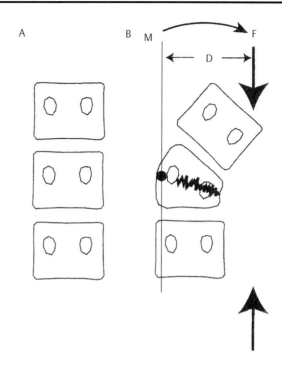

Fig. 6.20 (A) Eccentrically applied loads cause bending of the straight spine. **(B)** The bending occurs in the direction of the eccentrically applied load (*F*, *large arrow*) with respect to the IAR (*dot*). If failure of the vertebral body occurs, it will be oriented in the same direction. *Abbreviations: D*, length of moment arm (from IAR to plane of *F*). M, bending moment. (From Benzel EC, ed. Biomechanics of Spine Stabilization. New York: Thieme; 2001:76, with permission.)

injuries, many coexist with a sagittal plane fracture component (**Fig. 6.22**).

Flexion with Distraction: Flexion-Distraction (Chance) Fractures

Although axial loading is one of the most common force vectors applied to the subaxial spine, distraction is relatively uncommon. A mechanism of injury that involves distraction is associated with deceleration in a motor vehicle accident, with the patient wearing a lap belt without a shoulder harness. The belt restricts the pelvis and lumbosacral movement. This, in turn, results in forward flexion (flexion bending moment) and unrestricted distraction of the remainder of the spine. Thus, the mechanism of injury with this type of trauma is flexion and distraction of the lumbar spine.[1,45–48] This injury was first described by Chance[45] and is of two basic types. One involves a pure bony cleavage plane, and the other involves the vertebral end plate (**Fig. 6.23**). Although there are variations of Chance fractures, the injury mechanism is the same. These fractures are considered overtly unstable because they involve both the ventral and dorsal columns.

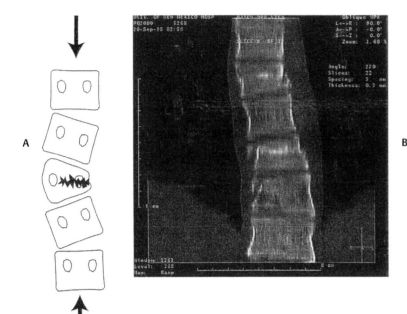

Fig. 6.21 **(A)** A depiction of spine buckling secondary to axial load application as a cause of a wedge compression fracture. **(B)** This is also depicted with a coronal computed tomography reconstruction. (From Benzel EC, ed. Biomechanics of Spine Stabilization. New York: Thieme; 2001:77, with permission.)

Axial Force Vectors Dorsal to the Instantaneous Axis of Rotation: Dorsal Element Fractures

Axial force vectors applied dorsal to the IAR result in a compressive force applied to the dorsal elements at the affected spinal level, increasing the chance of dorsal element failure (**Fig. 6.24**). Dorsal element fractures are relatively common, especially in the cervical spine where the vertebral segments are small and a lordotic posture is naturally assumed. In the cervical spine, with the relatively coronal orientation of the facets, extension forces the opposing facet surfaces together. This exposes the facets and pars interarticularis to significant stress, resulting in laminar, spinous process, or facet fractures. With rotation, the facets can slide past each other.

Like the cervical spine, the lumbar spine assumes a lordotic posture. There is a lower incidence of dorsal fractures in the lumbar spine because of the relatively larger vertebral size and the sagittal orientation of the facet

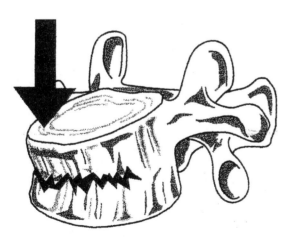

Fig. 6.22 The mechanism of injury of a combination ventral and lateral wedge compression fracture. The *arrow* depicts an eccentrically applied load. (From Benzel EC, ed. Biomechanics of Spine Stabilization. New York: Thieme; 2001:76, with permission.)

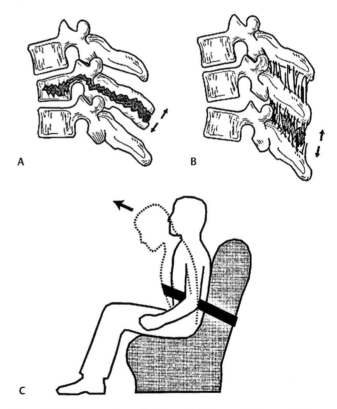

Fig. 6.23 There are two fundamental types of Chance (flexion-distraction) fracture. **(A)** Diastasis fracture through the pedicles and vertebral body. **(B)** Fracture through the vertebral end plate or disk. **(C)** The mechanism of injury. (From Benzel EC, ed. Biomechanics of Spine Stabilization. New York: Thieme; 2001:77, with permission.)

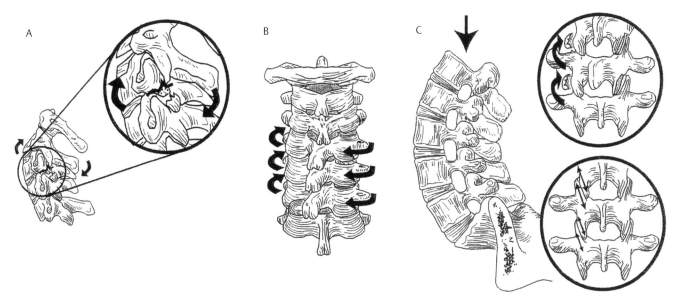

Fig. 6.24 The mechanism of injury of dorsal element fractures. **(A)** Cervical spine extension forcibly approximates the facet joints or the laminae. **(B)** Cervical rotation causes the coronally oriented facet joints to slide past each other. The former may produce fracture; the latter may produce isolated ligamentous disruption or dislocation. **(C)** In the lumbar region, the facet joints are able to slide past each other during extension, thus abutting against the other. This results in facet fracture if the force is substantial (*upper inset*). Conversely, extension or flexion causes the sagittally oriented facet joint to slide past each other (*lower inset*). (From Benzel EC, ed. Biomechanics of Spine Stabilization. New York: Thieme; 2001:78, with permission.)

joints. Because of this sagittal orientation, hyperextension results in the facet joints sliding past each other. The relative lack of flexibility and the sagittal orientation of the lumbar facets result in fractures of the facets being a relatively uncommon event (**Fig. 6.24**). Fractures of the lamina and pars interarticularis, however, may result.[49] Because the orientation of the lumbar facets restricts rotation, the likelihood that rotation will cause injury is minimized.

Other spine injuries are associated with dorsal element lumbar spine fractures, including compression fractures, translational injuries, and rotational injuries. If the rotatory force vector is of significant magnitude, dorsal element injuries may occur by forcing the opposing inferior and superior articulating facet joint against each other (**Fig. 6.24**). With this significant force, vertebral body fractures or disk interspace disruption may occur as well as disruption of the integrity of the ventral axial-load-resisting substructure.[50]

Spinous process and laminar fractures may occasionally result from extreme flexion or extension. Extreme lateral bending may also cause transverse process fractures on the convex side of the bend (**Fig. 6.25**).

Ligamentous Injuries

The spinal ligaments provide passive stabilization and both tension-band and translational support of the vertebral column. The contribution of a spinal ligament to spinal stability is related to the ligament's tensile strength (**Fig. 6.26**), as well as to the moment arm through which it acts. The amount of resistance a ligament provides is proportional to the distance from the IAR to its point of attachment (**Fig. 6.27**). Thus, although the interspinous ligament is not as strong as the posterior longitudinal ligament when tested in isolation, because its insertion site is farther from the IAR, the interspinous ligament provides a significant contribution to flexion resistance in selected regions of the

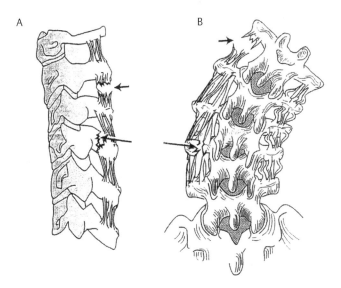

Fig. 6.25 **(A)** Extreme flexion may cause spinous process fracture (*long arrow*) or ligamentous disruption (*short arrow*). **(B)** Extreme lateral bending may cause a transverse process fracture (*long arrow*) or ligamentous disruption (*short arrow*). (From Benzel EC, ed. Biomechanics of Spine Stabilization. New York: Thieme; 2001:79, with permission.)

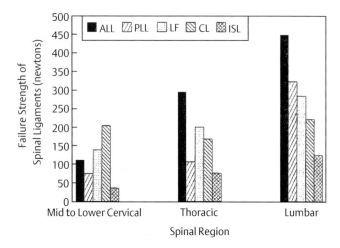

Fig. 6.26 Failure strength of spinal ligaments versus spinal region. *Abbreviations*: ALL, anterior longitudinal ligament; PLL, posterior longitudinal ligament; LF, ligamentum flavum; CL, capsular ligament; ISL, interspinous ligament. (From Benzel EC, ed. Biomechanics of Spine Stabilization. New York: Thieme; 2001:8, with permission.)

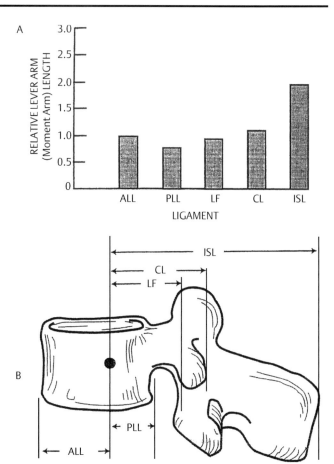

Fig. 6.27 (A) The relative lever arm (moment arm) length of ligaments causing flexion (or resisting extension). **(B)** The ligaments and their effective moment arms. Note that this length depends on the location of the IAR (*dot*). An "average" location is used in this illustration. *Abbreviations*: ALL, anterior longitudinal ligament; PLL, posterior longitudinal ligament; LF, ligamentum flavum; CL, capsular ligament; ISL, interspinous ligament. (From Benzel EC, ed. Biomechanics of Spine Stabilization. New York: Thieme; 2001:9, with permission.)

spine. Isolated ligamentous injuries are more common in the cervical spine and are caused, in part, by the increased flexibility of the cervical spine. This results in a greater strain placed on the ligaments (**Fig. 6.25**). Ligament injuries are thought by many to be the anatomical/pathologic correlate of the whiplash syndrome.[51–57] These ligamentous injuries of the cervical[21,58,59] and thoracic spine[60] can be identified with MRI and are often not detected with radiographs or CT. Although the T2-weighted image with fat suppression is the most useful MRI sequence to detect ligamentous lesions, MRI is also useful for the evaluation of the spinal cord, for vascular injuries,[61] and for a limited evaluation of the bone.[62] Because activities of daily living expose the cervical spine ligaments to stresses that are greater than most whiplash injuries,[63] the evaluation of patients with neck pain is difficult, and the diagnosis of whiplash is likely made too frequently.[64] Care must be taken when considering the significance of neck pain following an injury, particularly when the neck pain is the result of an accident in which there was little or no damage to the vehicle. With most whiplash injuries, optimal clinical results are achieved with early activity and early resumption of work.[65,66] The injury mechanisms of cervical whiplash injuries have been well characterized.[52]

Isolated ligamentous injuries of the lumbar spine are less common because the more massive and less flexible lumbar spine does not rely as much on ligamentous support. Indeed, the dorsal ligaments, particularly the interspinous and supraspinous ligaments (especially in the low lumbar region) are weak or essentially nonexistent. When ligamentous injuries do occur in the lumbar spine, they are often associated with other bony injuries.

Facet Dislocation

The incidence of facet dislocation is highest in the cervical spine, less frequent in the thoracic spine, and rare in the lumbar spine. The increased incidence in the cervical and thoracic spine is because of the more coronal orientation of the facet joints in these regions. With the application of an exaggerated flexion force vector, the normal limits of mobility of the facet joint can be overcome, and the facets may perch, lock (**Fig. 6.28**), or fracture. Spine stability is compromised with these injuries.

The applied force vectors affect the injury pattern. When a true flexion moment is applied, a bilateral facet dislocation may occur. When a flexion moment is combined with a rotational component, a unilateral facet dislocation can occur (**Fig. 6.29**). Hyperextension with an axial load may cause facet fractures (**Fig. 6.24**).

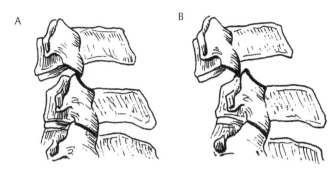

Fig. 6.28 Cervical spine facet injuries: **(A)** perched and **(B)** locked. (From Benzel EC, ed. Biomechanics of Spine Stabilization. New York: Thieme; 2001:79, with permission.)

Stability of Subaxial Spine Fractures

Stability of the spine may be characterized and defined as the ability of the spine under physiologic loads to limit patterns of displacement so as not to damage or irritate the spinal cord or nerve roots and, in addition, to prevent incapacitating deformity or pain caused by structural changes.[17] Instability has been divided into acute and chronic types. Although trauma generally causes acute instability, chronic instability may occur if acute instability is left unattended. Acute instability can be described as overt or limited.

Overt instability is the inability of the spine to support the body during normal activity. This generally occurs when loss of vertebral column and dorsal element integrity occurs, resulting in a circumferential loss of spine integrity. Although vertebral column integrity can be readily determined with plain radiographs, CT, or MRI, the documentation of dorsal element integrity is more challenging. Clinical examination may reveal pain on palpation of the dorsal element structures or loss of midline soft tissue definition (**Fig. 6.30**). Although plain radiographs and CT may demonstrate splaying of the spinous processes or frank dorsal element fractures, MRI may be the most sensitive in assessing dorsal ligamentous integrity.[58] The use

of sagittal T2-weighted images with fat suppression or short tau inversion recovery (STIR) sequences may offer greater specificity regarding the determination of the dorsal ligamentous and soft tissue element injuries.[67] With overt instability, operative stabilization is required and often involves surgical management.

With limited instability, there is loss of either ventral or dorsal spinal integrity, usually with preservation of the other. With this type of instability, most normal activities are supported. Examples of isolated loss of ventral spinal integrity include isolated wedge or burst vertebral fractures with preservation of the integrity of dorsal elements. Examples of loss of dorsal spinal integrity include isolated laminar fractures or ligamentous disruption with intact ventral elements. Because of the difficulty in determining the loss of dorsal ligamentous integrity, overt instability may be mistaken for limited instability. MRI and dynamic flexion/extension radiographs may assist with this differentiation. Care must be taken with the interpretation of dynamic radiographs. If guarding is present, and the excursion between flexion and extension is limited, dynamic radiographs may not accurately portray the extent of dorsal ligament laxity or failure. With limited instability, management usually involves nonoperative bracing. If a significant risk of chronic instability exists, surgical management may be required.

Classification of Subaxial Spine Fractures

Several classification schemes have been developed to assess the stability of subaxial spine injuries. They all incorporate the concept of columns. Louis[68] suggested that the spine bears loads through three columns: the vertebral body and both facet joint complexes. This scheme addresses axial load transmission. It is, however, limited in its ability to assess distraction, flexion, and extension components of injury and the integrity of ligamentous structures.

Holdsworth[28] and Kelly and Whitesides[31] proposed a two-column concept that assisted with the assessment of angular deformations. Kelly and Whitesides defined the

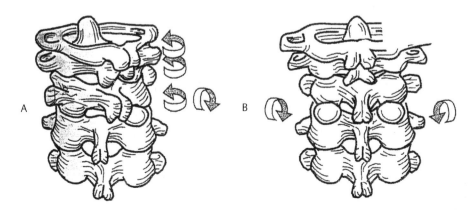

Fig. 6.29 (A) Flexion plus rotation (*curved arrows*) causes unilateral cervical facet joint dislocation. **(B)** Pure flexion (*curved arrows*) causes bilateral cervical facet joint dislocation. (From Benzel EC, ed. Biomechanics of Spine Stabilization. New York: Thieme; 2001:79, with permission.)

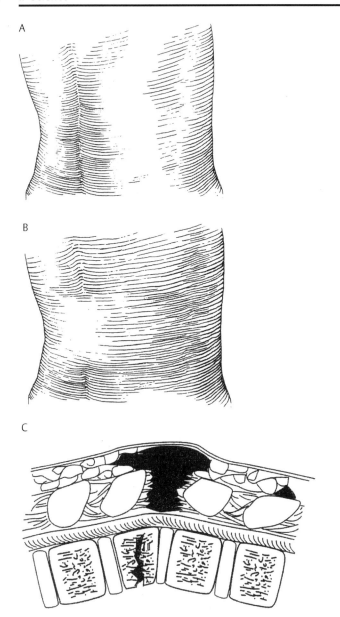

two columns as involving the vertebral bodies and the neural arches, respectively. They highlighted the importance of the dorsal ligamentous complex in the assessment of spine stability.

The three-column theory was introduced by Denis[14] and is still used today. With this scheme, the anterior column includes the anterior longitudinal ligament and the ventral vertebral body, and the middle column includes the dorsal vertebral body, posterior longitudinal ligament, and dorsal anulus fibrosus. The posterior column includes the pedicles, the facet joints, and the supraspinous ligaments. The inclusion of a middle column in this classification scheme allows for the assessment of the neutral axis. The neutral axis is the longitudinal region of the spinal column that bears a significant axial load and usually contains the IAR. Within the neutral axis, spinal element distraction or compression does not excessively occur with physiologic flexion or extension. With the Denis scheme, compromise of any two of the three columns increases the concern for an unstable fracture. Four major fracture types were described by Denis: compression, burst, seat-belt type, and fracture-dislocation (**Table 6.1**).

Another spinal fracture classification scheme is that of the Arbeitsgemeinschaft für Osteosynthesefragen (AO, Association for the Study of Internal Fixation),[69] in which fractures are first divided into types and are further subdivided into groups, subgroups, and specifications. This classification is extensive and covers the majority of spine fractures. Plain radiographs and CT are used to determine the mechanism of injury, and attention is paid to both bony and ligamentous integrity. It also includes an indirect assessment of the dorsal ligamentous complex and interprets it as being intact or deficient. The first level of the classification divides fractures into types A, B, and C. Type A fractures are ventral column injuries that result from flexion with axial loading (**Table 6.2**). Type B fractures are ventral and dorsal column injuries that result from flexion or extension with distraction (**Table 6.3**). Type C fractures are ventral and dorsal column injuries and include rotational forces (**Table 6.4**).

Type A injuries are further subdivided into impaction fractures (wedge), split fractures (including pincer), and burst

Fig. 6.30 Dorsal instability in the thoracic and lumbar region can be suggested, particularly in thin patients, by physical examination. The presence of tenderness over the spinous processes or the absence of the normal midline crease **(A)**, on account of swelling or hematoma formation below the skin **(B)**, suggests underlying soft tissue injury **(C)**. This, in turn, suggests but does not prove the presence of dorsal spinal instability. (From Benzel EC, ed. Biomechanics of Spine Stabilization. New York: Thieme; 2001:34, with permission.)

Table 6.1 Basic Modes of Failure of the Three Columns in the Four Types of Spinal Injuries[14]

Types of Fracture	Columns		
	Anterior	**Middle**	**Posterior**
Compression	Compression	None	None or severe distraction
Burst	Compression	Compression	None
"Seat belt"	None or compression	Distraction	Distraction
Fracture-dislocation	Compression rotation shear		Distraction rotation shear

Table 6.2 AO Classification: Type A Injuries

Type A: Vertebral body compression

A1 Impaction fractures

  A1.1 End-plate impaction

  A1.2 Wedge impaction features

  A1.3 Vertebral body collapse

A2 Split fractures

  A2.1 Sagittal split fracture

  A2.2 Coronal split fracture

  A2.3 Pincer fracture

A3 Burst fractures

  A3.1 Incomplete burst fracture

  A3.2 Burst-split fracture

  A3.3 Complete split fracture

Table 6.3 AO Classification: Type B Injuries

Type B: Anterior and posterior element injury with distraction

B1 Posterior disruption predominantly ligamentous (flexion-distraction injury)

  B1.1 With transverse disruption of the disk

  B1.2 With type A fracture of the vertebral body

B2 Posterior disruption predominantly osseous (flexion-distraction injury)

  B2.1 Transverse bicolumn fracture

  B2.2 With disruption of the disk

  B2.3 With type A fracture of the vertebral body

B3 Anterior disruption through the disk (hyperextension-shear injury)

  B3.1 Hyperextension-subluxations

  B3.2 Hyperextension-spondylolysis

  B3.3 Posterior dislocation

fractures. Type B injuries are subdivided into ligamentous flexion distraction, bony flexion distraction, and hyperextension shear injuries. Type C injuries are subdivided into type A with rotation and type B with rotation and rotational shear. Only with type A fractures are the dorsal bony and ligamentous integrity considered to be intact. Although the additional use of MRI may improve the reproducibility of the AO classification,[70,71] classification based solely on MRI findings correlates poorly with the classification scheme.[70]

Table 6.4 AO Classification: Type C Injuries

Type C: Anterior and posterior element injury with rotation

C1 Type A injuries with rotation (compression injuries with rotation)

  C1.1 Rotational wedge fracture

  C1.2 Rotational split fracture

C2 Type B injuries with rotation

  C2.1 B1 injuries with rotation (flexion-distraction injuries with rotation)

  C2.2 B2 injuries with rotation (flexion-distraction injuries with rotation)

  C2.3 B3 injuries with rotation (hyperextension-shear injuries with rotation)

C3 Rotational-shear injuries

  C3.1 Slice fracture

  C3.2 Oblique fracture

Although the detailed inclusion of most fracture types in the AO classification provides a basis for research, it may be difficult to apply in day-to-day clinical decision making. Classification systems have been designed with point systems to assess spine stability and guide in treatment.

White and Panjabi[17] developed a point system (**Table 6.5**) in which a score of 5 or more is suggestive of overt instability, and a score of 2 to 4 is suggestive of limited instability. The translation and angulation cut-off values for resting and dynamic films have been compiled in **Table 6.6** for cervical, thoracic and lumbar levels. These values are derived from cadaveric biomechanical studies, and meta-analyses of normal physiologic values.[17]

More modern points classification systems have been developed that incorporate the use of MRI. These systems are also designed to incorporate the current understanding of the biomechanics of thoracolumbar injuries, and to be relatively simple to achieve high inter- and intraobserver reliability.[60] The Thoracolumbar Injury Classification and Severity Score (TLICS) was developed[72] not only to classify injuries, but also to give general guidelines of treatment. In this system, points are given within three major categories: the morphology of injury, the integrity of the posterior ligamentous complex, and the neurologic status of the patient. In this classification system, patients with ≤ 3 total points are considered nonoperative candidates, and patients with ≥ 5 points are operative candidates. If the total score is 4, either nonoperative or operative treatment may be considered. The details of the subcategories and their point assignment are listed in **Tables 6.7** and **6.8**. Validity and reliability testing of this system has yet to be fully assessed.[73]

Table 6.5 Quantitation of Acute Instability for Subaxial Cervical, Thoracic, and Lumbar Injuries[17]

Condition	Points Assigned
Loss of integrity of anterior (and middle) column	2
Loss of integrity of posterior column(s)	2
Acute resting translational deformity	2
Acute resting angulation deformity	2
Acute dynamic translational deformity exaggeration	2
Acute dynamic angulation deformity exaggeration	2
Neural element injury	3
Acute disk narrowing at level of suspected pathology	1
Dangerous loading anticipated	1

Table 6.6 Resting and Dynamic Radiologic Guidelines[17]

	Resting	Dynamic
Subaxial cervical spine	> 3.5 mm displacement	> 3.5 mm translation
	> 11 degree angulation	> 20 degree angulation
Thoracic spine	> 2.5 mm displacement	
	> 5 degree angulation	
Lumbar spine	> 4.5 mm displacement	> 4.5 mm translation
	> 22 degree angulation	> 15 degree L1-L4
		> 20 degree L4-L5
		> 25 degree L5-S1

Table 6.7 Thoracolumbar Injury Classification and Severity Score (TLICS)[72]

Parameter	Points
Morphology	
Compression fracture	1
Burst fracture	2
Translational/rotational	3
Distraction	4
Neurologic involvement	
Intact	0
Nerve root	2
Cord, conus medullaris	
Incomplete	3
Complete	2
Cauda equina	3
Posterior ligamentous complex	
Intact	0
Injury suspected/indeterminate	2
Injured	3

Sacral Injuries

Isolated injuries of the sacrum are rare, and sacral fractures are usually associated with pelvic ring disruption in at least one additional location.[74] Biomechanical studies have determined that with axial loads, the sacral alae bear the most significant loads in the sacrum, with the principal strain direction being obliquely aligned from the vertical, resulting in predominantly compressive strain in the superior sacrum and tensile strain inferiorly.[75] The resulting fractures have been divided into two basic types: vertical and horizontal. They have been classified according to

Table 6.8 Management as Per TLICS Score[72]

Management	Points
Nonoperative	0–3
Nonoperative or operative	4
Operative	≥ 5

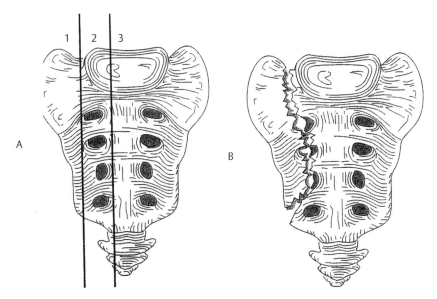

Fig. 6.31 **(A)** Sacral fractures and the three zones of injury. **(B)** An example of a type II fracture. (From Benzel EC, ed. Biomechanics of Spine Stabilization. New York: Thieme; 2001:80, with permission.)

the three zones of the sacrum that are involved (**Fig. 6.31**). Zone 1 injuries do not involve the neural foramina and are usually vertical fractures through the ala. These fractures usually involve lateral compression forces and are relatively stable if no significant translation component is present. Zone 2 injuries are generally vertical and involve the ventral neural foramina. Zone 3 injuries are vertical or horizontal and involve the sacral spinal canal. Neurologic injuries (particularly bladder dysfunction) have been associated with these fractures.[76]

■ Conclusion

The application of biomechanical principles to spine injury aids in the understanding of the fracture patterns that occur. The study of biomechanics and spine injury, however, is not static. With better understanding of the causes underlying spine injury, improved preventative and treatment strategies can be developed, with the ultimate goal of eliminating spine injury altogether.

References

1. Bucholz RW, Burkhead WZ. The pathological anatomy of fatal atlanto-occipital dislocations. J Bone Joint Surg Am 1979;61:248–250
2. Burke JT, Harris JH Jr. Acute injuries of the axis vertebra. Skeletal Radiol 1989;18:335–346
3. Effendi B, Roy D, Cornish B, et al. Fractures of the ring of the axis: a classification based on the analysis of 131 cases. J Bone Joint Surg Br 1981;63-B:319–327
4. Francis WR, Fielding JW, Hawkins RJ, et al. Traumatic spondylolisthesis of the axis. J Bone Joint Surg Br 1981;63-B:313–318
5. Mouradian WH, Fietti VG Jr, Cochran GV, et al. Fractures of the odontoid: a laboratory and clinical study of mechanisms. Orthop Clin North Am 1978;9:985–1001
6. Williams TG. Hangman's fracture. J Bone Joint Surg Br 1975;57:82–88
7. Levine AM, Edwards CC. Treatment of injuries in the C1–C2 complex. Orthop Clin North Am 1986;17:31–44
8. Wood-Jones F. The ideal lesion produced by judicial hanging. Lancet 1913;1:53
9. Yarbrough BE, Hendey GW. Hangman's fracture resulting from improper seat belt use. South Med J 1990;83:843–845
10. Haralson RH III, Boyd HB. Posterior dislocation of the atlas on the axis without fracture: report of a case. J Bone Joint Surg Am 1969;51: 561–566
11. Patzakis MJ, Knopf A, Elfering M, et al. Posterior dislocation of the atlas on the axis: a case report. J Bone Joint Surg Am 1974;56:1260–1262
12. Spence KF Jr, Decker S, Sell KW. Bursting atlantal fracture associated with rupture of the transverse ligament. J Bone Joint Surg Am 1970;52:543–549
13. Heggeness MH, Doherty BJ. Was Jefferson wrong? A biomechanical study of fractures of the atlas. Presented at the 14th annual meeting, Baylor College of Medicine, Houston, TX, 1999
14. Denis F. The three column spine and its significance in the classification of acute thoracolumbar spinal injuries. Spine 1983;8:817–831
15. Anderson LD, D'Alonzo RT. Fractures of the odontoid process of the axis. J Bone Joint Surg Am 1974;56:1663–1674
16. Benzel EC, Hart BL, Ball PA, et al. Fractures of the C-2 vertebral body. J Neurosurg 1994;81:206–212
17. White AA, Panjabi MM. Clinical Biomechanics of the Spine, 2nd ed. Philadelphia: Lippincott, 1990:130–342
18. Starr JK, Eismont FJ. Atypical hangman's fractures. Spine 1993;18:1954–1957
19. Matsui H, Imada K, Tsuji H. Radiographic classification of os odontoideum and its clinical significance. Spine 1997;22: 1706–1709
20. Noble ER, Smoker WR. The forgotten condyle: the appearance, morphology, and classification of occipital condyle fractures. AJNR Am J Neuroradiol 1996;17:507–513
21. Anderson PA, Montesano PX. Morphology and treatment of occipital condyle fractures. Spine 1988;13:731–736
22. Ide C, Nisolle JF, Misson N, et al. Unusual occipitoatlantal fracture dissociation with no neurological impairment: case report. J Neurosurg 1998;88:773–776

23. Sun PP, Poffenbarger GJ, Durham S, et al. Spectrum of occipitoatlantoaxial injury in young children. J Neurosurg 2000;93:28–39

24. Montane I, Eismont FJ, Green BA. Traumatic occipitoatlantal dislocation. Spine 1991;16:112–116

25. Garber JN. Abnormalities of the atlas and axis vertebrae–congenital and traumatic. J Bone Joint Surg Am 1964;46:1782–1791

26. Subach BR, McLaughlin MR, Albright AL, et al. Current management of pediatric atlantoaxial rotatory subluxation. Spine 1998;23:2174–2179

27. Fielding JW, Cochran GB, Lawsing JF III, et al. Tears of the transverse ligament of the atlas: a clinical and biomechanical study. J Bone Joint Surg Am 1974;56:1683–1691

28. Holdsworth F. Fractures, dislocations, and fracture-dislocations of the spine. J Bone Joint Surg Am 1970;52:1534–1551

29. Jelsma RK, Kirsch PT, Rice JF, et al. The radiographic description of thoracolumbar fractures. Surg Neurol 1982;18:230–236

30. Keene JS. Radiographic evaluation of thoracolumbar fractures. Clin Orthop Relat Res 1984;58–64

31. Kelly RP, Whitesides TE Jr. Treatment of lumbodorsal fracture-dislocations. Ann Surg 1968;167:705–717

32. Atlas SW, Regenbogen V, Rogers LF, et al. The radiographic characterization of burst fractures of the spine. AJR Am J Roentgenol 1986;147:575–582

33. Castillo M, Mukherji SK. Vertical fractures of the dens. AJNR Am J Neuroradiol 1996;17:1627–1630

34. Cope R, Kilcoyne RF, Gaines RW. The thoracolumbar burst fracture with intact posterior elements: implications for neurologic deficit and stability. Neuro-Orthopedics 1989;7:83–87

35. Court-Brown CM, Gertzbein SD. The management of burst fractures of the fifth lumbar vertebra. Spine 1987;12:308–312

36. McAfee PC, Yuan HA, Fredrickson BE, et al. The value of computed tomography in thoracolumbar fractures: an analysis of one hundred consecutive cases and a new classification. J Bone Joint Surg Am 1983;65:461–473

37. McEvoy RD, Bradford DS. The management of burst fractures of the thoracic and lumbar spine: experience in 53 patients. Spine 1985;10:631–637

38. Tran NT, Watson NA, Tencer AF, et al. Mechanism of the burst fracture in the thoracolumbar spine: the effect of loading rate. Spine 1995;20:1984–1988

39. Patwardhan AG, Havey RM, Ghanayem AJ, et al. Load-carrying capacity of the human cervical spine in compression is increased under a follower load. Spine 2000;25:1548–1554

40. Hashimoto T, Kaneda K, Abumi K. Relationship between traumatic spinal canal stenosis and neurologic deficits in thoracolumbar burst fractures. Spine 1988;13:1268–1272

41. Das De S, McCreath SW. Lumbosacral fracture-dislocations: a report of four cases. J Bone Joint Surg Br 1981;63-B:58–60

42. Cantor JB, Lebwohl NH, Garvey T, et al. Nonoperative management of stable thoracolumbar burst fractures with early ambulation and bracing. Spine 1993;18:971–976

43. Chow GH, Nelson BJ, Gebhard JS, et al. Functional outcome of thoracolumbar burst fractures managed with hyperextension casting or bracing and early mobilization. Spine 1996;21:2170–2175

44. Ching RP, Watson NA, Carter JW, et al. The effect of post-injury spinal position on canal occlusion in a cervical spine burst fracture model. Spine 1997;22:1710–1715

45. Chance GQ. Note on a type of flexion fracture of the spine. Br J Radiol 1948;21:452–453

46. Gertzbein SD, Court-Brown CM. Flexion-distraction injuries of the lumbar spine: mechanisms of injury and classification. Clin Orthop Relat Res 1988;227:52–60

47. Rennie W, Mitchell N. Flexion distraction fractures of the thoracolumbar spine. J Bone Joint Surg Am 1973;55:386–390

48. Smith WS, Kaufer H. Patterns and mechanisms of lumbar injuries associated with lap seat belts. J Bone Joint Surg Am 1969;51:239–254

49. Bucholz RW, Gill K. Classification of injuries to the thoracolumbar spine. Orthop Clin North Am 1986;17:67–73

50. Whitesides TE Jr. Traumatic kyphosis of the thoracolumbar spine. Clin Orthop Relat Res 1977;78–92

51. Jonsson H Jr, Cesarini K, Sahlstedt B, et al. Findings and outcome in whiplash-type neck distortions. Spine 1994;19:2733–2743

52. Kaneoka K, Ono K, Inami S, et al. Motion analysis of cervical vertebrae during whiplash loading. Spine 1999;24:763–769 discussion 770

53. Panjabi MM, Cholewicki J, Nibu K, et al. Simulation of whiplash trauma using whole cervical spine specimens. Spine 1998;23:17–24

54. Panjabi MM, Cholewicki J, Nibu K, et al. Capsular ligament stretches during in vitro whiplash simulations. J Spinal Disord 1998;11:227–232

55. Pettersson K, Karrholm J, Toolanen G, et al. Decreased width of the spinal canal in patients with chronic symptoms after whiplash injury. Spine 1995;20:1664–1667

56. Winkelstein BA, Nightingale RW, Richardson WJ, et al. The cervical facet capsule and its role in whiplash injury: a biomechanical investigation. Spine 2000;25:1238–1246

57. Zabel DD, Tinkoff G, Wittenborn W, et al. Adequacy and efficacy of lateral cervical spine radiography in alert, high-risk blunt trauma patient. J Trauma 1997;43:952–956 discussion 957–958

58. Benzel EC, Hart BL, Ball PA, et al. Magnetic resonance imaging for the evaluation of patients with occult cervical spine injury. J Neurosurg 1996;85:824–829

59. Dickman CA, Mamourian A, Sonntag VK, et al. Magnetic resonance imaging of the transverse atlantal ligament for the evaluation of atlantoaxial instability. J Neurosurg 1991;75:221–227

60. Lee HM, Kim HS, Kim DJ, et al. Reliability of magnetic resonance imaging in detecting posterior ligament complex injury in thoracolumbar spinal fractures. Spine 2000;25:2079–2084

61. Weller SJ, Rossitch E Jr, Malek AM. Detection of vertebral artery injury after cervical spine trauma using magnetic resonance angiography. J Trauma 1999;46:660–666

62. Klein GR, Vaccaro AR, Albert TJ, et al. Efficacy of magnetic resonance imaging in the evaluation of posterior cervical spine fractures. Spine 1999;24:771–774

63. AO ASIF Principles in Spine Surgery. Berlin: Springer-Verlag, 1998

64. Freeman MD, Croft AC, Rossignol AM. "Whiplash associated disorders: redefining whiplash and its management" by the Quebec Task Force. A critical evaluation. Spine 1998;23:1043–1049

65. Borchgrevink GE, Kaasa A, McDonagh D, et al. Acute treatment of whiplash neck sprain injuries: a randomized trial of treatment during the first 14 days after a car accident. Spine 1998;23:25–31

66. Rosenfeld M, Gunnarsson R, Borenstein P. Early intervention in whiplash-associated disorders: a comparison of two treatment protocols. Spine 2000;25:1782–1787

67. Saifuddin A. MRI of acute spinal trauma. Skeletal Radiol 2001;30: 237–246

68. Louis R. Spinal stability as defined by the three-column spine concept. Anat Clin 1985;7:33–42

69. Magerl F, Aebi M, Gertzbein SD, et al. A comprehensive classification of thoracic and lumbar injuries. Eur Spine J 1994;3: 184–201

70. Oner FC, van Gils AP, Dhert WJ, et al. MRI findings of thoracolumbar spine fractures: a categorisation based on MRI examinations of 100 fractures. Skeletal Radiol 1999;28:433–443

71. Saifuddin A, Noordeen H, Taylor BA, et al. The role of imaging in the diagnosis and management of thoracolumbar burst fractures: current concepts and a review of the literature. Skeletal Radiol 1996;25:603–613

72. Vaccaro AR, Lehman RA Jr, Hurlbert RJ, et al. A new classification of thoracolumbar injuries: the importance of injury morphology, the integrity of the posterior ligamentous complex, and neurologic status. Spine 2005;30:2325–2333

73. Lee JY, Vaccaro AR, Lim MR, et al. Thoracolumbar injury classification and severity score: a new paradigm for the treatment of thoracolumbar spine trauma. J Orthop Sci 2005;10:671–675

74. Schmidek HH, Smith DA, Kristiansen TK. Sacral fractures. Neurosurgery 1984;15:735–746

75. Kayanja M, Tsai E, Takeuchi Y, et al. The biomechanics of insufficiency fractures and augmentation of the sacrum. Presented at the North American Spine Society, Seattle, Washington, 2006

76. Bents RT, France JC, Glover JM, et al. Traumatic spondylopelvic dissociation: a case report and literature review. Spine 1996;21: 1814–1819

III Management

7 Prehospital Management of Spinal Injuries

Paul Park and Kevin T. Foley

Spinal cord injury (SCI) is a devastating event. In addition to the significant morbidity associated with SCI, there is a high mortality rate. The most common causes of mortality are respiratory and cardiac-related illnesses, accounting for 28 and 23% of deaths, respectively.[1,2] Mortality is highest during the first year following injury and tends to decrease after the first year of survival. Young adults are most commonly afflicted with SCI. In the United States, the average age at injury was 28.7 years in the 1970s; however, the average age since the year 2000 has been 38.0 years, likely due to an aging population.[3] By far the most common cause of SCI is motor vehicle accidents.[3–6] Other causes include pedestrian trauma, falls, penetrating wounds, sports injuries, and industrial and agricultural accidents.[7] Recent data suggest that violence-related injuries have increased significantly, and violence is now the second most common cause after motor vehicle accidents. Cervical injuries represent 54% of all SCIs, and complete injuries are more common in the young (**Fig. 7.1**).[8] Men are also four times more likely to suffer SCI than women (**Table 7.1**).

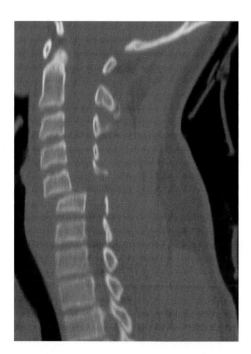

Fig. 7.1 Sagittal view of a reformatted computed tomography scan from a 15-year-old boy who sustained a C5-C6 fracture and a partial spinal cord injury in a diving accident.

In the individual with a spinal column injury without SCI or with partial SCI, the primary goal is to prevent development or progression of neurologic injury. In 1971, the emergency medical service (EMS) and the Spinal Cord Injury Model Systems (SCIMS) (**Table 7.2**) were established.[9] In relation to spinal injury, EMS was designed to save lives and prevent further neurologic injury after the initial traumatic event. The goal of the federally sponsored SCIMS was to provide comprehensive care for patients with SCI. Five components comprise the SCIMS: prevention, prehospital care, acute care, rehabilitation, and follow-up. Prehospital care consists of emergency care, including evaluation, resuscitation, immobilization, retrieval (extrication), and transport.[9,10] Since the 1970s, there has been a decrease in the number of patients with spinal injuries who present to the emergency department with complete SCI. This decrease has been attributed to EMS and the principles of prehospital care.[7,11]

■ Prehospital Management

In contrast to many European countries, emergency medical technician–ambulances (EMT-As), –paramedics (EMT-Ps), and, in certain instances, nurses, not physicians, provide the majority of prehospital medical care in the

Table 7.1 Spinal Cord Injury (SCI) Overview

- Respiratory-related illnesses account for 28% of SCI deaths[1,2]
- Cardiac-related illnesses account for 23% of SCI deaths[1,2]
- Mortality is highest during the first year following injury and tends to decrease after the first year of survival
- Most common cause of SCI is motor vehicle accidents
- Violence-related injuries have increased significantly, and violence is now the second most common cause after motor vehicle accidents[3–6]
- Average age of SCI since the year 2000 has been 38.0 years[3]
- Cervical injuries represent 54% of all SCIs, and complete injuries are more common in the young[8]
- Men are four times more likely to suffer SCI than women

Table 7.2 Spinal Cord Injury Model Systems (SCIMS)

- Five components comprise the SCIMS: prevention, prehospital care, acute care, rehabilitation, and follow-up

- Prehospital care consists of five phases: evaluation, resuscitation, immobilization, retrieval (extrication), and transport[9,10]

- Since 1970, there has been a decrease in the number of patients with complete SCI; this decrease has been attributed to EMS and the principles of prehospital care[7,11]

United States.[10,12] EMT-As are trained in basic life support, immobilization, and extrication techniques, whereas EMT-Ps are skilled in advanced cardiac life support, including neurologic assessment, intubation, defibrillation, and administration of intravenous medication.[7] These specially trained personnel are responsible for the five phases of prehospital management of SCI: (1) evaluation, (2) resuscitation, (3) immobilization, (4) extrication, and (5) transport.

Evaluation

In accordance with advanced trauma life support/advanced cardiac life support guidelines, the initial evaluation consists of a primary and then more thorough secondary survey.[11] The primary survey assesses the "ABCDEs": airway, breathing, circulation, disability (neurologic status), and exposure/environmental control.[13] Although ordered in sequence of importance, the ABCDEs of trauma are typically assessed and treated simultaneously. Initial evaluation should confirm airway patency. In the patient with an obstructed airway, the establishment of an airway should be made while protecting the cervical spine. It is important to note that a conscious patient with SCI may or

may not convey neck or back pain, and the unconscious patient is always assumed to have SCI. The assessment of breathing should include visual inspection, palpation, percussion, and auscultation of the chest for potential injuries (e.g., tension pneumothorax) that can impact ventilation. In evaluating the circulation, the level of consciousness, skin color, and pulse can assist in determining if the patient is hypovolemic. External bleeding is controlled with manual pressure. After the ABC of the ABCDEs have been assessed, a rapid neurologic assessment is performed (the D of ABCDE). Potential signs and symptoms of SCI include motor weakness/paralysis, sensory alterations, bowel/bladder incontinence, and tenderness to palpation along the spine.[7] Deformities of the spine or abrasions/lacerations over the spine are also associated with SCI. Typically performed in the emergency department, exposure and environmental control (the E of ABCDE) entail completely undressing the patient for a more thorough examination and prevention of hypothermia[13] (**Table 7.3**).

Resuscitation

Supplemental oxygen should be provided for any patient with suspected or confirmed SCI.[10] In the conscious patient with a patent airway, a cut-off standard airway or a tongue blade wrapped in tape can be used as a "bite-stick" to prevent gagging.[7] When an obstruction is present, establishment of a patent airway is critical. Any obvious foreign body should be removed. The chin lift and jaw thrust maneuver can help to open an airway, and a standard oral or nasopharyngeal airway can be used to maintain patency.[13,14] Because aggressive use of the chin lift and jaw thrust can exacerbate cervical instability, in-line stabilization should always be used in conjunction with these maneuvers. In addition, the nasopharyngeal airway appears to minimize the risk of exacerbating spinal instability as compared with the esophageal obturator or standard oral airway[14] (**Table 7.4**).

Table 7.3 Prehospital Management: Evaluation

- Nurses, not physicians, provide the majority of prehospital medical care in the United States[10,12]

- Emergency medical technician–ambulances (EMT-As) are trained in basic life support, immobilization, and extrication techniques[7]

- Emergency medical technician–paramedics (EMT-Ps) are skilled in advanced cardiac life support, including neurologic assessment, intubation, defibrillation, and administration of intravenous medication[7]

- The primary survey assesses the "ABCDE's": airway, breathing, circulation, disability (neurologic status), and exposure/environmental control[13]

- The conscious patient with SCI may or may not convey neck or back pain, and the unconscious patient is always assumed to have SCI

- Assessment of breathing should include visual inspection, palpation, percussion, and auscultation of the chest for potential injuries (e.g., tension pneumothorax) that can impact ventilation

- The level of consciousness, skin color, and pulse can assist in determining if the patient is hypovolemic

- Potential signs and symptoms of SCI include motor weakness/paralysis, sensory alterations, bowel/bladder incontinence, and tenderness to palpation along the spine[7]

Table 7.4 Prehospital Management: Resuscitation

- Supplemental oxygen should be provided for any patient with suspected or confirmed SCI

- Because aggressive use of the chin lift and jaw thrust can exacerbate cervical instability, in-line stabilization should always be used in conjunction with these maneuvers

- Nasopharyngeal airway appears to minimize the risk of exacerbating spinal instability as compared with the esophageal obturator or standard oral airway[14]

- If breathing is impaired with a patent airway, the patient requires intubation

- Cadaveric studies have shown that nasotracheal intubation can cause less motion to the unstable subaxial cervical spine than orotracheal intubation[14,15]

- Orotracheal intubation with in-line cervical stabilization also limits motion to the unstable cervical spine and appears to be a safe alternative[17,18]

- Nasotracheal intubation is strongly contraindicated in the apneic patient and is relatively contraindicated in the patient with significant facial or skull-base fractures[13]

- For C1-C2 injuries, both nasotracheal and orotracheal techniques can result in narrowing of the spinal canal during intubation[16]

- Cardiovascular stabilization not only is necessary for systemic health but also is important to prevent neurologic injury via ischemia and hypotension[11]

- In the prehospital setting, active hemorrhage should be treated with direct manual pressure and placement of a pressure dressing[7,10]

- Hypertonic saline has also been advocated as an alternative solution for volume resuscitation

If breathing is impaired with a patent airway, the patient should be intubated. Options include nasotracheal or orotracheal intubation. Nasotracheal intubation is absolutely contraindicated in the apneic patient and is relatively contraindicated in the patient with significant facial or skull-base fractures.[13] Cadaveric studies have shown that nasotracheal intubation can cause less motion to the unstable subaxial cervical spine than orotracheal intubation.[14,15] For C1-C2 injuries, however, both nasotracheal and orotracheal techniques can result in narrowing of the spinal canal during intubation.[16] As an alternative to blind nasotracheal intubation, which can be unreliable, studies have shown that orotracheal intubation with in-line cervical stabilization also limits motion to the unstable cervical spine and appears to be a safe alternative.[17,18]

Cardiovascular stabilization not only is crucial to the overall health of the patient but also helps to prevent progression of neurologic injury.[11] Ischemia related to vascular alterations ranging from systemic hypotension to changes in local autoregulation and spinal cord blood flow have been postulated to be secondary mechanisms of SCI after the primary insult.[19] In one clinical study, early volume resuscitation and elevation of the mean arterial blood pressure to greater than 85 mm Hg resulted in improvement in neurologic outcome after SCI.[20]

In the prehospital setting, active hemorrhage should be treated with direct manual pressure and placement of a pressure dressing.[7,10] Intravenous (IV) access is usually obtained, but if rapid transport to a definitive care facility is available, prolonged delay for placement of an IV may not be warranted.[11] Typically, however, at least one IV is

placed, and Ringer lactated solution is infused. Hypertonic saline has also been advocated as an alternative solution for volume resuscitation. However, a recent randomized trial of hypertonic saline versus Ringer lactate in patients with hypotension and traumatic brain injury found no difference in neurologic outcome.[21] If indicated, measures including defibrillation and administration of cardiogenic medication are instituted to reestablish a normal cardiac rate and rhythm.

Patients with SCI may develop hemorrhagic shock. In those with injury above T4, neurogenic shock as well as hemorrhagic shock or a combination of the two may occur. Low blood pressure and body temperature are present in either hemorrhagic or neurogenic shock. The distinguishing characteristic is the heart rate, which is typically bradycardic with neurogenic shock and tachycardic and irregular with hemorrhagic shock. In neurogenic shock, the loss of the sympathetic nervous system causes decreased peripheral vascular tone and ultimately results in decreased cardiac return of blood from the periphery. Bradycardia occurs due to the lack of sympathetic tone to the heart, which results in increased parasympathetic activity. Placement of the patient in the Trendelenburg position is helpful in either type of shock.[7,11] Fluid resuscitation is used to treat hemorrhagic shock, but care must be taken in the patient with neurogenic shock because the problem is not volume loss. Excessive volume resuscitation in cases of neurogenic shock can cause congestive heart failure.[11] Although their efficacy is unclear in neurogenic shock, military antishock trousers may also be used.[10] As a temporizing measure, 0.4 mg of atropine or dopamine may be

Table 7.5 Spinal Cord Injury Shock

- Patients with SCI may develop hemorrhagic shock

- For injuries above T4, neurogenic shock, hemorrhagic shock, or a combination of the two may occur; low blood pressure and body temperature are present in either hemorrhagic or neurogenic shock

- The distinguishing characteristic is the heart rate, which is typically bradycardic with neurogenic shock and tachycardic and irregular with hemorrhagic shock

- Excessive volume resuscitation in cases of neurogenic shock can cause congestive heart failure[11]

- Although their efficacy is unclear in neurogenic shock, military antishock trousers may also be used[10]

administered in cases of neurogenic shock until the patient is transported for definitive care[7] (**Table 7.5**).

Immobilization

In the patient with a suspected or known SCI, the chief concern is to prevent further neurologic impairment from an unstable spine. Because as many as 20% of SCIs involve multiple levels, the entire spine requires immobilization.[11] The best method for immobilization is the rigid, straight board in conjunction with a cervical stabilization device.[7] The use of a semirigid cervical collar and bilateral sandbags joined with tape across the forehead attached to a board has been shown to be most effective in limiting motion compared with the soft collar, hard collar, extrication collar, semirigid (Philadelphia) collar, or bilateral sandbags and tape alone.[22] Sandbags, however, are difficult and impractical to use. Therefore, the use of a rigid cervical collar with some type of bilateral bolstering device alongside the head and neck with the patient secured to a rigid board appears to be the best alternative.[13,23]

Although it has become standard practice to immobilize all patients having a potential mechanism for SCI, immobilization in a cervical collar while strapped to a rigid board is not without adverse effects. Patient discomfort can be significant, and pressure sores can develop.[24] Pulmonary function can also be significantly restricted.[25,26] Selective

spinal immobilization, as a consequence, has been advocated. Specifically, it has been proposed that immobilization should be reserved for those patients having a potential mechanism for SCI and with specific prehospital findings of altered mental status, neurologic deficit, spinal pain, intoxication, or distracting injury (e.g., extremity fracture).[27] In a retrospective study of 331 patients, each of these prehospital findings was associated with a significant cervical spinal injury.[28] A subsequent prospective study using these criteria found 94.9% sensitivity and 35.0% specificity for a finding of spinal injury. The positive predictive value was only 4.7%; however, the negative predictive value was 99.5%.[29] Although these findings suggest that a patient can be cleared clinically in the prehospital setting, further research is needed prior to universal acceptance of this practice (**Table 7.6**).

Extrication

Multiple factors can impact extrication, including accessibility to the patient, the local environment, and the condition of the patient.[10] In general, EMT-As, EMT-Ps, and firefighters are specially trained in extrication techniques. Given the variability of the trauma scene, a common-sense approach has been advocated. Manual stabilization of the head and neck in the neutral position is recommended during extrication rather than use of a cervical collar. Movement of the patient to a neutral supine position

Table 7.6 Prehospital Management: Immobilization

- Chief concern is to prevent further neurologic injury from an unstable spine

- Twenty percent of SCIs involve multiple levels, the entire spine requires immobilization[11]

- Best method for immobilization is the rigid, straight board in conjunction with a cervical stabilization device[7]

- Adverse effects associated with proper immobilization include patient discomfort and the development of pressure sores[24]

- Pulmonary function can also be significantly restricted[25,26]

- To minimize adverse effects, it has been proposed that spinal immobilization be reserved for patients with a potential mechanism for SCI in addition to specific prehospital findings of altered mental status, neurologic deficit, spinal pain, intoxication, or distracting injury (i.e., extremity fracture)[27]

Table 7.7 Prehospital Management: Extrication

- Multiple factors can impact extrication, including accessibility to the patient, the local environment, and the condition of the patient[10]

- Manual stabilization of the head and neck in the neutral position is recommended during extrication rather than use of a cervical collar

- Movement of the patient to a neutral supine position rapidly and safely achieves the goal of a successful extrication[7]

- Selection of the most appropriate transport is dependent on the patient's condition, availability, geography, and distance[30,31]

rapidly and safely achieves the goal of a successful extrication[7] (**Table 7.7**).

Transport

Once the SCI patient is stabilized, early transfer to a specialized SCI center results in decreased complications and better neurologic outcomes.[9,30,31] Modes of transportation include ambulance, helicopter, or fixed wing aircraft. Selection of the most appropriate transport is dependent on the patient's condition, availability, geography, and distance.[30,31]

■ Conclusion

Prehospital management of SCI consists of five phases, each designed to prevent neurologic progression of SCI and optimize recovery. The recent decline in the number of emergency department patients presenting with complete SCI is likely the result of the establishment of EMS combined with implementation of the principles of prehospital management for SCI.

References

1. Weaver FM, Smith B, Evans C, et al. Outcomes of outpatients visits for acute respiratory illness in veterans with spinal cord injuries and disorders. Am J Phys Med Rehabil 2006;85:718–726
2. DeVivo MJ, Krause JS, Lammertse DP. Recent trends in mortality and causes of death among persons with spinal cord injury. Arch Phys Med Rehabil 1999;80:1411–1419
3. Spinal Cord Injury. Facts and Figures at a Glance. National Spinal Cord Injury Statistical Center, The University of Alabama at Birmingham. June 2006. http://www.spinalcord.uab.edu/show.asp?durki=21446
4. Donovan WH, Kopaniky D, Stolzmann E, Carter RE. The neurological and skeletal outcome in patients with closed cervical spinal cord injury. J Neurosurg 1987;66:690–694
5. Prasad VS, Schwartz A, Bhutani R, Sharkey PW, Schwartz ML. Characteristics of injuries to the cervical spine and spinal cord in polytrauma patient population: experience from a regional trauma unit. Spinal Cord 1999;37:560–568
6. Surkin J, Gilbert BJ, Harkey HL III, Sniezek J, Currier M. Spinal cord injury in Mississippi: findings and evaluation, 1992–1994. Spine 2000;25:716–721
7. Green BA, Eismont FJ, O'Heir JT. Spinal cord injury–a systems approach: prevention, emergency medical services, and emergency room management. Crit Care Clin 1987;3:471–493
8. Nobunaga AI, Go BK, Karunas RB. Recent demographic and injury trends in people served by the Model Spinal Cord Injury Care Systems. Arch Phys Med Rehabil 1999;80:1372–1382
9. Waters RL, Meyer PR Jr, Adkins RH, Felton D. Emergency, acute, and surgical management of spine trauma. Arch Phys Med Rehabil 1999;80:1383–1390
10. Soderstrom CA, Brumback RJ. Early care of the patient with cervical spine injury. Orthop Clin North Am 1986;17:3–13
11. Dyson-Hudson TA, Stein AB. Acute management of traumatic cervical spinal cord injuries. Mt Sinai J Med 1999;66:170–178
12. Benitez FL, Pepe PE. Role of the physician in prehospital management of trauma: North American perspective. Curr Opin Crit Care 2002;8:551–558

13. American College of Surgeons Committee on Trauma. Advanced Trauma Life Support Program for Doctors. 6th ed. Chicago: ACSC; 1997
14. Aprahamian C, Thompson BM, Finger WA, Darin JC. Experimental cervical spine injury model: evaluation of airway management and splinting techniques. Ann Emerg Med 1984;13:584–587
15. Donaldson WR, Towers JD, Doctor A, Brand A, Donaldson VP. A methodology to evaluate motion of the unstable spine during intubation techniques. Spine 1993;18:2020–2023
16. Donaldson WR, Heil BV, Donaldson VP, Silvaggio VJ. The effect of airway maneuvers on the unstable C1–C2 segment: a cadaver study. Spine 1997;22:1215–1218
17. Holley J, Jorden R. Airway management in patients with unstable cervical spine fractures. Ann Emerg Med 1989;18:1237–1239
18. Majernick TG, Bieniek R, Houston JB, Hughes HG. Cervical spine movement during orotracheal intubation. Ann Emerg Med 1986; 15:417–420
19. Sekhon LH, Fehlings MG. Epidemiology, demographics, and pathophysiology of acute spinal cord injury. Spine 2001;26(suppl): S2–S12
20. Vale FL, Burns J, Jackson AB, Hadley MN. Combined medical and surgical treatment after acute spinal cord injury: results of a prospective pilot study to assess the merits of aggressive medical resuscitation and blood pressure management. J Neurosurg 1997;87:239–246
21. Cooper DJ, Myles P, McDermott F, et al. Prehospital hypertonic saline resuscitation of patients with hypotension and severe traumatic brain injury: a randomized controlled trial. JAMA 2004;291:1350–1357
22. Podolsky S, Baraff LJ, Simon RR, Hoffman JR, Larmon B, Ablon W. Efficacy of cervical spine immobilization methods. J Trauma 1983;23:461–465
23. Hadley MN, Walters BC, Grabb PA, et al. Cervical spine immobilization before admission to the hospital. Neurosurgery 2002; 50(suppl):S7–S17

24. Cordell WH, Hollingsworth JC, Olinger ML, Stroman SJ, Nelson DR. Pain and tissue-interface pressures during spine-board immobilization. Ann Emerg Med 1995;26:31–36

25. Bauer D, Kowalski R. Effect of spinal immobilization devices on pulmonary function in the healthy, nonsmoking man. Ann Emerg Med 1988;17:915–918

26. Schafermeyer RW, Ribbeck BM, Gaskins J, Thomason S, Harlan M, Attkisson A. Respiratory effects of spinal immobilization in children. Ann Emerg Med 1991;20:1017–1019

27. Domeier RM. Indications for prehospital spinal immobilization. National Association of EMS Physicians Standards and Clinical Practice Committee. Prehosp Emerg Care 1999;3:251–253

28. Domeier RM, Evans RW, Swor RA, Rivera-Rivera EJ, Frederiksen SM. Prehospital clinical findings associated with spinal injury. Prehosp Emerg Care 1997;1:11–15

29. Domeier RM, Swor R, Evans R, et al. Multicenter prospective validation of prehospital clinical spinal clearance criteria. J Trauma 2002;53:744–750

30. Hadley MN, Walters BC, Grabb PA, et al. Transportation of patients with acute traumatic cervical spine injuries. Neurosurgery 2002; 50(suppl):S18–S20

31. Hachen HJ. Emergency transportation in the event of acute spinal cord lesion. Paraplegia 1974;12:33–37

8 Timing of Surgery for Spinal Injuries

Gordon K. T. Chu and Michael G. Fehlings

A 24-year-old man was admitted to our institution following a blunt assault. On admission, the patient had complete injury at the C6 level. He had an admission American Spinal Injury Association (ASIA) grade of A, and he sustained no other injuries. His admission computed tomography (CT) and magnetic resonance imaging (MRI) are shown in **Figs. 8.1** and **8.2**. The MRI showed no evidence of disk herniation. He was then taken to the operating room for a closed reduction under fluoroscopic guidance followed by posterior fixation. This was achieved between 12 and 24 hours after arrival. A repeat MRI revealed some continued cord compression secondary to a disrupted disk (**Fig. 8.3**), and the patient underwent an anterior diskectomy and fusion the following day.

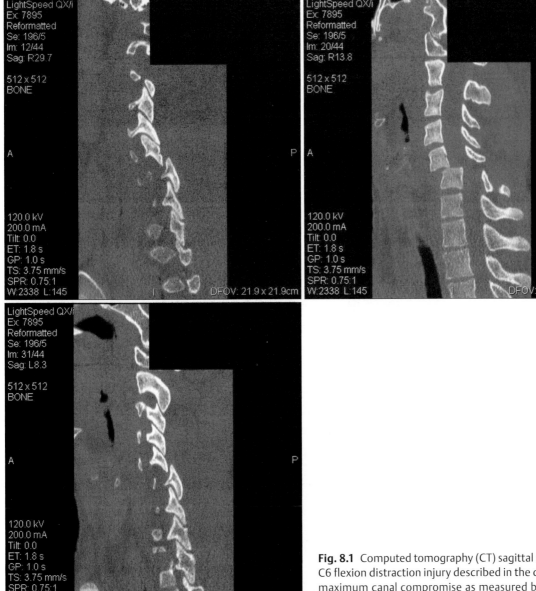

Fig. 8.1 Computed tomography (CT) sagittal reconstruction of the C5-C6 flexion distraction injury described in the case study. There is a 60% maximum canal compromise as measured by both CT and magnetic resonance imaging (MRI).[1,2]

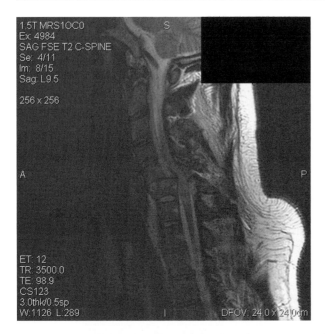

Fig. 8.2 T2-weighted MRI with sagittal image. There is increased signal in the spinal cord at the C5-C6 level, indicative of possible hematoma formation. There is no disk herniation noted.

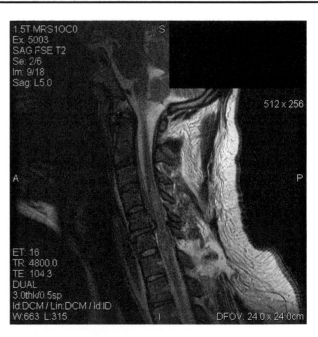

Fig. 8.3 T2-weighted MRI after reduction and posterior fixation. There is some continued cord compression from a disrupted disk, which necessitated an anterior diskectomy.

Although a major effort was made to intervene urgently, the extent of the trauma resulted in some continued cord compression that was not completely resolved until at least 48 hours after injury (**Fig. 8.4**). Twelve months later, his ASIA grade had improved to B. This case illustrates one of the most important unresolved questions in the operative management of spinal cord injuries (SCIs), namely, the timing of surgery to decompress the spinal cord.

A

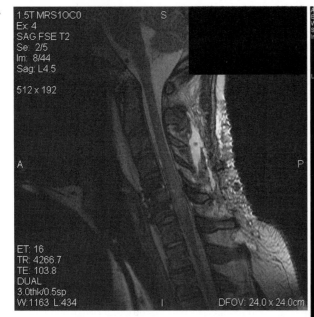

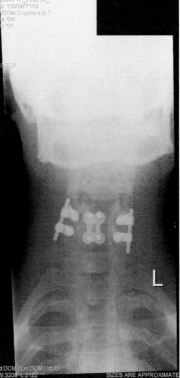

B

Fig. 8.4 (A) T2-weighted MRI midsagittal image and **(B)** the final construct of the patient after decompression and stabilization approximately 1 week after the injury. There is a high-intensity signal at the C6 level, indicative of ongoing edema and early cystic changes.

Table 8.1 Spinal Cord Injury Characteristics

Treatment	Currently no adequate treatment to restore function
Cases	> 12,000 per year in North America
Affected individuals	300,000 live with SCI (many being young or middle-aged)
Costs	• > $7 billion in 1995
	• Increased life span = increased cost of care

Table 8.2 Treatment Data

Class of Evidence	Type of Study
I	Randomized controlled clinical trial
II	Prospective, nonrandomized study
III	Retrospective study, case series, expert opinion

Would earlier intervention in this case (i.e., less than 24 hours after injury or sooner) have resulted in increased recovery? Despite advancements in imaging, critical care, operative technique, and instrumentation, it is still unknown if there is an advantage to early decompression of the spinal cord and what the time window is after injury for decompression to have the maximal benefit. This chapter discusses the controversy surrounding this topic and examines the latest data on the subject.

Spinal cord injury has been acknowledged as a severe injury since ancient Egyptian times, yet there is still no adequate treatment to restore function. Every year in North America, there are over 12,000 cases of SCI. Currently, close to 300,000 people live with SCI, of which many are still young or middle-aged.[3–5] The costs directly associated with SCI was in excess of $7 billion in 1995. With improving medical and surgical techniques, the life span of SCI patients will lengthen; therefore, the costs related to their ongoing care can only increase (**Table 8.1**).[6] It is imperative that we in the medical community find a way to change the limited prognosis of these patients.

There is currently no definitive standard for the surgical and medical management of SCI. This is due to an incomplete understanding of the pathophysiology underlying SCI[5,7,8] and a scarcity of class I data (**Table 8.2**)

with regard to treatment. Careful scientific studies of SCI have categorized the injury as primary or secondary (**Table 8.3**). The primary injury mechanism consists of a physical deformation and destruction of spinal cord tissue at the time of injury. It is not amenable to treatment. The primary injury triggers a secondary cascade of events, resulting in continued destruction of the spinal cord; this cascade is known as the secondary injury. Secondary injury resulting in further deterioration of the spinal cord is due to (1) vascular abnormalities, (2) biochemical and electrolyte shifts, and (3) cellular and molecular changes. There is ischemia, loss of autoregulation, and hemorrhage after SCI, as well as calcium and sodium influx and increased extracellular concentration of potassium and excitatory neurotransmitters, such as glutamate, serotonin, and catecholamines. Cellular and molecular changes include infiltration of inflammatory cells, loss of mitochondrial potential, and activation of caspase proteins leading to forms of programmed cell death, including apoptosis. These secondary events can occur from seconds to days to possibly weeks after the primary injury and therefore would afford physicians a chance to intervene and perhaps improve recovery.

The National Acute Spinal Cord Injury Study (NASCIS) II and III showed that methylprednisolone therapy may improve the neurologic outcome modestly if started within 8 hours of injury (**Table 8.4**).[9,10] NASCIS III suggests that treatment started within 3 hours of injury need only be for 24 hours, as opposed to 48 hours when started

Table 8.3 Spinal Cord Injury Categorized

Primary (immediate)	• Defined: physical deformation and destruction of cord tissue at the time of injury
	• Not amenable to treatment
	• Triggers cascade of events resulting in progressive destruction of cord (secondary injury)
Secondary (days to weeks)	Further deterioration of spinal cord, due to
	1. Vascular abnormalities: ischemia, loss of autoregulation, and hemorrhage
	2. Biochemical and electrolyte shifts: calcium and sodium influx, increased extracellular concentration of potassium, and increased concentration of excitatory neurotransmitters, such as glutamate, serotonin, and catecholamines
	3. Cellular and molecular changes: infiltration of inflammatory cells, loss of mitochondrial potential, caspase activation resulting in apoptosis

Table 8.4 Methylprednisolone Therapy in Improving Neurologic Outcomes

NASCIS	National Acute Spinal Cord Injury Study
NASCIS II and III[9,10]	• Showed methylprednisolone therapy may modestly improve neurologic outcomes if given within 8 hours of injury
	• If given within 3 hours of injury, the duration of treatment required is 24 hours
	• If given after 3 hours but within 8 hours of injury, the duration of treatment required is 48 hours
Treatment effects	• Halt several of the secondary injuries seen in SCI
	• Remain controversial

later than 3 hours and up to 8 hours after injury. Treatment with methylprednisolone is aimed at arresting several of the above-mentioned mechanisms. This treatment remains controversial due to the analysis of the data from these randomized trials. One important aspect to these studies is that they are the very first randomized controlled trials to imply a potential therapeutic time window for SCI. This partly validates the secondary injury hypothesis. However, this concept of a therapeutic time window not only is attractive for medical therapies but may also apply to surgical treatment.[11–15]

■ The Role of Nonsurgical Management Alone in Spinal Cord Injury (Table 8.5)

The uniformly poor outcomes of SCI have led physicians and surgeons universally to have a fatalistic approach to the treatment of these patients. Patients with SCI secondary to burst fractures and dislocations were routinely untreated surgically in the past. This belief was strengthened by studies demonstrating poorer outcomes in patients whose

spinal cords were decompressed with laminectomies and higher complication rates, including neurologic injury following surgery.[16–19] Therefore, to justify surgical intervention at all in these patients, the outcomes of nonoperative treatment must be carefully assessed. Class I evidence (**Table 8.2**) comparing outcomes of operative versus nonoperative patients is lacking. There is only class III evidence from retrospective studies in which to analyze outcomes. Frankel et al,[20] in their study of 612 conservatively managed patients, found that 29% of the Frankel A grade patients improved at least one neurologic grade. Instability was noted in only four patients. Others have also shown neurologic improvement with conservative management. In contrast, Katoh et al[21] demonstrated that 10% of patients with incomplete cervical cord injury deteriorated with nonsurgical treatment. A prospective nonrandomized case-controlled study of 208 patients by Tator et al[22] showed that surgery resulted in a lower mortality than conservative management despite an increased incidence of thromboembolic events. However, no difference in neurologic recovery between the groups could be determined, and the issue of timing of surgery was not examined. Given the absence of class I evidence, nonoperative management cannot be excluded as a valid treatment option, especially

Table 8.5 Nonoperative Approach to Spinal Cord Injury

History	• Poor outcomes of SCI led physicians to take fatalistic approach to SCI patients	
	• Approach supported by studies showing poorer outcomes in surgical approach to SCI	
Contradictory studies	Frankel et al[20]	29% of 612 nonoperative patients improved one neurologic grade
	Katoh et al[21]	10% of patients deteriorated in nonoperative approach
	Tator et al[22]	• In 208 patients, surgery lowered mortality but increased thromboembolic events
		• No difference in neurologic recovery discerned
Future approach	• Nonoperative treatment cannot be excluded	
	• Advances in neuroanesthesia, critical care, instrumentation, and surgical technique allowing spinal stabilization have led many spinal surgeons to take the surgical approach with minimal morbidity, compared with in the past	
	• For those with central cord syndrome, nonoperative approach may still be considered but is no longer the preferred treatment option	

for medically unstable patients. However, it is the opinion of most spinal surgeons that advances in neuroanesthesia, critical care, instrumentation, and surgical technique have allowed spinal stabilizations and not just laminectomies to be performed safely with minimal morbidity when compared with how they were performed in the past. These stabilization procedures enable earlier mobilization and easier respiratory care for the patient. Nonoperative management may still be warranted for patients with central cord syndrome; however, nonoperative treatment of SCI is no longer the preferred treatment option.[23]

■ Experimental Studies of Early Decompression (Table 8.6)

Early surgery following SCI has been shown to be of benefit in animal models.[24–27] Dimar et al,[27] using a rat model of SCI whereby the cord was injured with a weight drop and subsequent compression maintained by epidural spacers, demonstrated that minimizing the time of compression results in improved recovery. They had compressed the cord for 0, 2, 6, 24, and 72 hours after the weight drop and assessed hind limb recovery over a 6-week period. The functional recovery was better the shorter the time of compression throughout the 6-week period. Using a dog model, Carlson et al[26] concluded that greater neurologic improvement occurred with earlier decompression. They used a hydraulic piston to produce spinal cord compression for 30 or 180 minutes. Following the compression, somatosensory evoked potentials and motor tests were conducted for 28 days. The dogs with the shorter period of compression were able to recover the evoked potentials within 1 hour following decompression compared with no recovery in the 180-minute group. The motor recovery

was also much improved in the early decompression group. Two weeks after the injury, the 30-minute compression group had significantly better results with balance, cadence, stair climbing, and climbing an inclined plane. Furthermore, histologic evaluation of the spinal cords revealed that increased compression time resulted in increased lesion volumes of the spinal cords.

■ Clinical Studies of Early Decompression in Spinal Cord Injury (Table 8.7)

Though animal data have shown the potential for early decompression, human trials have yet to show a definitive answer. There is no class I evidence demonstrating a superior outcome with early decompression. In fact, there have been no class I studies at all with respect to this issue. This is due to a variety of factors; chief among them is the pervasive belief of many surgeons that recovery after SCI cannot be improved. This belief stems from past studies that demonstrated surgery's worsened outcome (as described earlier in this chapter). Pollard et al,[28] in a retrospective review of 412 patients with traumatic, incomplete cervical SCIs with an average follow-up time of 2 years, concluded that the most important prognostic factor for improved recovery was the completeness of the original injury. They also found that younger patients with incomplete injury or either a central cord or Brown-Séquard syndrome had a favorable prognosis. However, they did not find any data to support early surgical intervention or high-dose steroid administration.

The controversy surrounding methylprednisolone administration and the general lack of dramatic effect from other medical therapies may also have added to this

Table 8.6 Experimental Decompression Studies

Dimar et al[27] (rat model)	• Minimizing compression time results in improved recovery
	• Compressed cord for 0, 2, 6, 24, and 72 hours; hind limb recovery was then assessed over a 6-week period
	• Results: better functional recovery in group with shorter compression time
Carlson et al[26] (dog model)	• Showed greater neurologic improvement with early decompression
	• Compressed cord for 30 or 180 minutes
	• Results:
	• Somatosensory and motor tests done showed dogs with shorter decompression were able to recover evoked potentials and motor function within 1 hour, whereas those with 180-minute decompression showed no recovery
	• 2 weeks postinjury: 30-minute decompression group showed better balance, cadence, stair climbing, and climbing inclined plane
	• Histologically: increased compression time = increased spinal cord lesion volumes

Table 8.7 Early Decompression Clinical Studies

Class I studies	• Yet to be done, mainly because of pervasive opinion of surgeons that recovery after SCI cannot be improved	
	• There is no agreement as to what constitutes early decompression	
Class II studies	Some have shown feasibility of early decompression[31,32]	
	Ng et al[31]	Surgical decompression within 8 hours was feasible in 8% without increased complications
	Papadopoulos et al[32]	Patients with closed reduction within 6 hours had better results than open reduction within 12 hours, but with increased risk in closed reduction (8.1% of 585 closed reduction cases showed worsening neurologic functions)
	Pointillant et al[35]	No outcome difference in patients operated within 8 hours versus > 8 hours
	Vaccaro et al[34]	No difference in neurologic outcomes in early (< 72 hours) versus delayed (75 days) decompression

overall poor attitude regarding recovery from SCI. NASCIS has numerous detractors and the GM1 ganglioside (Sygen) study, despite showing promising initial results, ultimately did not show a significant improvement over methylprednisolone.[29,30] There is also no agreement as to what constitutes early decompression in humans. Is the time window 8 hours, as it is with methylprednisolone therapy, or is it 12 hours, or is it earlier? This concept of what constitutes early decompression is controversial. It is uncertain whether any animal studies can be directly translatable, given that clinical SCI is so varied with respect to mechanisms and force when compared with experimental models. Several class II studies have shown the feasibility of early decompression.[31,32] Using less than 25 hours as the definition of early surgery and drawing from the NASCIS II database, Duh et al[33] concluded that early decompression was beneficial compared with nonsurgical management, although there was no statistical significance. They also noted that surgery after 200 hours (delayed) may also improve outcomes. Another study on 91 patients with cervical SCI demonstrated that a greater percentage of patients with early surgery (< 10 hours) had better neurologic recovery than the control group.[32] However, this was a prospective nonrandomized trial, though the authors did demonstrate the achievability of early surgery, as all but one patient underwent surgery within 9 hours of arrival at the hospital. In contrast, Vaccaro et al[34] reported in a prospective, randomized clinical trial that early decompression (< 72 hours) resulted in no difference in neurologic outcome compared with delayed surgery (> 5 days). However, there are two main criticisms with this study. First, nearly one third of the patients were lost to follow-up. Second, the authors defined early surgery as < 72 hours, but it has been argued that 72 hours is too long a delay to constitute early decompression. Given these reasons, this study should be considered class II evidence.

Another prospective nonrandomized study conducted by Pointillart et al[35] could not find a difference in outcomes for patients operated within 8 hours and for those operated after 8 hours. The study had 106 patients, 49 of whom were operated early. The intent of that study, however, was to examine differences between methylprednisolone, nimodipine, and no medical treatment but not early surgery. In a retrospective study, Aebi et al[36] reported that 75% of patients who recovered from SCI were reduced by closed or open reduction within 6 hours.

Papadopoulos et al[30] noted that patients with closed reduction (within 6 hours) had better results than open reduction within 12 hours. However, closed reduction is not without risks, as there was worsening of neurologic function in 8.1% of 585 cases of closed reduction.[15]

La Rosa et al[37] reviewed studies from 1966 to 2000 that focused on early versus late decompression (**Table 8.8**). The goal of the study was to draw definitive conclusions regarding neurologic recovery from early surgical decompression (within 24 hours), as opposed to late surgery or no surgery, in patients after a traumatic SCI. If there was

Table 8.8 Larosa et al[37] (1966–2000)

Study	Early vs late decompression
Goal	Draw definitive conclusions on neurologic recovery from
	• Early surgical decompression (< 24 hours)
	• Late surgical decompression (≥ 24 hours)
	• Conservative approach (no surgery)
Conclusions	1. Statistically, patients with early surgery showed better recovery
	2. Due to heterogeneous nature of study, only results from patients with incomplete neurologic deficits were reliable; thus, no definitive recommendations regarding early surgery could be made

Table 8.9 Evidence for the Timing of Surgery

Level of Recommendation	Class of Evidence	Details
Standards	I	There are no standards regarding the role and timing of decompression in acute SCI
Guidelines	II	• Early surgery (< 72 hours) can be done safely in patients with SCI if they are hemodynamically optimized
		• There are data to support a recommendation for urgent reduction of bilateral locked facets in a patient with incomplete tetraplegia
		• There are data to support a recommendation for urgent decompression in a patient with SCI experiencing neurologic deterioration
Options	III	• Decompression is a reasonable practice option in acute cervical SCI; when possible (excluding patients with life-threatening multisystem trauma) it is recommended that urgent decompression be performed within 24 hours of SCI
		• There is class III evidence that early (< 24 hours) surgery reduces length of stay in patients with acute SCI and may reduce postinjury medical complications

Source: Modified from Fehlings MG, Perrin R. The timing of surgical intervention in the management of spinal cord injury: a systematic review of recent clinical evidence. Spine 2006;31(suppl):S28–35.

an effect with early decompression, the authors also wished to quantify it. There was a total number of 1687 patients who were categorized into early (within 24 hours), late (more than 24 hours), and conservative (no surgery) groups. The authors concluded statistically that patients who had early surgery had better recovery than those who had late surgery. However, due to the heterogeneous nature of the studies that were reviewed, only results from patients with incomplete neurologic deficits would be reliable. Therefore, the authors could not make definitive recommendations regarding early surgery.

Curiously, class III evidence comes mainly from retrospective studies, which have also reported that late decompression may be beneficial.[38] Duh et al[33] had noted a similar finding. In contrast, Waters et al[39] reported that delayed surgery (more than 14 days) did not improve outcome. However, delayed surgery continues to be practiced for fear of the increased morbidity from early surgery that has been reported by various authors.[33,40–43]

Though class I data are lacking for early surgery in many types of traumatic SCI, there is sufficient evidence to support a recommendation of early reduction of bilateral locked facets in patients with incomplete injury. A study of 76 patients, half of whom were admitted under 8 hours, showed that early reduction improved outcomes in patients with incomplete SCI.[44] Other studies with class II evidence have also had similar findings.

The evidence for early reduction of bilateral facet dislocations, notwithstanding the evidence that early surgery increases recovery from traumatic SCI, is still unsubstantiated. At present, the University of Toronto and Thomas Jefferson University, in conjunction with the Spine Trauma Study Group, are collaborating on a multicenter, prospective trial to resolve this issue. The Surgical Timing in Acute Spinal Cord Injury Study (STASCIS) trial requires 450 patients and is currently open for enrollment.

■ Conclusion

Animal studies demonstrate that traumatic SCI results in tissue damage that persists and increases with time following the initial injury. This prolonged destruction of spinal cord tissue leaves open the possibility that a time window exists in which treatments given in a delayed fashion may rescue the tissue and improve the outcome. This may explain why treatments such as methylprednisolone can have some effect on outcome. Accordingly, this may be extrapolated to include surgical therapy. Animal studies have shown that early decompression can have similar results. Whether these results from experimental laboratories can be directly translated to clinical practice remains to be determined. It is clear that early surgery is feasible and can be performed safely. However, most evidence for early decompression remains class III, so at this time it can only be considered as a surgical option and not a standard of care (**Table 8.9**).

References

1. Fehlings MG, Furlan JC, Massicotte EM, et al. Interobserver and intraobserver reliability of maximum canal compromise and spinal cord compression for evaluation of acute traumatic cervical spinal cord injury. Spine 2006;31:1719–1725

2. Fehlings MG, Rao SC, Tator CH, et al. The optimal radiologic method for assessing spinal canal compromise and cord compression in patients with cervical spinal cord injury: 2. Results of a multicenter study. Spine 1999;24:605–613

3. Sekhon LH, Fehlings MG. Epidemiology, demographics, and pathophysiology of acute spinal cord injury. Spine 2001;26(suppl): S2–S12

4. Tator CH, Duncan EG, Edmonds VE, Lapczak LI, Andrews DF. Neurological recovery, mortality and length of stay after acute spinal cord injury associated with changes in management. Paraplegia 1995;33:254–262

5. Tator CH, Fehlings MG. Review of the secondary injury theory of acute spinal cord trauma with emphasis on vascular mechanisms. J Neurosurg 1991;75:15–26

6. Povlishock JT, Christman CW. The pathobiology of traumatically induced axonal injury in animals and humans: a review of current thoughts. J Neurotrauma 1995;12:555–564

7. Bracken MB, Shepard MJ, Collins WF, et al. A randomized, controlled trial of methylprednisolone or naloxone in the treatment of acute spinal-cord injury: results of the Second National Acute Spinal Cord Injury Study. N Engl J Med 1990;322:1405–1411

8. Bracken MB, Shepard MJ, Holford TR, et al. Administration of methylprednisolone for 24 or 48 hours or tirilazad mesylate for 48 hours in the treatment of acute spinal cord injury: results of the Third National Acute Spinal Cord Injury Randomized Controlled Trial. JAMA 1997;277:1597–1604

9. Fehlings MG, Perrin RG. The timing of surgical intervention in the management of spinal cord injury: a systematic review of recent clinical evidence. Spine 2006;31(suppl):S28–S36

10. Fehlings MG, Perrin RG. The role and timing of early decompression for cervical spinal cord injury: update with a review of recent clinical evidence. Injury 2005;36(suppl 2):B13–B26

11. Fehlings MG, Sekhon LH, Tator C. The role and timing of decompression in acute spinal cord injury: what do we know? What should we do? Spine 2001;26(suppl):S101–S110

12. Fehlings MG, Tator CH. An evidence-based review of decompressive surgery in acute spinal cord injury: rationale, indications, and timing based on experimental and clinical studies. J Neurosurg 1999;91(suppl):1–11

13. Tator CH, Fehlings MG, Thorpe K, et al. Current use and timing of spinal surgery for management of acute spinal surgery for management of acute spinal cord injury in North America: results of a retrospective multicenter study. J Neurosurg 1999; 91(suppl):12–18

14. Bedbrook GM. Spinal injuries with tetraplegia and paraplegia. J Bone Joint Surg Br 1979;61-B:267–284

15. Collins WF. A review and update of experiment and clinical studies of spinal cord injury. Paraplegia 1983;21:204–219

16. Bedbrook GM, Sedgley GI. The management of spinal injuries–past and present. Int Rehabil Med 1980;2:45–61

17. Bedbrook GM, Sakae T. A review of cervical spine injuries with neurological dysfunction. Paraplegia 1982;20:321–333

18. Frankel HL, Hancock DO, Hyslop G, et al. The value of postural reduction in the initial management of closed injuries of the spine with paraplegia and tetraplegia. Paraplegia 1969;7: 179–192

19. Katoh S, el Masry WS, Jaffray D, et al. Neurologic outcome in conservatively treated patients with incomplete closed traumatic cervical spinal cord injuries. Spine 1996;21:2345–2351

20. Tator CH, Duncan EG, Edmonds VE, Lapczak LI, Andrews DF. Comparison of surgical and conservative management in 208 patients with acute spinal cord injury. Can J Neurol Sci 1987;14:60–69

21. Yamazaki T, Yanaka K, Fujita K, Kamezaki T, Uemura K, Nose T. Traumatic central cord syndrome: analysis of factors affecting the outcome. Surg Neurol 2005;63:95–99

22. Kobrine AI, Evans DE, Rizzoli HV. Experimental acute balloon compression of the spinal cord: factors affecting disappearance and return of the spinal evoked response. J Neurosurg 1979;51:841–845

23. Brodkey JS, Richards DE, Blasingame JP, Nulsen FE. Reversible spinal cord trauma in cats: additive effects of direct pressure and ischemia. J Neurosurg 1972;37:591–593

24. Carlson GD, Gorden CD, Oliff HS, Pillai JJ, LaManna JC. Sustained spinal cord compression: 1. time-dependent effect on long-term pathophysiology. J Bone Joint Surg Am 2003;85-A:86–94

25. Dimar JR II, Glassman SD, Raque GH, Zhang YP, Shields CB. The influence of spinal canal narrowing and timing of decompression on neurologic recovery after spinal cord contusion in a rat model. Spine 1999;24:1623–1633

26. Pollard ME, Apple DF. Factors associated with improved neurologic outcomes in patients with incomplete tetraplegia. Spine 2003; 28:33–39

27. Geisler FH, Coleman WP, Grieco G, Poonian D; Sygen Study Group. The Sygen multicenter acute spinal cord injury study. Spine 2001;26(suppl):S87–S98

28. Geisler FH, Dorsey FC, Coleman WP. Recovery of motor function after spinal-cord injury–a randomized, placebo-controlled trial with GM-1 ganglioside. N Engl J Med 1991;324:1829–1838

29. Ng WP, Fehlings MG, Cuddy B, et al. Surgical treatment for acute spinal cord injury study pilot #2: evaluation of protocol for decompressive surgery within 8 hours of injury. Neurosurg Focus 1999;6:article 3

30. Papadopoulos SM, Selden NR, Quint DJ, Patel N, Gillespie B, Grube S. Immediate spinal cord decompression for cervical spinal cord injury: feasibility and outcome. J Trauma 2002;52:323–332

31. Duh MS, Shepard MJ, Wilberger JE, Bracken MB. The effectiveness of surgery on the treatment of acute spinal cord injury and its relation to pharmacological treatment. Neurosurgery 1994;35:240–248

32. Vaccaro AR, Daugherty RJ, Sheehan TP, et al. Neurologic outcome of early versus late surgery for cervical spinal cord injury. Spine 1997;22:2609–2613

33. Pointillart V, Petitjean ME, Wiart L, et al. Pharmacological therapy of spinal cord injury during the acute phase. Spinal Cord 2000; 38:71–76

34. Aebi M, Mohler J, Zäch GA, Morscher E. Indication, surgical technique, and results of 100 surgically-treated fractures and fracture-dislocations of the cervical spine. Clin Orthop Relat Res 1986;(203):244–257

35. La Rosa G, Conti A, Cardali S, Cacciola F, Tomasello F. Does early decompression improve neurological outcome of spinal cord injured patients? Appraisal of the literature using a meta-analytical approach. Spinal Cord 2004;42:503–512

36. Larson SJ, Holst RA, Hemmy DC, Sances A Jr. Lateral extracavitary approach to traumatic lesions of the thoracic and lumbar spine. J Neurosurg 1976;45:628–637

37. Waters RL, Meyer PR Jr, Adkins RH, Felton D. Emergency, acute, and surgical management of spine trauma. Arch Phys Med Rehabil 1999;80:1383–1390

38. Anderson PA, Bohlman HH. Anterior decompression and arthrodesis of the cervical spine: long-term motor improvement: 2. Improvement in complete traumatic quadriplegia. J Bone Joint Surg Am 1992;74:683–692

39. Bohlman HH, Anderson PA. Anterior decompression and arthrodesis of the cervical spine: long-term motor improvement: 1. Improvement in incomplete traumatic quadriparesis. J Bone Joint Surg Am 1992;74:671–682

40. Transfeldt EE, White D, Bradford DS, Roche B. Delayed anterior decompression in patients with spinal cord and cauda equina injuries of the thoracolumbar spine. Spine 1990;15:953–957

41. Brodkey JS, Miller CF Jr, Harmody RM. The syndrome of acute central cervical spinal cord injury revisited. Surg Neurol 1980;14:251–257

42. Burke DC, Berryman D. The place of closed manipulation in the management of flexion-rotation dislocations of the cervical spine. J Bone Joint Surg Br 1971;53:165–182

43. DeVivo MJ. Causes and costs of spinal cord injury in the United States. Spinal Cord 1997;35:809–813

44. Kraus JF, Franti CE, Riggins RS, Richards D, Borhani NO. Incidence of traumatic spinal cord lesions. J Chronic Dis 1975;28:471–492

9 Management of Cervical Injuries

David O. Okonkwo, Rod J. Oskouian Jr., and Christopher I. Shaffrey

Cervical spinal injury occurs in 4 to 10% of patients who sustain traumatic brain injuries due to blunt force trauma. Cervical spinal injury should be suspected in any trauma patient with loss of consciousness. All of the following patients should undergo a radiographic search for a cervical spinal injury: patients who present awake with neck pain or tenderness, patients with a neurologic deficit, patients who have sustained a traumatic brain injury, patients with a distracting injury that clouds the cervical spine examination, and patients who present following a sufficient mechanism of injury.

This chapter discusses the presentation, classification, radiographic characteristics, and management options for cervical spinal injuries, grouped by injuries of the craniocervical junction and injuries of the subaxial cervical spine.

■ Craniocervical Junction

Occipital Condyle Fractures

Occipital condyle fractures were first described by Bell[1] in 1817, and the association of occipital condyle fractures and severe head trauma was initially drawn in autopsy series, with an incidence as high as 4% in fatal head injuries.[2] However, the clinical diagnosis and management of occipital condyle fractures are principally phenomena of the computed tomography (CT) era.

Conventional cervical spine plain films miss between 50 and 93% of occipital condyle fractures,[3,4] which are the most common cervical spine fracture missed by radiology residents.[5] With the advent of routine CT scanning in high-energy blunt trauma, the spectrum of this disease has become much better elucidated.

Occipital condyle fractures should be suspected in trauma patients with lower cranial nerve palsies, upper cervical spine mobility restriction, or persistent neck pain. The 12th cranial nerve is most commonly involved, due to the proximity of the hypoglossal canal, but palsies of cranial nerves VI, IX, and X also occur with occipital condyle fractures. Cranial nerve palsies resulting from occipital condyle fractures may occur acutely or in a delayed fashion. Prognosis is more favorable with cranial nerve palsies with delayed presentation; acute cranial nerve palsies rarely heal completely.

Brainstem compression from displaced fracture fragments, torticollis, and retropharyngeal hematoma with acute respiratory distress have also been reported following occipital condyle fractures.[1,6,7] These fractures can also precipitate rotatory subluxation. Full clinical assessment is often difficult because many patients have concomitant traumatic brain injury and altered level of consciousness. Brainstem compression from displaced occipital condyle fractures is rare, reported only five times in the literature, but surgical decompression is indicated.

Anderson and Montesano[8] first classified occipital condyle fractures in 1988 based on the vector of force precipitating the injury (**Table 9.1** and **Fig. 9.1**):

- Type I fractures result from axial loading. The fractured condyle is comminuted with minimal or no displacement.
- Type II fractures result from direct trauma to the skull. Type II fractures occur in conjunction with basilar skull fractures (**Fig. 9.1A**).

Table 9.1 Occipital Condyle Fracture Classification Systems

Classification System	Type	Description	Stability	Treatment Options
Anderson and Montesano[8]	I	Comminuted fracture with no or minimal displacement	Stable	C-collar
	II	Direct trauma with basilar skull fracture	Stable	C-collar
	III	Avulsion fracture from alar ligament	Unstable	Halo or surgical fixation
Tuli et al[9]	1	Nondisplaced	Stable	No treatment or C-collar
	2A	Displaced with intact ligaments	Stable	C-collar, halo
	2B	Displaced and craniocervical instability	Unstable	Halo or surgical fixation

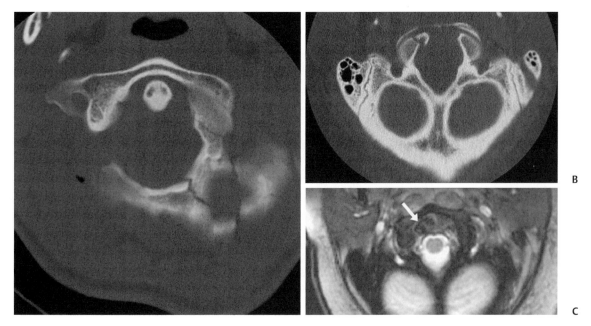

Fig. 9.1 Occipital condyle fractures. **(A)** Axial computed tomography (CT) image of Anderson and Montesano type II and Tuli type 1 occipital condyle fracture. Note the associated basilar skull fracture. **(B)** Axial CT and **(C)** T2-weighted axial magnetic resonance imaging (MRI) of an Anderson and Montesano type III and Tuli type 2A occipital condyle fracture. An intact transverse ligament (*arrow*) has avulsed the tip of the right occipital condyle.

- Type III fractures are avulsion fractures that occur from lateral flexion or rotatory forces with resultant pulling by the alar ligament (**Fig. 9.1B**).

  Anderson and Montesano concluded that type I and II fractures were stable, whereas type III fractures were unstable and require rigid immobilization.

  In 1997, Tuli et al[9] proposed an alternative classification scheme for occipital condyle fractures (**Table 9.1**):

- Type 1 fractures are nondisplaced and stable (**Fig. 9.1A**).
- Type 2A are displaced fractures with intact ligaments (**Fig. 9.1B**).
- Type 2B fractures are displaced occipital condyle fractures with craniocervical junction instability.

  In this context, craniocervical junction instability is determined via evidence from MRI demonstrating ligamentous injury or CT with coronal reconstructions revealing joint misalignment in the occiput-C1-C2 complex.

  Tuli et al[9] proposed that type 1 fractures be managed without intervention, type 2A fractures be managed with C-collar immobilization, and type 2B fractures require halo traction or surgical immobilization. Contemporary reports advise C-collar immobilization for both type 1 and 2A fractures.[10,11] At the conclusion of the period of immobilization, flexion-extension views should be obtained to confirm the absence of craniocervical junction instability.

Atlanto-Occipital Dislocation

The recognition of atlanto-occipital dislocation, as with occipital condyle fractures, has increased with the advent of routine CT evaluation of the cervical spine in the trauma survey. Atlanto-occipital (AO) dislocations are high-velocity, high-force injuries. Typically, AO dislocation results from distraction with extreme hyperextension and rupture of the tectorial membrane (the cranial extension of the posterior longitudinal ligament).

Atlanto-occipital dislocation accounts for 8 to 35% of fatalities from motor vehicle accidents and 10% of cervical spine injury fatalities.[12] Classically, AO dislocation was considered fatal. Survival is now common, perhaps related to increased sensitivity of detection during the trauma survey. Twenty percent of survivors have normal neurology; 10% have lower cranial nerve palsies, 34% hemiparesis or hemiplegia, and 38% quadriparesis or quadriplegia.[13]

Death from AO dislocation results most commonly from respiratory depression secondary to neurogenic shock.[2] Patients surviving AO dislocation frequently have neurologic deficits secondary to injuries other than the AO dislocation, such as traumatic brain injury (24%), carotid or vertebral artery injury, or brachial plexus injury.[14,15]

Both type I and type II odontoid fractures increase the risk for AO dislocation due to weakening or rupture of the alar ligament, apical ligaments, or tectorial membrane. The more classic association is with type I odontoid fractures;

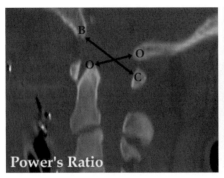 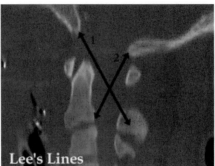 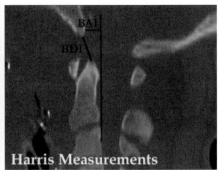

A–C

Fig. 9.2 Three methods for measuring atlanto-occipital dislocation are depicted. **(A)** The Power's ratio is the ratio of the distance from the tip of the basion to the posterior arch of C1 (B-C) divided by the distance of from the tip of the opisthion to the tip of the odontoid (O-O). Ratios greater than 1 are consistent with the diagnosis of anterior atlanto-occipital dislocation. **(B)** For Lee's lines, two intersecting lines are drawn, one from the tip of the basion to the anterior aspect of the posterior ring of C2 and a second from the tip of the opisthion to the posteroinferior aspect of the C2 body. The first line should pass across the superior-posterior aspect of the odontoid process, and the second should pass just anterior to the posterior portion of the ring of C1. **(C)** Harris's measurements involve two calculations: the basion-dens interval (BDI), the distance between the inferior and posterior tip of the basion and the superior tip of the odontoid; and the basion-posterior axial interval (BAI), the distance from the posterior axial line to the inferior and posterior tip of the basion. For both the BDI and BAI, a value greater than 12 mm is indicative of an anterior atlanto-occipital dislocation.

in fact, any type I odontoid fracture diagnosis should prompt an evaluation for AO dislocation.

The diagnosis of AO dislocation is frequently delayed or missed in patients who present neurologically intact or with incomplete neurologic syndromes.[13] The radiographic evaluation of AO dislocation involves the calculation of Power's ratio, Lee's line measurements, or Harris's measurements. Power's ratio is the distance from the tip of the basion to the posterior arch of C1 (B-C) divided by the distance from the tip of the opisthion to the tip of the odontoid (O-O) (**Fig. 9.2A**). Ratios greater than 1 suggest anterior AO dislocation. Ratios less than 1 are normal unless a posterior AO dislocation is present. Caution must be used employing Power's ratio in the setting of congenital anomalies of the craniocervical junction or with C1 fractures such as Jefferson fractures.

The X-line method, or Lee's lines, involves assessment of relationships of bony elements at the craniocervical junction. Two intersecting lines are drawn, one from the tip of the basion to the anterior aspect of the posterior ring of C2 and a second from the tip of the opisthion to the posteroinferior aspect of the C2 body (**Fig. 9.2B**). The first line should pass across the superior-posterior aspect of the odontoid process, and the second should pass just anterior to the posterior portion of the ring of C1.

Lee's method sought to improve the sensitivity of plain film radiographs in the diagnosis of AO dislocation, because proper identification of the midpoint of the posterior arch of C1 for calculation of Power's ratio can be difficult on lateral x-rays.

Harris's measurements, or the rule of 12s, involve two calculations: the basion-dens interval (BDI) and the basion-posterior axial interval (BAI) (**Fig. 9.2C**). The BDI is

the distance between the inferior and posterior tip of the basion and the superior tip of the odontoid. To calculate the BAI, a vertical line is drawn along the posterior aspect of the odontoid, extending above the level of the foramen magnum (the posterior axial line). A perpendicular line is drawn from this posterior axial line to the inferior and posterior tip of the basion, and the distance is measured. For both the BDI and BAI, a value greater than 12 mm is indicative of an anterior atlanto-occipital dislocation (hence, the rule of 12s).

With modern continuous slice acquisition CT and three-dimensional reconstructions of the spine and head, Power's ratio, Lee's method, or Harris's measurements may be employed with reliability and accuracy for evaluation for AO dislocation.[16]

Spontaneous reduction of AO dislocation can occur such that any of the aforementioned measurement techniques no longer detect it. An increased distance between the posterior elements of C1 and C2 may be the only clue on CT, with subsequent magnetic resonance (MR) evaluation revealing substantial ligamentous injury at the craniocervical junction. Retropharyngeal hematomas occur in all AO dislocations and, if noted on CT or plain film radiographs, should prompt MR evaluation of the cervical spine (**Fig. 9.3**).

Traynelis and colleagues[17] classified three types of AO dislocations (**Table 9.2**):

- Type I: anterior displacement of the occiput relative to the atlas (**Fig. 9.3**)
- Type II: longitudinal distraction with separation of the occiput and atlas
- Type III: posterior displacement of the occiput with respect to the atlas

Table 9.2 Traynelis Atlanto-Occipital Dislocation Classification System

Type	Description	Stability	Treatment Options
I	Anterior displacement of occiput over atlas	Unstable	• Gentle traction under fluoroscopy may be indicated to realign the spine followed by immediate immobilization with a halo vest if possible, especially if there is a neurologic deficit
			• Surgical stabilization is indicated when spine is realigned
II	Distraction with longitudinal separation of occiput and atlas	Unstable	• Gentle traction under fluoroscopy may be indicated to realign the spine followed by immediate immobilization with a halo vest if possible, especially if there is a neurologic deficit
			• Surgical stabilization is indicated
III	Posterior displacement of occiput over atlas	Unstable	• Gentle traction under fluoroscopy may be indicated to realign the spine followed by immediate immobilization with a halo vest if possible, especially if there is a neurologic deficit
			• Surgical stabilization is indicated when spine is realigned

Note that Power's ratio may be falsely negative in detecting type III (posterior) AO dislocations.

Patients with AO dislocation should be treated to avoid progression of neurologic deficits due to the highly unstable nature of these fractures. Occipital-cervical fusion is the treatment of choice, although halo ring-vest orthosis is an alternative for patients where occipital-cervical fusion is contraindicated. Early surgical intervention does not increase risk of neurologic worsening or late instability. In most case of AO dislocations, traction results in longitudinal distraction. It would therefore not be indicated in patients whose spinal column was in good alignment and whose primary pathology was longitudinal distraction (type II). For type II AO dislocations, traction is controversial and is associated with a 10% risk of neurologic deterioration because it could increase the distraction distance.[18]

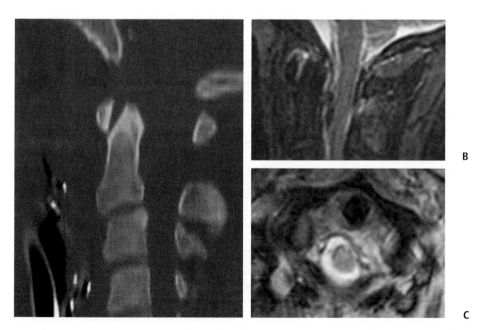

Fig. 9.3 Radiographic images of a patient with anterior atlanto-occipital dislocation. **(A)** Sagittal CT reconstruction at presentation demonstrates a clear dissociation of bony elements at the craniocervical junction and a Power's ratio greater than 1. **(B)** Sagittal T2-weighted MRI obtained hours later demonstrates interval decrease in the basion-dens interval, indicating spontaneous reduction of the atlanto-occipital (AO) dislocation. However, associated disruption in the posterior ligamentous complex is seen. **(C)** Axial T2-weighted MRI reveals an epidural hematoma adjacent to the upper cervical spinal cord. The patient had a left hemiparesis.

Table 9.3 Classification of Isolated C1 (Atlas) Fractures

Type I: Fractures of a single arch
Type II: Burst fracture (classic Jefferson fracture with a four-point burst fracture of the ring of C1)
Type III: Lateral mass fractures of the atlas

Source: From Landells CD, Van Peteghem PK. Fractures of the atlas: classification, treatment and morbidity. Spine 1988;13:450–452.

For type I and III AO dislocations, if the spine is not in alignment, then gentle traction at the bedside but without weights can be warranted, especially if there is a neurologic deficit present to realign the spine. Most often just by changing the head position the alignment can be normalized.

Isolated C1 Fractures

Isolated fractures of C1 rarely cause neurologic sequelae. Improper management of these fractures, however, can lead to delayed neurologic deficit. Atlas fractures may involve the lateral mass (13–37%), the anterior or posterior ring (31–45%), or a Jefferson fracture of both the anterior and posterior ring (37–51%) (**Table 9.3**).

The critical clinical feature to discern in isolated C1 fractures is integrity of the transverse ligament. Integrity of the transverse ligament may be assessed on anteroposterior (AP) or open-mouth odontoid plain film radiography or coronal reconstruction CT by measuring the lateral mass displacement. If the cumulative displacement of the lateral masses is ≥ 7 mm, then the transverse ligament is considered incompetent (the rule of Spence).[19] Panjabi's group[20] found that an atlanto-dens interval (ADI) greater than 3.5 mm on flexion radiographs was the most reliable predictor of transverse ligament disruption. Transverse ligament disruption can also be diagnosed on magnetic resonance imaging (MRI).

There is no class I or class II evidence regarding treatment for isolated C1 fractures. Fractures of the C1 lateral mass, which are unlikely to be associated with disruption of the transverse ligament or an increase in the ADI, can be treated with external cervical immobilization. There is no evidence to support the use of a halo orthosis over rigid cervical collars. External immobilization for 8 to 12 weeks is sufficient, and healing should be assessed with flexion-extension plain film radiographs to exclude pseudarthrosis and craniocervical instability. Some clinicians advocate use of a halo orthosis for comminuted lateral mass fractures to increase fusion rates over rigid cervical collar immobilization, but this decision should be multifactorial and take into consideration the overall medical condition, as older patients with significant medical comorbidities do not tolerate external immobilization well.

Fractures of either the anterior or posterior arch should be assessed for concomitant instability or disruption of the transverse ligament. Instability is characterized by an ADI > 3.5 mm, lateral mass displacement > 7 mm, or MR evidence of transverse ligament avulsion or disruption. Isolated C1 ring fractures of either the anterior or posterior arch may be treated with cervical collar immobilization, sternal occipital mandibular immobilization (SOMI) brace, or halo for up to 3 months. There is no evidence to support the use of one option over the others.[21,22]

Fractures of both the anterior and posterior arch carry special treatment considerations. Sir Geoffrey Jefferson[23] in 1920 initially described his fracture of the C1 ring as bilateral fractures of the junction of the lateral masses and the anterior and posterior arches. This fracture of both the anterior and posterior arch is also referred to as a C1 burst fracture. Treatment of C1 burst fractures is dictated by the presence or absence of instability, defined as either an ADI > 3.5 mm or lateral mass displacement > 7 mm on CT or disruption of the transverse ligament on MRI. A C1 burst fracture with an intact transverse ligament may be treated with external cervical immobilization (rigid cervical collar or halo vest orthosis) for up to 3 months. An unstable burst fracture may be treated with either a halo device for 3 months or C1-C2 internal fixation and fusion, with postoperative immobilization dictated by the fusion procedure chosen.

Surgical options for C1-C2 fusion for unstable C1 burst fractures include the Harms technique (C1 lateral mass and the C2 pedicle, pars interarticularis or translaminar fixation with cervical polyaxial screws and rods),[24] C1-C2 transarticular screw fixation,[25,26] or a Brooks, Gallie, or Sonntag posterior wiring fusion.

Dickman and Sonntag[27] reported their long-term results for C1-C2 transarticular screw fixation and noted a substantially higher fusion rate for C1-C2 transarticular screws over Brooks, Gallie, or Sonntag posterior wiring techniques.[27] The Harms technique of C1-C2 fixation was described in 2001, but large case series with long-term data are not yet available.[24] However, the Harms C1-C2 fusion has biomechanical advantages over the Magerl technique of transarticular screw fixation, is less likely to injure the vertebral artery, does not require structural bone graft or wiring, and is less likely to be contraindicated by anatomy. In addition, Harms and Melcher[24] reported a 100% fusion rate in their initial series of 37 patients. Postoperative external cervical immobilization is not necessary following a Harms C1-C2 fusion, in contradistinction to Sonntag's original description of his modification of the posterior wiring technique, further limiting postoperative morbidity of the Harms C1-C2 fusion.

More recently, Harms described a transoral reduction and C1 osteosynthesis technique for young patients as an alternative function-preserving option for unstable Jefferson fractures.[28]

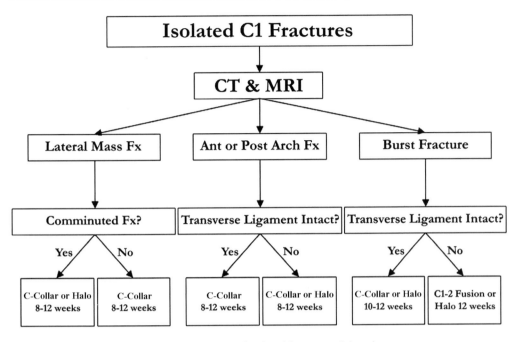

Fig. 9.4 Treatment algorithm for management of isolated fractures of the atlas.

Figure 9.4 depicts an evidence-based treatment algorithm for management of isolated fractures of the atlas. Treatment choice must be weighed in the context of other traumatic injuries, medical comorbidities, and patient preference.

Isolated C2 Fractures

Approximately 20% of all cervical spine trauma cases involve C2. The spectrum of C2 fractures includes hangman's fractures (bilateral traumatic spondylolisthesis of the atlas), odontoid fractures, and miscellaneous fractures of the C2 vertebral body. The incidence of neurologic deficit in surviving patients is low (7.5% in one series), likely due to the larger spinal canal diameter at this level.[29] C2 fractures are common in the elderly and carry a significant in-hospital mortality rate, perhaps as high as 25%.[30,31] However, recent evidence suggests that surgical management of C2 fractures

among the elderly is associated with acceptable rates of morbidity and lower mortality for this group of fractures, arguing for more routine use of surgical management in appropriate patients in this population.[32]

Odontoid Fractures

Odontoid fractures are the most common traumatic injuries of the axis and account for 7 to 14% of all cervical spine injuries. The most common symptom is high cervical pain, as neurologic deficits are infrequent. However, spinal cord compression may result from subluxation of the fracture dens, and maintenance of spinal alignment must be a primary goal of the evaluation and management of these fractures.

Anderson and D'Alonzo[33] proposed a classification system for odontoid fractures in 1974 that is still in use today (**Table 9.4**). Type I fractures are oblique fractures

Table 9.4 Anderson and D'Alonzo Classification of Odontoid Fractures

Type	Description	Stability	Treatment Options
I	Fracture through tip of dens	Stable	C-collar
	In association with atlanto-occipital dislocation	Unstable	Surgical fixation, C-collar, halo
II	Through base of dens	Often unstable	Surgical fixation, C-collar, halo
IIA	Through base of dens with comminuted fragments	Unstable	Surgical fixation
III	Fracture extends through body of C2	Usually stable	C-collar, halo if unstable

through the tip of the odontoid process. Type I fractures are rare, representing less than 1% of odontoid fractures, but may occur during atlanto-occipital dislocation.[34,35] Type I fractures may lead to os odontoideum due to resorption of the lower dens from avascular necrosis. Type II fractures are those occurring at the base of the odontoid process at the junction with the body of C2. Type III odontoid fractures extend through the dens and into the body of C2. Anderson and D'Alonzo themselves stated that type III odontoid fractures should be considered fractures of the body of C2. In fact, later authors argued that type III odontoid fractures should be grouped with other, miscellaneous fractures of C2. Nevertheless, the designation of type III odontoid fracture remains in clinical use today.

Mark Hadley and colleagues[36] modified the Anderson and D'Alonzo classification scheme to distinguish comminuted fractures with free fragments of the base of the odontoid. These fractures are termed type IIA fractures. Although rare (only 5% of the Hadley series of type II fractures), the type IIA fracture is unstable, and early surgical intervention is recommended.

The distinction between type II and type III fractures can be difficult because no clear definition exists to distinguish a "high" type III from a "low" type II fracture.[37] Grauer and colleagues[38] proposed an alternative modification to the Anderson and D'Alonzo classification scheme to better define suitability of treatment options such as anterior odontoid placement. The authors defined type IIA fractures as minimally or nondisplaced type II fractures with no comminution, type IIB fractures as displaced fractures extending anterior-superior to posterior-inferior or traverse fractures, and type IIC fractures as fractures extending from anterior-inferior to posterior-superior. The authors report that type IIA fractures can often be managed conservatively, type IIB fractures were suitable for anterior odontoid screw placement, and type IIC fractures are treated with posterior atlantoaxial stabilization.

No treatment intervention is considered inappropriate for any type of odontoid fracture except in extreme circumstances (e.g., age > 100, low Karnofsky score, hospice patients).[39] Type I odontoid fractures, unless in association with atlanto-occipital dislocation, may be managed with cervical collar alone, with fusion rates of 100% reported (**Table 9.3**).[33,40]

Type II odontoid fractures are the most common subtype and have presented the greatest treatment dilemmas to the spine surgeon. Nonunion rates for conservative management of type II odontoid fractures are as high as 75%. Risk factors associated with nonunion of type II odontoid fractures include age > 50 and dens displacement ≥ 6 mm. Lennarson and colleagues[41] in Iowa provided class II evidence (case-control study) that substantiates surgical treatment for type II odontoid fractures in patients over age 50. Seybold and Bayley[42] reached a similar conclusion, in that patients over age 60 had high symptomatic nonunion rates (19.5%) and lower cervical range of motion

when treating type II and III odontoid fractures with halo immobilization. Pepin et al[43] noted poor halo tolerance in elderly patients and argued for early surgical intervention in older patients with type II odontoid fractures. Andersson and colleagues[44] noted poor union rates in elderly patients treated nonsurgically for type II odontoid fractures and further noted that posterior approaches were superior to anterior odontoid screw in this patient population. Surgical intervention for type II odontoid fractures should also be considered if there is failure to maintain spinal alignment following traction and external immobilization. As mentioned above, type IIA fractures should be treated with early surgical intervention when clinically feasible.[36]

Type III odontoid fractures may be treated with cervical immobilization with a fusion rate over 80%. Although type III (and type II) odontoid fractures have historically been treated with halo vest immobilization, cervical collars are equivalent to halo devices in prevention of late nonunion or late need for surgical stabilization.[45,46] Surgical fixation for type III odontoid fractures may be reserved for patients with nonunion/late instability following attempted nonsurgical management with cervical immobilization or failure to maintain spinal alignment with external immobilization. Our preference is rigid cervical collar over halo orthosis; however, patient compliance and confounding factors such as smoking history and other traumatic injuries must be considered.

Surgical options for odontoid fractures include posterior atlantoaxial wiring techniques (Brooks, Gallie, or Sonntag methods), the Magerl C1-C2 transarticular screw techniue,[25] the Harms C1-lateral mass-C2 pedicle screw technique,[24] or an anterior odontoid screw in certain cases. Posterior C1-C2 fusion procedures result in greater loss of motion of the atlantoaxial joint but higher fusion rates and fewer contraindications than an anterior odontoid lag screw fusion.[24,44]

Traumatic Spondylolisthesis of the Axis (Hangman's Fracture)

A hangman's fracture is the colloquial name given to a fracture of the pedicles or pars interarticularis (isthmus) of the axis (C2 vertebra). Schneider et al[47] coined the term "hangman's fracture" in 1965 in their series of eight patients whose injuries mimicked the fracture pattern of judicial hanging described by Wood-Jones[48] in the first volume of *Lancet* in 1913.

Traumatic bilateral spondylolisthesis of the pars interarticularis of the axis is a hyperextension and compression with axial loading that is often seen with motor vehicle accidents, falls, and diving accidents. The classic scenarios are that of an unrestrained occupant in a motor vehicle accident who is thrown forward and hits the windshield, or a swimmer who dives and hits the bottom of a shallow

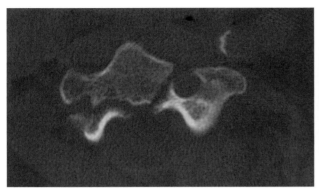 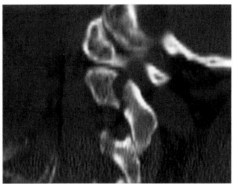

A B

Fig. 9.5 Radiographic images of a patient with an atypical hangman's fracture. **(A)** Axial and **(B)** sagittal reconstruction CT images demonstrate a fracture through the posterior aspect of the verte-bral body with bilateral continuity of the posterior cortex or pedicle. A typical hangman's fracture occurs through the pars interarticu-laris itself.

pool. In both instances the combined forces of hyperex-tension and axial compression occur. The fracture seen in trauma is similar to that induced by judicial hangings; however, the true judicial "hangman's fracture" results from distraction and hyperextension, not compression and hyperextension. There is often anterior subluxation of C2 on C3, and it is usually stable, with neurologic deficits being rare. Instability can usually be identified if there is ≥ 4 mm of subluxation of C2 on C3 or ≥ 50% sub-luxation of C2 on C3, excessive angulation, or significant motion on flexion-extension films

Multiple classification systems for traumatic spondy-lolisthesis of the axis exist, though none is in routine clin-ical use. Pepin and Hawkins[49] described two types: type I is a nondisplaced fracture of the posterior elements, and type II is a displaced fracture of the posterior elements and the dens. Francis and colleagues[50] described five grades of hangman's fractures on the basis of displace-ment of the C2 body (less than or greater than 3.5 mm) and the angulation of C2 on C3 (less than or greater than 11 degrees). Effendi and colleagues[51] describe three types on the basis of mechanism of injury (type I, axial loading; type II, hyperextension and rebound flexion; type III, hy-perflexion and rebound extension). Levine and Edwards[52] modified the Effendi classification such that type I in-juries resulted from a hyperextension-axial loading force, type II injuries from an initial hyperextension-axial load-ing force followed by severe flexion, type IIa injuries from flexion-distraction, and type III injuries from flexion-com-pression.

Starr and Eismont[53] drew attention to the atypical hangman's fracture, defined as canal-compressive trau-matic spondylolisthesis of the axis with significant neuro-logic deficit. Atypical hangman's fractures occur through the posterior aspect of the vertebral body, with uni- or bilateral continuity of the posterior cortex or pedicle (**Fig. 9.5**). These fractures have higher rates of spinal canal compromise because of the fracture pattern and degree of

subluxation; hence the higher rates of neurologic deficit with the atypical hangman's fracture.

No class I or II studies have been performed regarding management of traumatic spondylolisthesis of the axis. Multiple large case series (class III evidence) have been published, which report that almost all hangman's frac-tures heal with traction, when necessary, followed by 12 weeks of external cervical immobilization with a rigid cervical collar or, more commonly, halo orthosis.[50,54] Fusion rates with halo orthosis alone are as high as 95%.[50]

Li et al[55] published a systematic review of 32 papers on the management of hangman's fractures. The authors recommend that most stable Effendi types I and Levine-Edwards type II injuries be managed with cervical collar, unstable Effendi types I and II and Levine-Edwards type II fractures be managed with traction and external cervical immobilization, Levine-Edwards types IIa and III fractures be managed with rigid immobiliza-tion, and Levine-Edwards types IIa and III fractures with significant dislocation be managed with surgical stabilization (**Table 9.5**).

Surgery for hangman's fractures should be reserved for significant C2-C3 disk disruption, failure to induce or maintain reduction, or nonunion following halo immobi-lization. Though clinicians in most series employed halo ring-vest orthoses, a Philadelphia cervical collar for 12 weeks is likewise effective for nondisplaced traumatic spondylolisthesis of the axis with less device-associated morbidity.[56,57] When surgery is indicated, options include C2-C3 anterior cervical fusion and C1-C3 posterior fusion techniques. No study has demonstrated the superiority of anterior versus posterior approaches, and an anterior approach does spare rotation at C1-C2.

Figure 9.6 depicts an evidence-based treatment algo-rithm for management of traumatic spondylolisthesis of the axis. The treatment choice must be weighed in the context of other traumatic injuries, medical comorbidities, and patient preference.

Table 9.5 Classification System of Hangman's Fractures

Type	Description	Radiology	Mechanism	Stability and Treatment
I	Vertical pars interarticularis fracture	≤ 3 mm subluxation of C2 on C3 and no angulation	Axial loading and extension	Stable on flexion and extension x-rays Neurologic deficit is rare Hard collar is recommended
IA	Fracture lines through the pars interarticularis on each side are not parallel	C2 may be subluxed 2–3 mm on C3	May be rotational during hyperextension	Know as the "atypical hangman's fracture" with a 30% incidence of neurologic injury Fracture can extend through the foramen transversum
II	Vertical fracture through pars with disruption of C2-C3 disk and posterior longitudinal ligament	Subluxation of C2 on C3 > 3 mm	Axial loading and extension	Usually reduces with traction, and neurologic deficit is rare
IIA	Oblique fracture	Very little subluxation (usually < 3 mm) but can have more angulation of C2 on C3	Flexion distraction (posterior arch fails in tension)	Traction can make angulation and widening of disk space worse
III	Vertical pars fracture with C2-C3 facet capsules disrupted with anterior longitudinal ligament disruption	C2–C3 facets may be locked or unstable	Unclear (flexion and compression?)	Traction may be dangerous Open reduction and stabilization are indicated

Source: Adapted from Greenberg MS. Handbook of Neurosurgery. 6th ed. New York: Thieme, 2006; Effendi B, Roy D, Cornish B, Dussault RG, Laurin CA. Fractures of the ring of the axis: a classification based on the analysis of 131 cases. J Bone Joint Surg Br 1981;63-B:319–327; Levine AM, Edwards CC. Fractures of the atlas. J Bone Joint Surg Am 1991;73:680–691; Dickman CA, Sonntag VK. Posterior C1–C2 transarticular screw fixation for atlantoaxial arthrodesis. Neurosurgery 1998;43:275–280.

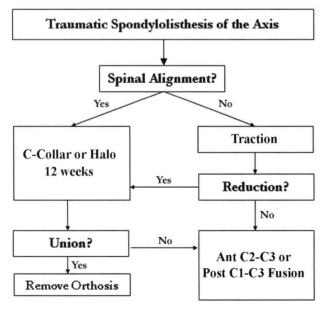

Fig. 9.6 Treatment algorithm for management of traumatic spondylolisthesis of the axis.

Miscellaneous C2 Fractures

C2 vertebral body fractures occur that are neither odontoid fractures nor a part of traumatic spondylolisthesis of the axis. They represent a diverse group of fractures. Several investigators argue that type III odontoid fractures are misleading and, in fact, belong categorized with other nonodontoid C2 body fractures.[33,58] In several series of miscellaneous C2 body fractures,[54,58–60] all fractures healed with external cervical immobilization (either rigid cervical collar or halo device) with the possible exception of C2 burst fractures.[60] Surgery is reserved for cases of nonunion, the rare C2 burst fractures with spinal cord compromise, or the rare miscellaneous C2 body fracture that fails to reduce with traction.

Combined C1-C2 Injuries

The description of combined fractures of the atlas and axis goes back to the original published series of Jefferson,[23] from which the C1 burst fracture became characterized as Jefferson fractures. Fractures of C1 occur in up to 53% of

Table 9.6 Combined C1-C2 Injuries

Injury Type	Modifier	Stability	Treatment Options
C1–type II odontoid fracture	ADI < 5 mm	Stable	C-collar, halo, surgical fixation
	ADI ≥ 5 mm	Unstable	Halo, surgical fixation
C1–type III odontoid fracture		Unstable	Halo, surgical fixation
C1–hangman's fracture	C2-C3 angulation < 11 degrees	Stable	C-collar, halo
	C2-C–3 angulation ≥ 11 degrees	Unstable	Halo, surgical fixation
C1–miscellaneous C2 fracture		Stable	C-collar, halo

type II or III odontoid fractures. Similarly, odontoid fractures are noted in up to 50% of patients with C1 fractures, and C1 fractures are seen in up to 26% of hangman's fractures. In a large review of almost 800 patients with upper cervical injuries, the incidence of C1-C2 combination injuries in patients with either a C1 or C2 injury was 27%, and combined C1-C2 fractures represented 4% of all cervical spine injuries.[61]

Combined C1-C2 injuries have higher rates of death and neurologic deficit than isolated fractures of C1 or C2, consistent with the presumed higher degrees of force necessary to precipitate combination fractures.[21,62,63]

The management of C1-C2 combination injuries is dictated principally by the characteristics of the C2 fracture. As such, these injuries fall into four groups: C1–type II odontoid combination fractures, C1–type III odontoid combination fractures, C1–hangman's combination fractures, and C1–miscellaneous C2 combination fractures (**Table 9.6**).[62] Hence, most C1-C2 combination injuries can be treated with external immobilization as discussed above for the specific C2 injury involved. Surgery for combined C1-C2 injuries is reserved for ADI > 5 mm, C2-C3 angulation greater than 11 degrees, or nonunion after nonsurgical management. In patients requiring surgery, again, the surgical approach is dictated by the appropriate approach for the C2 injury. When the injury to the ring of C1 does not permit instrumentation, occipital-cervical fusion or C1-C2 transarticular screw fixation are viable options.

■ Subaxial Cervical Spine (Based on AO Classification)

Biomechanical Considerations

The two-column concept of the cervical spine was proposed in Holdsworth's[64] landmark paper in 1963. The anterior column consists of the vertebral body, anterior and posterior longitudinal ligaments, and intervertebral disks, whereas the posterior column consists of the facet joints, capsular ligaments, spinous process, lamina, and interspinous ligament. Holdsworth contended that instability occurs with injury to the posterior ligamentous complex in association with an anterior column injury. The determinants of cervical spinal column injury are the magnitude, vector, and rate of force application sustained by the cervical spine.[65–67] White and Panjabi[68] defined instability as "loss of the ability of the spine under physiologic loads to maintain its pattern of displacement so that there is no initial or additional neurologic deficit, no major deformity, and no incapacitating pain." It may result from ligamentous injury with or without associated bony injury.

More recently, the Cervical Spine Injury Severity Score was proposed for measuring stability after cervical spine trauma.[69] The scoring system evaluates the extent of bony and ligamentous disruption in the anterior, posterior, left, and right columns, and the summated score is a valid, reliable indicator of spinal instability. It is validated for injuries from C2 to T1. The system is a useful adjunct in the decision-making process during evaluation and management of the patient with cervical spine trauma.

The most common subaxial cervical level injured is C5-C6, believed to be due to the higher degree of flexion-extension motion (**Table 9.7**) at this level compared with the rest of the cervical spine.

Classification

Argenson et al[70] in Nice, France, built upon the schemata of Allen et al[71] and Harris et al[72] to classify subaxial cervical spine injuries on the principal force vectors producing specific patterns of injury (**Table 9.6**). The first of these force vectors is compression injury, which may occur in association with flexion or extension.

Compression Injuries

Pure axial loading as a cause of cervical spine injury is relatively rare below C2, described in only 7% of subaxial injuries in the Nice series. (Axial loading in atlantoaxial injuries was discussed above.) Pure axial compression results

Table 9.7   Degrees of Motion in the Cervical Spine

Level	Motion			
	Flexion-Extension[56]	Axial Rotation[57]	Lateral Bending[58]	Translation*[59]
C3-C4	15.2 ± 3.8	4.5 ± 1.1	3.5 ± 1.4	0.6 ± 0.2
C4-C5	17.1 ± 4.5	4.6 ± 1.1	3.3 ± 1.0	0.9 ± 0.3
C5-C6	17.1 ± 3.9	4.0 ± 1.1	4.3 ± 1.4	0.9 ± 0.2
C6-C7	18.1 ± 6.1	1.6 ± 1.8	5.7 ± 1.9	0.6 ± 0.3
Overall	(60 to 75)[60]	134.2 ± 17.1[61]	64.2 ± 6.8[62]	N/A

*Translation does not occur in the absence of axial rotation.

in comminuted fractures, which may or may not push back into the spinal canal to endanger neural elements.

The most common force producing traumatic spinal cord injuries and unstable cervical spinal fractures is compression with flexion (**Table 9.8**). Force vectors directed in flexion will result in distraction of posterior elements and compression of anterior elements. Clinically, axial loading plus flexion vectors direct force at the anterior column (anterior aspect of the vertebral body and the intervertebral disk). Less severe degrees of axial loading produce wedge fractures, whereas severe forces result in unstable teardrop fractures.

Compression Fractures

True compression (pure axial loading) injuries of the cervical spine can only occur with loss of cervical lordosis. As such, compression or wedge fractures typically result from axial loading in combination with some degree of flexion or extension. Compression fractures, by definition, involve only the anterior column, and there is no retropulsion of bony fragments into the canal. Compression fractures heal with external immobilization alone, with an overall 5% nonunion rate.[73,74]

Burst Fractures

Burst fractures are, like compression fractures, the result of axial loading forces, typically in combination with flexion. Failure of both the anterior and posterior columns occurs, and neurologic injury may result from retropulsion of bony fragments into the canal (**Fig. 9.7**). Subaxial cervical burst fractures may occur with or without disruption of the posterior ligamentous complex. Burst fractures in patients with normal or incomplete neurologic functioning should be treated with surgical intervention to decompress the neural elements and fuse these unstable injuries. Rigid external immobilization may be considered in patients with complete spinal cord injuries.

Table 9.8   Classification of Subaxial Cervical Spine Injuries

Type	Injury Mechanism	%	Injury Pattern	%	Characteristics
A	Compression injuries		I: anterior compression (wedge) fracture	3	Principally bony damage; often associated with flexion forces
		33	II: comminuted fracture	7	
			III: teardrop fracture	23	
B	Flexion/extension/ distraction injuries	28	I: moderate whiplash with neurologic injury	5	Principally disk and ligamentous damage
			II: severe whiplash (sprain)	14	
			III: bilateral facet fracture-dislocation	9	
C	Rotation injuries		IV: unilateral facet fracture	20	Asymmetric lesions; rotation is always associated with lateral flexion
		39	II: fracture separation of the articular pillar	10	
			III: unilateral dislocation	9	

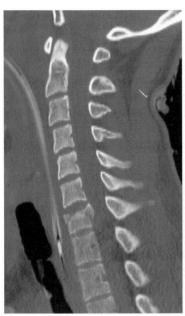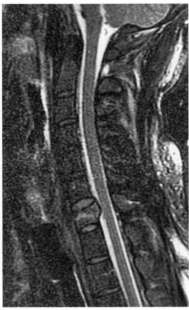

Fig. 9.7 **(A)** Sagittal CT and **(B)** T2-weighted MRI of a C5 burst fracture in a 19-year-old man involved in a high-speed motor vehicle accident with ejection. Note the retropulsion of bony fragments into the canal on CT and disruption of the posterior ligamentous complex on MRI. Spinal cord impingement was mild, and the patient had no deficits referable to the burst fracture.

A–B

Teardrop Fractures

Teardrop fractures result from hyperflexion-compression injuries. These fractures can be misleading in that they appear as small chip fractures of the anteroinferior margin of the vertebral body, but true teardrop fractures are biomechanically unstable and frequently associated with devastating neurologic injuries. Instability results from disruption of the disk and anterior and posterior ligaments. MRI demonstrating disk or ligament disruption distinguishes teardrop fractures from simple avulsion fractures.

Teardrop fractures are unstable injuries that require surgical intervention. Teardrop fractures in the absence of canal compromise may be treated via a posterior approach. If canal compromise exists, a combined anterior and posterior approach is usually necessary to decompress neural elements and achieve fusion.

Rotation Injuries

A rotational injury manifests itself clinically in the form of asymmetric lesions such as unilateral locked or fractured facets or fractures of the articular pillar (the facets absorb half of the load resulting from rotational forces applied to the cervical spine). Rotational injuries are designated type C injuries in the Nice classification (**Table 9.8**). Rotational injury always occurs with lateral flexion vectors superimposed on rotation. Spinal column alignment, in general, is maintained following rotational injuries. Rotational injuries are typically stable, with the exception of the unilateral "perched facet," in which ligamentous injury (and attendant spinal instability) results from avulsion of ligaments from bony attachments during the rotational event itself.

Unilateral Facet Dislocations

Unilateral facet dislocation is the prototypical asymmetric rotation-flexion injury. The inferior articulating facet of the upper vertebral level becomes perched anterior to the superior articulating facet of the lower vertebra. Anterolisthesis may occur and is typically less than 25% of the diameter of the vertebral body.

Both nerve root and spinal cord injury may occur secondary to unilateral facet dislocations. Treatment is closed reduction with traction followed by halo orthosis or open surgical fixation. Closed reduction, discussed in more detail below, is unsuccessful in up to 26% of cases. If closed reduction fails, open reduction in the operating room is warranted.

Flexion-Extension-Distraction Injuries

The final group of injury force vectors to consider is flexion-extension injuries, the less severe versions of which are commonly known as "whiplash" injuries. These injuries are characterized by disproportionate injury to the spinal ligaments and intervertebral disks compared with the bony elements.

The physiologic movements of flexion and extension are modulated by the posterior longitudinal ligament, which is strong in the cervical spine. Thus, when the posterior longitudinal ligament remains intact after whiplash injury (with mild or moderate force magnitude), the transverse axis of the spine remains intact, and neurologic injury is rare. However, when the posterior longitudinal ligament is disrupted in more severe injuries, often in association with failure of the posterior annulus, unstable spinal lesions are produced (type BII and BIII, **Table 9.8**). Unstable lesions happen when failure of the posterior longitudinal ligament and posterior annulus occurs in combination with anterolisthesis, end-plate angulation > 10 degrees, facet malalignment, or distracted vertebral segments due to posterior ligamentous complex injury.[75]

Whiplash

In mild and moderate flexion-extension injuries, static and dynamic radiographs may be normal, but subclinical ligamentous injury and delayed deformity may arise. This is supported experimentally by work that has demonstrated on microscopic analysis multilevel disk and anterior longitudinal ligament injury in spines that are radiographically normal with exaggerated, though subpathologic, motion at multiple levels on motion segment.[76]

Management of whiplash injuries is controversial. Patients with persistent neck pain following trauma, despite normal plain films or CT scans of the cervical spine, should be evaluated with MRI. Mild soft tissue injury in the absence of instability may be treated with physical therapy or C-collar immobilization, with meta-analysis indicating more rapid recovery, less pain, and improved cervical range of motion in patients treated with physical therapy without immobilization.[77] The medicolegal climate in the United States clouds management of whiplash injuries.

Bilateral Facet Fracture-Dislocations

Bilateral fracture-dislocation (or jumped facets, **Fig. 9.8**) occurs when the traumatizing force of distraction with flexion or extension persists in the setting of posterior longitudinal ligament failure and disruption of the posterior ligamentous complex (supra/interspinous ligaments). This ligamentous injury has important implications for clinical management of flexion-compression injuries: traction with larger weights may be dangerous; halo fixation is more likely to fail with ligamentous injury; and anterior approaches may jeopardize the remaining intact anterior ligaments, worsening stability and increasing the likelihood of pseudarthrosis.

Extension-distraction injuries are far less common than flexion-distraction injuries, but their consequences tend to be more severe with spinal instability and neurologic deficit.[78]

Closed reduction is controversial. The reports of neurologic worsening with closed reduction led to the argument that closed reduction should not be attempted in patients with normal function or incomplete spinal cord injury prior to MR evaluation for herniated disk. Mortality with closed reduction is as high as 7%, although most of these reports were prior to the ready availability of MRI for the trauma patient.[73,79–81] More modern reports indicate the safety of closed reduction, even in the setting of disk herniation.[82] Closed reduction is successful in approximately three fourths of facet dislocation cases. When closed reduction fails or is contraindicated, open reduction is almost always successful whether via an anterior or posterior approach. The medicolegal climate and the ready availability of MRI in most major trauma centers in the United States lead a majority of spine surgeons to obtain MRI before attempting closed reduction.

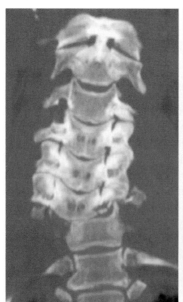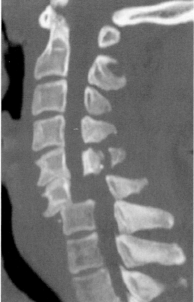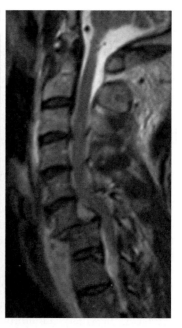

A–C

Fig. 9.8 (A) Coronal and **(B)** sagittal CT reconstructions of a patient with bilateral facet fracture-dislocations at C6-C7. Degree of anterolisthesis is greater than 50%. **(C)** T2-weighted sagittal MRI demonstrates distortion of the spinal cord. Patient suffered an incomplete spinal cord injury, American Spinal Injury Association (ASIA) class B.

Bilateral facet dislocation injuries are unstable, and reduction should be followed by internal fixation and fusion. Either anterior or posterior approaches are appropriate, and the presence or absence of disk herniation causing neural element compression may help guide the choice of the surgical approach. Anterior approaches alone have a slightly higher rate of delayed instability (6%)[83,84] than posterior alone approaches (3%).[73,85,86] Timing of surgery, whether or not early intervention improves outcome, remains controversial.

Cervicothoracic Junction Injuries

The cervicothoracic junction is a transitional zone. The incidence of cervicothoracic junction injury is significantly less than other cervical injuries or thoracolumbar junction injuries. These injuries were frequently missed due to inadequate plain film radiographs (in approximately 25% of all trauma patients, the C7-T1 disk space is not adequately visualized on the three-view x-ray series) (**Fig. 9.9A**), but the CT era has improved the detection of cervicothoracic junction trauma.

The cervicothoracic region has unique anatomy where the lordotic, mobile cervical spine transitions to the kyphotic, rigid thoracic spine. Upper thoracic spine rigidity comes from rib articulation with the sternum (the so-called fourth column of the thoracic spine). Recent CT kinematics studies demonstrate the cervicothoracic junction is twice as stiff as compared with its cervical neighbor.[87] However, the angular motion is similar in this region in comparison to the subaxial cervical spine.

The patterns of injury seen in the cervicothoracic junction include rotatory subluxation of C7 on T1, fracture-dislocations, unilateral and bilateral facet dislocations, and burst fractures. Fractures involving T1 through T4 are rare. The incidence of complete spinal cord injury from cervicothoracic junction trauma is high.

The principles of initial intervention involve immediate closed reduction of the fracture and establishing spinal alignment. Dislocations of the cervicothoracic junction require greater traction for prompt reduction, and weights up to 120 lb have been used to achieve closed reduction. Chapman et al[88] applied traction equal to 60% of the patient's body weight to achieve reduction. They did not notice any adverse outcome from the increased traction weight. If closed reduction is unsuccessful, then immediate operative reduction should be considered in cases of bilateral locked facets.

The selection criteria for surgical intervention for trauma involving the cervicothoracic junction are not well defined. There is no level I or level II evidence that delineates the selection criteria. Patients with progressive neurologic deficit or incomplete spinal cord injury require immediate closed reduction and realignment. If these measures fail and the patient demonstrates persistent neurologic deficit, then open reduction, decompression, and stabilization are warranted.

The goal of stabilization is to prevent progressive kyphosis and possibly diminish posttraumatic syrinx formation with a view toward preserving function above the level of the injury. Posttraumatic kyphotic deformity can cause spinal cord stretch and progressive neuronal injury to the anterior horn and motor neurons. Recent animal studies show that progressive kyphosis of the cervical spine results in demyelination of nerve fibers and neuronal loss in the anterior horn due to chronic

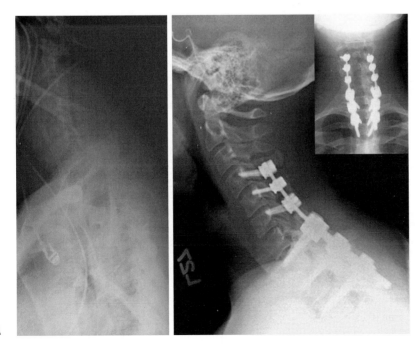

A

B

Fig. 9.9 (A) Inadequate visualization of the cervicothoracic junction during the trauma work-up of a patient involved in a high-speed motor vehicle accident who was later found to have a C7-T1 fracture dislocation. **(B)** C4-T4 posterior segmental instrumented fusion of the patient in **A** using a dual-diameter rod and screw system.

compression. As such, realignment remains one of the primary goals when addressing cervicothoracic junction trauma.

Stabilization of the cervicothoracic junction can be difficult, and a variety of techniques and approaches have been described for this procedure. One of the technical challenges has been that instrumentation constructs for the cervical spine are smaller than those for the thoracolumbar region. Newer dual diameter, or tapered, rod systems overcome this issue, allowing the surgeon to use a single rod, while placing the appropriate-sized instrumentation in each segment of the spinal column (**Fig. 9.9B**).

Cervicothoracic fixation of the unstable spine is challenging due to the transition of cervical lordosis to thoracic kyphosis. Stress and motion are important at the cervical level in contrast to the rigid upper thoracic spine. Rhee et al[89] compared the stiffness of several posterior fixation constructs. C7 and T1 pedicle screws are stronger than lateral mass screws at C7. This study also demonstrated that extension of the construct to C6 increased construct stiffness; wiring augmentation did not provide increased rigidity.

References

1. Bell C. Surgical observations. Middlesex Hosp J 1817;4:469–470
2. Bucholz RW, Burkhead WZ. The pathological anatomy of fatal atlanto-occipital dislocations. J Bone Joint Surg Am 1979;61:248–250
3. Hanson JA, Deliganis AV, Baxter AB, et al. Radiologic and clinical spectrum of occipital condyle fractures: retrospective review of 107 consecutive fractures in 95 patients. AJR Am J Roentgenol 2002;178:1261–1268
4. Diaz JJ Jr, Gillman C, Morris JA Jr, May AK, Carrillo YM, Guy J. Are five-view plain films of the cervical spine unreliable? A prospective evaluation in blunt trauma patients with altered mental status. J Trauma 2003;55:658–663
5. Goradia D, Blackmore CC, Talner LB, Bittles M, Meshberg E. Predicting radiology resident errors in diagnosis of cervical spine fractures. Acad Radiol 2005;12:888–893
6. Freeman BJ, Behensky H. Bilateral occipital condyle fractures leading to retropharyngeal haematoma and acute respiratory distress. Injury 2005;36:207–212
7. Bridgman SA, McNab W. Traumatic occipital condyle fracture, multiple cranial nerve palsies, and torticollis: a case report and review of the literature. Surg Neurol 1992;38:152–156
8. Anderson PA, Montesano PX. Morphology and treatment of occipital condyle fractures. Spine 1988;13:731–736
9. Tuli S, Tator CH, Fehlings MG, Mackay M. Occipital condyle fractures. Neurosurgery 1997;41:368–376
10. Capuano C, Costagliola C, Shamsaldin M, Maleci A, Di LN. Occipital condyle fractures: a hidden nosologic entity. An experience with 10 cases. Acta Neurochir (Wien) 2004;146:779–784
11. Caroli E, Rocchi G, Orlando ER, Delfini R. Occipital condyle fractures: report of five cases and literature review. Eur Spine J 2005;14:487–492
12. Davis D, Bohlman H, Walker AE, Fisher R, Robinson R. The pathological findings in fatal craniospinal injuries. J Neurosurg 1971;34:603–613
13. Fisher CG, Sun JC, Dvorak M. Recognition and management of atlanto-occipital dislocation: improving survival from an often fatal condition. Can J Surg 2001;44:412–420
14. Ferrera PC, Bartfield JM. Traumatic atlanto-occipital dislocation: a potentially survivable injury. Am J Emerg Med 1996;14:291–296
15. Lee C, Woodring JH, Walsh JW. Carotid and vertebral artery injury in survivors of atlanto-occipital dislocation: case reports and literature review. J Trauma 1991;31:401–407
16. Dziurzynski K, Anderson PA, Bean DB, et al. A blinded assessment of radiographic criteria for atlanto-occipital dislocation. Spine 2005;30:1427–1432
17. Traynelis VC, Marano GD, Dunker RO, Kaufman HH. Traumatic atlanto-occipital dislocation. Case report. J Neurosurg 1986;65:863–870
18. Dickman CA, Papadopoulos SM, Sonntag VK, Spetzler RF, Rekate HL, Drabier J. Traumatic occipitoatlantal dislocations. J Spinal Disord 1993;6:300–313
19. Spence KF Jr, Decker S, Sell KW. Bursting atlantal fracture associated with rupture of the transverse ligament. J Bone Joint Surg Am 1970;52:543–549
20. Oda T, Panjabi MM, Crisco JJ III, Oxland TR, Katz L, Nolte LP. Experimental study of atlas injuries: 2. Relevance to clinical diagnosis and treatment. Spine 1991;16(suppl):S466–S473
21. Fowler JL, Sandhu A, Fraser RD. A review of fractures of the atlas vertebra. J Spinal Disord 1990;3:19–24
22. Levine AM, Edwards CC. Fractures of the atlas. J Bone Joint Surg Am 1991;73:680–691
23. Jefferson G. Fractures of the atlas vertebra: report of four cases and a review of those previously reported. Br J Surg 1920;7:407–422
24. Harms J, Melcher RP. Posterior C1–C2 fusion with polyaxial screw and rod fixation. Spine 2001;26:2467–2471
25. Magerl F, Seeman PS. Stable posterior fusion of the atlas and axis by transarticular screw fixation. In: Kher, ed. Cervical Spine. New York: Springer-Verlag; 1987
26. Grob D, Magerl F. Surgical stabilization of C1 and C2 fractures. Orthopade 1987;16:46–54
27. Dickman CA, Sonntag VK. Posterior C1–C2 transarticular screw fixation for atlantoaxial arthrodesis. Neurosurgery 1998;43:275–280
28. Ruf M, Melcher R, Harms J. Transoral reduction and osteosynthesis C1 as a function-preserving option in the treatment of unstable Jefferson fractures. Spine 2004;29:823–827
29. Harrop JS, Sharan AD, Przybylski GJ. Epidemiology of spinal cord injury after acute odontoid fractures. Neurosurg Focus 2000;8:E4
30. Tashjian RZ, Majercik S, Biffl WL, Palumbo MA, Cioffi WG. Halovest immobilization increases early morbidity and mortality in elderly odontoid fractures. J Trauma 2006;60:199–203
31. Muller EJ, Wick M, Russe O, Muhr G. Management of odontoid fractures in the elderly. Eur Spine J 1999;8:360–365
32. Kuntz C, Mirza SK, Jarell AD, Chapman JR, Shaffrey CI, Newell DW. Type II odontoid fractures in the elderly: early failure of nonsurgical treatment. Neurosurg Focus 2000;8:e7
33. Anderson LD, D'Alonzo RT. Fractures of the odontoid process of the axis. J Bone Joint Surg Am 1974;56:1663–1674
34. Eismont FJ, Bohlman HH. Posterior atlanto-occipital dislocation with fractures of the atlas and odontoid process. J Bone Joint Surg Am 1978;60:397–399

35. Scott EW, Haid RW Jr, Peace D. Type I fractures of the odontoid process: implications for atlanto-occipital instability. Case report. J Neurosurg 1990;72:488–492

36. Hadley MN, Browner CM, Liu SS, Sonntag VK. New subtype of acute odontoid fractures (type IIA). Neurosurgery 1988;22(1 pt 1):67–71

37. Maak TG, Grauer JN. The contemporary treatment of odontoid injuries. Spine 2006;31(suppl):S53–S60

38. Grauer JN, Shafi B, Hilibrand AS, et al. Proposal of a modified, treatment-oriented classification of odontoid fractures. Spine J 2005;5:123–129

39. Clark CR, White AA III. Fractures of the dens: a multicenter study. J Bone Joint Surg Am 1985;67:1340–1348

40. Chiba K, Fujimura Y, Toyama Y, Fujii E, Nakanishi T, Hirabayashi K. Treatment protocol for fractures of the odontoid process. J Spinal Disord 1996;9:267–276

41. Lennarson PJ, Mostafavi H, Traynelis VC, Walters BC. Management of type II dens fractures: a case-control study. Spine 2000;25: 1234–1237

42. Seybold EA, Bayley JC. Functional outcome of surgically and conservatively managed dens fractures. Spine 1998;23:1837–1845

43. Pepin JW, Bourne RB, Hawkins RJ. Odontoid fractures, with special reference to the elderly patient. Clin Orthop Relat Res 1985;193:178–183

44. Andersson S, Rodrigues M, Olerud C. Odontoid fractures: high complication rate associated with anterior screw fixation in the elderly. Eur Spine J 2000;9:56–59

45. Polin RS, Szabo T, Bogaev CA, Replogle RE, Jane JA. Nonoperative management of types II and III odontoid fractures: the Philadelphia collar versus the halo vest. Neurosurgery 1996;38:450–456

46. Muller EJ, Schwinnen I, Fischer K, Wick M, Muhr G. Non-rigid immobilisation of odontoid fractures. Eur Spine J 2003;12:522–525

47. Schneider RC, Livingston KE, Cave AJ, Hamilton G. "Hangman's fracture" of the cervical spine. J Neurosurg 1965;22:141–154

48. Wood-Jones F. The ideal lesion produced by judicial hanging. Lancet 1913;1:53

49. Pepin JW, Hawkins RJ. Traumatic spondylolisthesis of the axis: hangman's fracture. Clin Orthop Relat Res 1981;157:133–138

50. Francis WR, Fielding JW, Hawkins RJ, Pepin J, Hensinger R. Traumatic spondylolisthesis of the axis. J Bone Joint Surg Br 1981;63-B:313–318

51. Effendi B, Roy D, Cornish B, Dussault RG, Laurin CA. Fractures of the ring of the axis: a classification based on the analysis of 131 cases. J Bone Joint Surg Br 1981;63-B:319–327

52. Levine AM, Edwards CC. The management of traumatic spondylolisthesis of the axis. J Bone Joint Surg Am 1985;67:217–226

53. Starr JK, Eismont FJ. Atypical hangman's fractures. Spine 1993;18:1954–1957

54. Greene KA, Dickman CA, Marciano FF, Drabier JB, Hadley MN, Sonntag VK. Acute axis fractures: analysis of management and outcome in 340 consecutive cases. Spine 1997;22:1843–1852

55. Li XF, Dai LY, Lu H, Chen XD. A systematic review of the management of hangman's fractures. Eur Spine J 2006;15:257–269

56. Grady MS, Howard MA, Jane JA, Persing JA. Use of the Philadelphia collar as an alternative to the halo vest in patients with C-2, C-3 fractures. Neurosurgery 1986;18:151–156

57. Coric D, Wilson JA, Kelly DL Jr. Treatment of traumatic spondylolisthesis of the axis with nonrigid immobilization: a review of 64 cases. J Neurosurg 1996;85:550–554

58. Benzel EC, Hart BL, Ball PA, Baldwin NG, Orrison WW, Espinosa M. Fractures of the C-2 vertebral body. J Neurosurg 1994;81:206–212

59. Burke JT, Harris JH Jr. Acute injuries of the axis vertebra. Skeletal Radiol 1989;18:335–346

60. Fujimura Y, Nishi Y, Kobayashi K. Classification and treatment of axis body fractures. J Orthop Trauma 1996;10:536–540

61. Gleizes V, Jacquot FP, Signoret F, Feron JM. Combined injuries in the upper cervical spine: clinical and epidemiological data over a 14-year period. Eur Spine J 2000;9:386–392

62. Dickman CA, Hadley MN, Browner C, Sonntag VK. Neurosurgical management of acute atlas-axis combination fractures: a review of 25 cases. J Neurosurg 1989;70:45–49

63. Fujimura Y, Nishi Y, Chiba K, Kobayashi K. Prognosis of neurological deficits associated with upper cervical spine injuries. Paraplegia 1995;33:195–202

64. Holdsworth H. Fractures, dislocations, and fractures-dislocations of the spine. J Bone Joint Surg Br 1963;45:6–20

65. Allen BL Jr, Ferguson RL, Lehmann TR, O'Brien RP. A mechanistic classification of closed, indirect fractures and dislocations of the lower cervical spine. Spine 1982;7:1–27

66. Pintar FA, Yoganandan N, Voo L. Effect of age and loading rate on human cervical spine injury threshold. Spine 1998;23:1957–1962

67. Yoganandan N, Pintar F, Butler J, Reinartz J, Sances A Jr, Larson SJ. Dynamic response of human cervical spine ligaments. Spine 1989;14:1102–1110

68. White A III, Panjabi M. Clinical Biomechanics of Spine. 2nd ed. Philadelphia: JB Lippincott; 1990

69. Moore TA, Vaccaro AR, Anderson PA. Classification of lower cervical spine injuries. Spine 2006;31(suppl):S37–S43

70. Argenson C, De Peretti F, Ghabris A, Eude P, Lovet J, Hovorka I. A scheme for the classification of lower cervical spine injuries. Maîtrise Orthopédique 2006

71. Allen BL Jr, Ferguson RL, Lehmann TR, O'Brien RP. A mechanistic classification of closed, indirect fractures and dislocations of the lower cervical spine. Spine 1982;7:1–27

72. Harris JH Jr, Edeiken-Monroe B, Kopaniky DR. A practical classification of acute cervical spine injuries. Orthop Clin North Am 1986;17:15–30

73. Bucholz RD, Cheung KC. Halo vest versus spinal fusion for cervical injury: evidence from an outcome study. J Neurosurg 1989;70: 884–892

74. Frankel H, Michaelis L, Paeslack V. Closed injuries of the cervical spine and spinal cord: results of conservative treatment of extension rotation injuries of the cervical spine with tetraplegia. Proc Veterans Adm Spinal Cord Inj Conf 1973;19:52–55

75. Louis R. Cervical sprains and cervical herniated discs [author's tranls]. Nouv Presse Med 1979;8:1843–1849

76. Stemper BD, Yoganandan N, Pintar FA, Rao RD. Anterior longitudinal ligament injuries in whiplash may lead to cervical instability. Med Eng Phys 2005;28:515–524

77. Spitzer WO, Skovron ML, Salmi LR, et al. Scientific monograph of the Quebec Task Force on Whiplash-Associated Disorders: redefining "whiplash" and its management. Spine 1995;20(suppl): 1S–73S

78. Cusick JF, Yoganandan N, Pintar F, Gardon M. Cervical spine injuries from high-velocity forces: a pathoanatomic and radiologic study. J Spinal Disord 1996;9:1–7

79. Burke DC, Berryman D. The place of closed manipulation in the management of flexion-rotation dislocations of the cervical spine. J Bone Joint Surg Br 1971;53:165–182

80. Hadley MN, Fitzpatrick BC, Sonntag VK, Browner CM. Facet fracture-dislocation injuries of the cervical spine. Neurosurgery 1992;30:661–666

81. Sonntag VK. Management of bilateral locked facets of the cervical spine. Neurosurgery 1981;8:150–152

82. Grant GA, Mirza SK, Chapman JR, et al. Risk of early closed reduction in cervical spine subluxation injuries. J Neurosurg 1999;90(suppl):13–18

83. Maiman DJ, Barolat G, Larson SJ. Management of bilateral locked facets of the cervical spine. Neurosurgery 1986;18:542–547

84. Wolf A, Levi L, Mirvis S, et al. Operative management of bilateral facet dislocation. J Neurosurg 1991;75:883–890

85. Fehlings MG, Cooper PR, Errico TJ. Posterior plates in the management of cervical instability: long-term results in 44 patients. J Neurosurg 1994;81:341–349

86. Pateder DB, Carbone JJ. Lateral mass screw fixation for cervical spine trauma: associated complications and efficacy in maintaining alignment. Spine J 2006;6:40–43

87. Simon S, Davis M, Odhner D, Udupa J, Winkelstein B. CT imaging techniques for describing motions of the cervicothoracic junction and cervical spine during flexion, extension, and cervical traction. Spine 2006;31:44–50

88. Chapman JR, Anderson PA, Pepin C, Toomey S, Newell DW, Grady MS. Posterior instrumentation of the unstable cervicothoracic spine. J Neurosurg 1996;84:552–558

89. Rhee JM, Kraiwattanapong C, Hutton WC. A comparison of pedicle and lateral mass screw construct stiffnesses at the cervicothoracic junction: a biomechanical study. Spine 2005;30:E636–E640

10 Classification, Diagnosis, and Management of Thoracolumbar Spinal Injuries

Steven C. Zeiller, Eli M. Baron, Neel Anand, Alan S. Hilibrand, and Alexander R. Vaccaro

The diagnosis and treatment of patients with thoracolumbar spine fractures has evolved over the last two decades. Advances have been made in the transportation of these patients from the field, as well as in imaging of the spine, diagnosis, classification, and nonoperative and operative techniques. At the same time, significant controversy has persisted regarding the most appropriate treatment of the most common of these fractures, the thoracolumbar burst fracture. However, regardless of the type of intervention employed, the fundamental principles that govern treatment include restoration of the mechanical stability of the spine with correction of deformity and protection of the neural elements. These principles apply whether the patient undergoes nonoperative or operative intervention. This chapter reviews the critical factors that apply to the evaluation of patients with thoracolumbar fractures and discusses the management of these injuries.

■ Etiology

Thoracolumbar fractures can result from a variety of different mechanisms acting on the spine. The most common is an axial load combined with varying degrees of flexion resulting in a burst fracture. Motor vehicle accidents are the source of the vast majority of these injuries.[1] Other common etiologies include falls from a height, sports injuries, and penetrating trauma. This type of injury is most commonly seen in young males between the ages of 15 and 29.[2,3] The geriatric population also is affected, due to the high incidence of osteoporosis among the elderly. Burst fractures in the elderly population are increasing, and they usually result from low-energy trauma. Thoracolumbar fractures in the osteoporotic spine present their own unique challenges with regard to treatment. Bracing is typically poorly tolerated in the elderly population. Additionally, surgical stabilization in patients with osteoporotic bone presents its own challenges due to limited internal fixation stability.

The thoracolumbar spine is particularly vulnerable to traumatic injury due to its unique anatomy. The thoracolumbar junction serves as the transition between the more rigid, less mobile kyphotic thoracic spine and the less rigid, more mobile lordotic lumbar spine. The thoracic spine has narrow disk spaces and coronally oriented facets, which limit motion, especially in the sagittal plane. Additional stability is provided by the ribs articulating with the spine and sternum. By comparison, the lumbar spine has larger disks with sagittally oriented facets, which promote mobility of the spine in flexion and extension. Consequently, high-energy injuries are transmitted through the thoracic spine and dissipated at the thoracolumbar junction, resulting in characteristic fracture types.

■ Classification Systems

There have been several classification systems for thoracolumbar fractures proposed over the last several decades. The classification systems to date have been a variety of morphologic, anatomical, and mechanistic descriptions of the identified injury. The primary objective of most of these classification systems was to define a specific fracture pattern that would prognostically identify the stability of the spinal column. However, the definition of "clinical instability" has remained a source of controversy regarding the treatment of these patients.

One of the earlier classification systems proposed was by Nicoll[4] in 1949. Nicoll studied 166 fractures and fracture-dislocations in a population of 152 coal miners. The most common mechanism was compression with varying degrees of flexion. Stability in the neurologically intact patients was based on the integrity of the posterior ligamentous complex (PLC). Patients without a PLC injury (stable group) received functional treatment, which consisted of bed rest for 3 to 4 weeks until the patient could participate in physical therapy. In the unstable patients with PLC injury, treatment consisted of casting with prolonged bed rest until bony consolidation was complete. In terms of the work capacity in the group treated with casting, 27% returned to the coal face, 10% performed light work underground, and 63% performed light work on the surface. In the group treated "functionally," 55% returned to the coal face, 27% performed light work underground, and 18% performed light work on the surface.

Anatomical classification systems that divide the spine into columns were first popularized by Holdsworth's[5] "two column" theory in 1963. Holdsworth defined the anterior and posterior columns of bone and soft tissue based on their location relative to the neural elements. The anterior column included the vertebral body and disks as well as the anterior longitudinal ligament (ALL) and the posterior longitudinal ligament (PLL). The posterior column consisted of the posterior elements and the PLC. This was later modified by Denis[6] some 20 years later with the advent of cross-sectional imaging. Denis divided the spine into three columns, introducing the middle column. According to Denis's system, the anterior column consisted of the ALL and the anterior half of the vertebral body. He defined a third, "middle" column, consisting of the posterior half of the vertebral body, the annulus, and the PLL. As per Holdsworth's classification system, the posterior column consisted of the posterior spinal elements. The key factor that Denis proposed that contradicted Holdsworth's theory was that isolated rupture of the posterior column was insufficient to establish instability. Injury to the PLL and posterior annulus was necessary to impart instability of the spinal column. As a result, Denis proposed that spinal instability required disruption of at least two of the three columns. This classification system has arguably been the most popular system employed by North American spine surgeons to date.

Denis[6] identified four types of fractures based on the three-column theory (**Fig. 10.1**): compression fractures, which consist of compression failure of the anterior column; burst fractures involving both anterior and middle columns; seat belt injuries, which consist of distraction failure of the posterior and middle columns; and fracture dislocations involving all three columns. Within Denis's classification system, four types of fractures (and more than 20 subtypes) were described. Denis also described varying degrees of instability, including first degree, which was mechanical instability with a possibility of progressive deformity developing; second degree or neurologic instability, in which an injury may predispose to neurologic compromise; and third degree, which included combined mechanical and neurologic disability.

Denis's classification was closely followed by the classification system of McAfee et al,[7] which divided thoracolumbar fractures into six types based on examination of the computed tomography (CT) scans of 100 patients (**Table 10.1** and **Fig. 10.2**). In the McAfee system, the status of the middle column was most important for subclassification. The six subtypes were as follows: (1) wedge compression fracture (an isolated anterior column injury); (2) stable burst fracture (an injury to both the anterior and middle columns but not to the posterior column); (3) unstable burst fracture (compression injury to the anterior and middle column as well as injury to the posterior ligamentous complex); (4) flexion-distraction injury

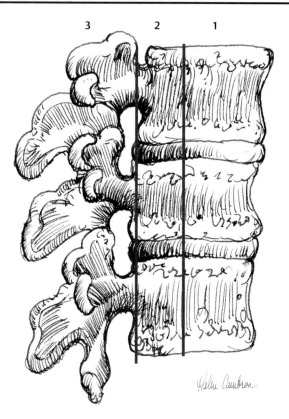

Fig. 10.1 Illustration of the Denis three-column theory. The anterior column includes the anterior longitudinal ligament, anulus fibrosus, and anterior one third of the vertebral body. The middle column includes the posterior two thirds of the vertebral body, posterior longitudinal ligament, and posterior anulus fibrosus. The posterior column includes the lamina, spinous processes, and all posterior elements in addition to the posterior ligamentous complex. (Courtesy of Helen Cambron, RN.)

(compression injury to the anterior column, tension injury of the middle column, and tension injury of the posterior column, where the mechanism of injury involved an anterior column fulcrum); (5) Chance-type fracture, where the anterior, middle, and posterior columns were all disrupted in tension via a flexion fulcrum anterior to the vertebral column, which differed from a flexion distraction injury, where the anterior column was disrupted via compression; and (6) translational injury, where shear forces were responsible for disruption of all three columns.

McCormack et al[8] subsequently devised a scoring mechanism that assisted in determining the need for adjunctive anterior column support following posterior short segment fixation of surgically treated thoracolumbar burst fractures. This scoring system addressed whether thoracolumbar fractures treated posteriorly alone via short segment fixation would be successfully treated in the long term or go on to instrumentation failure and spinal kyphosis. The scale consisted of three components: an assessment of the degree of fracture comminution, the degree of fracture fragment displacement, and the degree of required kyphosis correction.

Table 10.1 McAfee Classification System of Thoracolumbar Fractures

Wedge compression fracture	Isolated compression deformity of anterior vertebral body
Stable burst fracture	An isolated injury of anterior and posterior vertebral body
Unstable burst fracture	Injury to both anterior and posterior vertebral body but also to posterior elements
Flexion distraction injury	Anterior column compression, middle and posterior vertebral column disrupted in tension (anterior vertebral body served as a fulcrum for injury)
Chance-type fracture	Anterior and posterior vertebral body disrupted in tension, posterior elements disrupted in tension; the fulcrum here is anterior to the spinal column
Translational injury	Shear injury where all three columns of the spine are disrupted

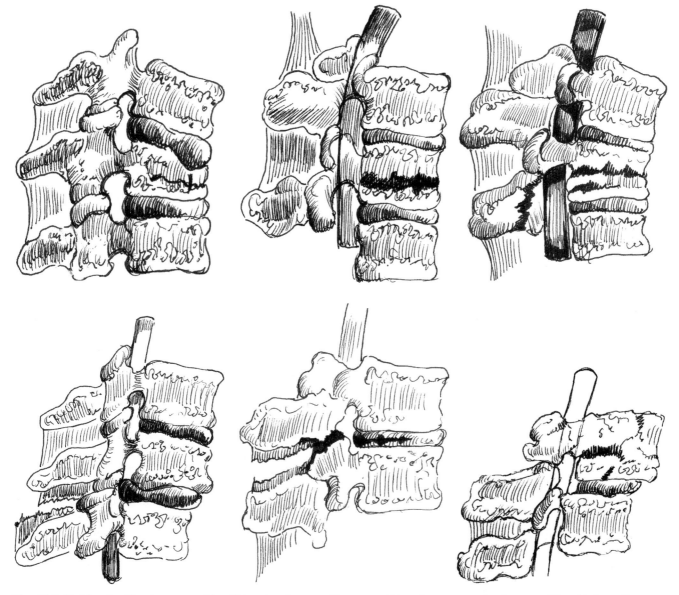

A–C

D–F

Fig. 10.2 McAfee classification system identifying six subtypes of fractures: **(A)** wedge compression fracture, **(B)** stable burst fracture, **(C)** unstable burst fracture, **(D)** flexion-distraction injury, **(E)** Chance fracture, and **(F)** translational injury. (Courtesy of Helen Cambron, RN.)

Magerl et al[9] proposed the Arbeitsgemeinschaft für Osteosynthesefragen (Association for the Study of Internal Fixation) (AO) classification system in 1994. This system was comprehensive in nature and employed both mechanistic and morphologic characteristics. The major categories of the system were based on the mechanism of injury (compression, distraction, translation). Within each major grouping, fracture subtypes were further categorized. This system is excellent for research purposes because it accounts for every fracture permutation, but due to its cumbersome nature (accounting for more than fracture subtypes), it has not been widely used clinically.

More recently, Vaccaro et al[10,11] proposed the Thoracolumbar Injury Classification and Injury Severity Score (TLICS). This system assesses three primary variables that dictate treatment of patients with thoracolumbar spine fractures: the morphology of the injury, the neurologic status of the patient, and the integrity of the PLC. Points in the scoring system are then assigned for each of the primary variables and their subtypes, creating a point total, the TLICS (**Table 10.2**). The total score is then used to dictate treatment based on a point scale. Injuries with 3 points or less are treated nonoperatively, whereas injuries with

5 points or more are treated operatively. Patients with 4 points may be treated in either fashion, based on other clinical parameters. To effectively use this scoring system, a few guidelines need to be followed. First, if there are multiple fractures present, the most severe injury is the only one that is scored. Fractures occurring at different spinal levels are not to be added together to determine the injury severity score. Second, only the morphology with the greatest point value is used. For instance, if a patient had a burst injury (2 points for the burst component) and a translational injury (3 points), only the points for translation would be counted because it has a higher value. The key to this system is that it provides a systematic approach to evaluate patients with thoracolumbar fractures using clinically relevant information.

■ Patient Evaluation

Initial Evaluation

Traumatized patients who have a sufficient mechanism should be treated as if they have a spinal fracture until proven otherwise. The patient should be collected in the field and transported while maintaining full spine precautions (use of cervical collar, log rolling, and transportation on a spine board). During the initial phase of the work-up in the emergency room, the patient should be managed according to the advanced trauma life support protocol. Once the patient's airway and hemodynamics have been stabilized, a more detailed examination can be performed. In the lucid patient a thorough neurologic examination (motor, sensory, rectal) can be performed. In addition, the spinal column can be palpated for pain and deformity. A detailed neurologic examination is crucial because the detection of a spinal cord injury or root injury (cauda equina) can have a major impact on the type and timing of the treatment of the patient. The neurologic status of the patient is one of the most important factors in determining whether the patient requires nonoperative or operative treatment. During the initial phase of the work-up of patients with suspected spinal trauma, it is important to keep track of how long the patient has been on the spine board. The patient should be taken off the board as soon as it is safe to do so, to ensure that there is no skin breakdown.

Radiographic Evaluation

The radiographic work-up of a patient suspected of having a spinal fracture typically begins with plain radiographs taken in the anteroposterior (AP) and lateral planes. The AP and lateral radiographs should be inspected for characteristic findings consistent with fractures in this region, including widened interpedicular distance and loss of vertebral body height. It is also critical to scrutinize the plain radiographs for evidence of any interspinous widening,

Table 10.2 Thoracolumbar Injury Classification and Severity Score (TLICS) System

Score is total of three components: injury morphology, neurologic status, and posterior ligamentary complex (PLC) disruption; a score of 3 or below suggests nonoperative treatment, 4 suggests operative or nonoperative treatment, and 5 or above suggests operative treatment.		
1. Description		**Points**
a. Compression fracture		1
b. Burst fracture		2
c. Translational/rotational		3
d. Distraction		4
2. PLC		**Points**
a. Intact		0
b. Suspected/indeterminate		2
c. Injured		3
3. Neurologic Status		
Involvement	**Qualifier**	**Points**
		0
Nerve root		2
Cord, conus medullaris	Incomplete	3
	Complete	2
Cauda equina		3

Source: Adapted from Lee JY, Vaccaro AR, Lim MR, et al. Thoracolumbar injury classification and severity score: a new paradigm for the treatment of thoracolumbar spine trauma. J Orthop Sci 2005;10(6):671–675.

thus implying a distraction mechanism. The fracture pattern should be analyzed to determine the morphology of injury (e.g., compression, distraction, translation). The determination of the fracture pattern provides a key piece of information regarding the amount of energy that caused the fracture and the resulting potential for instability. This also helps to stratify the patient with regard to treatment. Once a fracture is identified in the spinal column, it is mandatory to radiographically rule out contiguous and noncontiguous spinal fractures.

Plain films provide not only a useful method for screening for spinal fractures but also an assessment of both coronal and sagittal deformity in patients who have sustained thoracolumbar fractures. Traditionally, the kyphotic deformity that has warranted surgery was based on information obtained with the patient in the supine position with the spine in an unloaded position. Recently, the use of weight-bearing films in the subacute setting has been evaluated to see if they would alter management due to increased deformity in the loaded position. Mehta et al[12] performed a prospective study evaluating the use of weight-bearing films in patients with thoracolumbar fractures to see if they influenced management. Twenty-eight patients without neurologic deficits were evaluated. The mean Cobb angle in the supine position was 11 degrees, which increased to a mean of 18 degrees on weight-bearing films (either sitting or standing). The mean anterior vertebral body height compression changed from 36 to 46% when taken with the patient in the supine position and in the weight-bearing position, respectively. The authors of this study operated on patients with vertebral body collapse of 50% or more, the presence of a neurologic deficit or fracture-dislocation, or kyphosis of > 20 degrees. Based on their findings with regard to vertebral body collapse and kyphotic angle found on weight-bearing films, seven patients underwent operative stabilization who were initially going to be treated conservatively based on supine measurements. The authors concluded that in some patients a weight-bearing film might demonstrate a more significant injury that may have been missed using only supine plain film surveillance.

Computed tomography has played an integral role in the diagnostic work-up of patients with thoracolumbar fractures. The images generated in the axial plane when combined with the sagittal and coronal reconstructions allow the surgeon to clearly identify the fracture pattern. There are several factors that should be evaluated on CT images. First, is there disruption of the posterior vertebral body with retropulsed bone into the canal? This is the fundamental difference between a "compression" fracture, which rarely requires operative management, and a "burst" fracture, which is more likely to be associated with instability and a neurologic deficit. Second, is there a fracture of the lamina at these levels? If so, a posterior approach to address nerve root entrapment may be needed.

In addition, if operative treatment is indicated, the axial images provide information to allow the surgeon to determine if uninjured levels can accommodate pedicular fixation. Finally, the facet joints should be evaluated for any signs of subluxation suggesting a possible capsular or PLC injury. Injury to the PLC is an important finding because loss of this tension band places the patient at risk for developing a kyphotic deformity.

The use of CT in the polytraumatized patient as a screening tool has been studied. Hauser et al[13] evaluated 221 consecutive patients sustaining high-risk trauma that warranted plain films of the thoracolumbar spine. The accuracy of plain radiographs in diagnosing an injury was compared with CT of the chest, abdomen, and pelvis. The accuracy of CT for fractures in the thoracolumbar spine was 99% compared with 87% for plain films. Another important finding in the study was the time to spinal clearance. CT examination as a screening tool to clear the thoracolumbar spine took on average approximately 1 hour compared with 295 minutes for plain radiographs. Brandt et al[14] hypothesized that the data acquired from the thoracic and abdominal CT images were sufficient to screen for spinal fractures. They evaluated 207 polytraumatized patients in a retrospective fashion; 24% of patients had a spinal fracture on CT not recognized on plain films. Most of the missed fractures were transverse process fractures. The authors reported the average time required to perform a CT of the chest, abdomen, and pelvis was 55 minutes ± 32 minutes compared with 113 minutes ± 113 minutes for plain film screening for spinal fracture. The authors also noted that if only CT of the chest, abdomen, and pelvis had been ordered to screen for thoracolumbar fracture as opposed to plain films and a dedicated spinal CT, the cost savings would have been over $800 per patient.

The role of magnetic resonance imaging (MRI) in the evaluation of patients with thoracolumbar trauma is evolving. Although many clinicians reserve this imaging modality for patients with neurologic injury, valuable information can be obtained with regard to neural compression and edema patterns in both bony and soft tissue structures. Probably one of the most important roles in MRI is in evaluating the integrity of the PLC. Edema, denoted by hyperintensity of the posterior ligamentous structures on fat-suppressed T2-weighted images, is highly suggestive of a PLC injury (**Fig. 10.3**).

Lee et al[15] prospectively evaluated 34 patients with thoracolumbar fractures with MRI to compare its sensitivity, specificity, and reliability with physical examination, plain radiographs, and intraoperative findings when evaluating the integrity of the PLC. The sensitivity of detecting a PLC injury on physical examination (palpation of the spine) was 52.0%, specificity was 66.7%, and accuracy was 53.6%. The sensitivity, specificity, and accuracy of plain films were 66.7%. The sensitivity of MRI in evaluation of the supraspinous ligament was

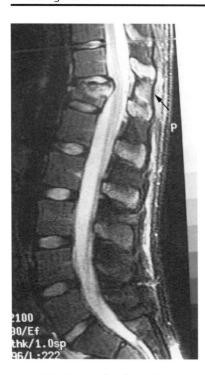

Fig. 10.3 T2-weighted sagittal magnetic resonance imaging demonstrating an unstable burst fracture. Note the evidence of posterior ligamentary complex disruption, where high signal is seen within the interspinous ligament (*arrow*).

92.9%, specificity was 80.0%, and accuracy was 90.9%. The sensitivity of MRI in evaluation of the interspinous ligament was 100%, specificity was 75%, and accuracy was 97%. The authors found a statistically significant relationship between MRI and intraoperative findings. The authors concluded that a fat-suppressed T2 was a highly sensitive, specific, and accurate method of evaluating the integrity of the PLC.

Oner et al[16] reported prospectively on 53 patients with 71 thoracolumbar fractures. The authors used MRI parameters developed in a previous study to predict complications associated with operative and nonoperative treatment.[17] These parameters included evaluating the integrity of the anterior and posterior longitudinal ligaments and end plates and noting the edema pattern in the vertebral body (edema pattern was determined on the sagittal MR images). Twenty-four patients were treated nonoperatively, and 29 patients were treated operatively (operative treatment consisted of segmental posterior pedicle screw fixation in 28 patients and one anterior decompression and stand-alone anterior fusion) with a 2-year follow-up. MRI scans were obtained within 1 week of the injury and at the 2-year follow-up. Based on the results of the study, the authors were able to make the following conclusions regarding the development of sagittal plane deformity. In the nonoperative group, involvement of more than one third of the vertebral body as evidenced by bone bruise on MRI in combination with cranial end-plate involvement resulted in more than a 50% chance of the kyphosis angle increasing. In the operative group, the authors noted that end-plate comminution, vertebral body involvement (edema involving more than one third of the body on sagittal MR images), injury to the PLC, and degree of correction were predictive of recurrent deformity. The authors concluded that MRI can be a useful adjunct in evaluation of patients with thoracolumbar fractures because it can demonstrate the extent of bony and soft tissue injuries. This information can in turn provide prognostic criteria on the likelihood of recurrent deformity in both operative and nonoperative patients.

■ Nonoperative Treatment

Most patients who sustain fractures in the thoracolumbar spine can be treated in a nonoperative fashion. The patient should have a detailed neurologic exam combined with careful scrutiny of all imaging studies. Ideal candidates for nonoperative treatment include those patients who are neurologically intact with either a compression or burst fracture and who do not have an injury to the PLC. Typically, these patients have a sagittal deformity of < 25 degrees, and the anterior column should be able to support the spinal column and upper body load.

If possible, the traumatized patient should be managed on a rotating bed to facilitate pulmonary function and prevent decubitus ulcer formation. Once the patient has been stabilized and is comfortable, he or she can be transferred to a regular hospital bed. At this point the patient either should be fitted with a custom-molded orthosis (thoracolumbar spinal orthosis, TLSO) or should be placed in a cast. Following mobilization, a standing radiograph on a 36-inch cassette with AP and lateral views should be obtained to ensure that overall coronal and sagittal alignments are acceptable.

There have been numerous studies in the literature reporting on the results of nonoperative treatment of thoracolumbar fractures in neurologically intact patients. Weinstein et al[18] performed a retrospective study that evaluated 42 patients who sustained traumatic burst fractures. The average follow-up was 20 years. At final follow-up, on a 10-point scale, with 0 being no pain and 10 representing severe pain, the average back pain score was 3.5. No patient had a deterioration in the neurologic exam at the final evaluation; 88% of patients were able to work at their preexisting level of activity. Radiographically, at final follow-up the average kyphosis in flexion was 26.4 degrees and in extension was 16.8 degrees. The authors found no correlation between the residual kyphotic deformity and the pain and functional scores at final follow-up.

Shen and Shen[19] retrospectively reviewed the outcome of patients with three-column thoracolumbar injuries. Thirty-eight patients had traumatic burst fractures and were evaluated with an average of 4-year follow-up. No reductions were performed. Patients were allowed to ambulate when comfortable. Twenty-nine patients did not wear any brace, whereas 9 patients wore a Jewett-type orthosis. All patients remained neurologically intact. The initial kyphosis angle averaged 20 degrees (range 10–35 degrees), and at follow-up it averaged 24 degrees (range 12–38 degrees). Thirty-two patients had none or mild pain, and 6 had moderate to severe pain at follow-up. The authors concluded that their less restrictive protocol of not enforcing brace wear provided results comparable to more formal bracing regimens.

■ Operative Treatment

Indications for the operative treatment of thoracolumbar fracture are based on whether a neurologic deficit is present, whether there is canal compromise or deformity, and whether there is disruption of the PLC. Depending on fracture type, surgical indications vary.

Compression fractures rarely require surgical intervention. In the elderly, osteoporotic compression fractures are very common. Those that continue to be painful and debilitating following 6 weeks of nonoperative treatment may be amenable to percutaneous cement stabilization procedures such as vertebroplasty or kyphoplasty. Compression fractures resulting in more than a 50% loss of height of the anterior vertebral body or an initial kyphosis of greater than 20 to 30 degrees may benefit from surgery.[12,20,21] As mentioned above, 36-inch cassette standing weight-bearing films may reveal considerably more kyphosis than supine films and may aid in the assessment of the neurologically intact patient who has no evidence of initial instability radiographically.[12]

Burst fractures are more likely to benefit from surgical intervention than compression fractures. Nevertheless, the majority of cases also may be treated nonoperatively. Wood et al,[22] in a controlled prospective randomized trial, found no benefit to surgical treatment versus conservative treatment for stable burst fractures in the absence of neurologic

deficit. Findings that may favor surgical treatment over conservative treatment include retropulsion of bony fragments into the canal with resultant neurologic deficit and evidence of a PLC disruption, including greater than 20 to 30 degrees of kyphotic angulation, subluxation of the facets, or an increase in intraspinous distance.[20,21,23–25] The management of flexion distraction injuries is based on the degree of bony versus soft tissue injury present. Typically in younger patients, primarily bony injury of the facet and posterior vertebral body occurs; thus body casting and a hyperextension cast may be useful.[26] When these injuries occur, however, in adults, these injuries typically involve the intervertebral disk and ligamentous complex. Thus, posterior operative reduction stabilization is usually the management of choice. Fracture-dislocation injuries of the thoracolumbar spine are extremely unstable and invariably will require operative stabilization.[20]

The Timing of Surgery

The timing of surgery for thoracolumbar spinal injuries remains controversial. Even though early surgery in patients who sustain polytrauma may be associated with fewer respiratory and medical complications and shorter hospital stays,[27] the timing of surgery has not yet been correlated with neurologic prognosis. In patients with complete injuries, early decompression has not been shown to be beneficial despite the theoretical advantage of earlier decompression resulting in neurologic improvement.[21] Additionally, the timing of surgery for incomplete injuries is controversial. Delayed surgery has been correlated with reduced perioperative blood loss compared with early surgery. An early posterior approach (less than 24 hours after injury) may allow improved sagittal alignment and improved canal clearance via a ligamentotaxis.[21,28,29]

Surgical Management Principles (Table 10.3)

For compression fractures where persistent pain remains despite bracing and conservative treatment, vertebroplasty or kyphoplasty may be beneficial. Vertebroplasty is very

Table 10.3 Surgical Strategies for Thoracolumbar Fractures

Vertebroplasty/kyphoplasty	Typically used for compression fractures; may be useful in select burst fracture cases; may have a role in the surgical management of patients with thoracolumbar fractures and osteoporosis
Ligamentotaxis	May be a useful strategy to reduce retropulsed bone fragments in the first few days after injury
Anterior decompression and fusion	Theoretically may result in a more satisfactory decompression over the posterior approach; additionally, allows for reconstruction of the anterior and middle columns; may be augmented with instrumentation; may need an additional posterior approach if the PLC is injured
Posterior fusion	The mainstay surgical strategy when the PLC has been injured; may be combined with transpedicular/lateral extracavitary approach for anterior decompression and provision of anterior column support; in posterior only constructs, without anterior column support, short segment fixation has a high failure rate, so the dictum has been extension of the fusion at two levels above and below the injury

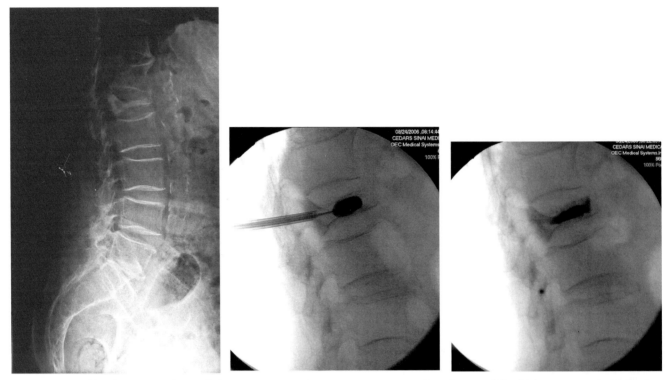

A–C

Fig. 10.4 Lateral lumbar spine radiograph demonstrating an L1 osteoporotic compression fracture **(A)**, which was treated with kyphoplasty where an inflatable bone tamp **(B)** is inserted through the pedicle followed by injection of polymethyl methacrylate cement **(C)**.

useful for patients with intense focal midline pain.[30] Kyphoplasty is also very useful for pain management and has demonstrated excellent results regardless of vertebral height restoration.[31] Additionally, kyphoplasty has a theoretical advantage of a controlled cavity being created by the surgeon using an inflatable bone tamp (**Fig. 10.4**). Kyphoplasty may be done in the thoracic spine via a unilateral or a bilateral approach. Recently, both vertebroplasty and kyphoplasty have been used for open vertebral cement augmentation for patients sustaining thoracolumbar osteoporotic burst fractures.[32] This allows for the treatment of the fracture with these modalities in the presence of retropulsed bone fragments.[20]

Burst fractures more commonly require surgical treatment than do compression fractures. This may be done via a posterior, anterior, or combined approach. Advantages of the posterior approach include its relative safety, anatomical familiarity for the majority of spine surgeons, and ability to reconstruct the posterior tension band. Additionally, canal decompression can be achieved via a transpedicular approach. In this manner the anterior column can be reconstructed even when there is significant structural disruption (**Fig. 10.5**).[21]

Short segment fixation in the setting of a thoracolumbar burst fracture has a high failure rate; as a result, multiple points of fixation have been advocated above and below the level of injury.[21] Additionally, within the first few days of the injury, retropulsed fragments may be more efficiently reduced via ligamentotaxis rather than on a delayed basis.[33–36]

In the presence of an incomplete neurologic deficit and anterior compressive pathology, an anterior approach is an efficient means of thoroughly decompressing the spinal canal. Anterior decompression and stabilization without a posterior procedure may be performed when there is no evidence of PLC injury.[37] Anterior surgery may also be useful to address the instability associated with severe anterior and middle column failure (**Fig. 10.6**). Without anterior column support, posterior instrumentation is subject to strong cantilever bending moments and thus may be predisposed to failure.[38] Nevertheless, prospective studies fail to demonstrate that an anterior approach is more likely to result in neurologic improvement in a neurologically compromised individual.[1,37,39–41] Additionally, a recent study found anterior surgery to have similar outcomes to posterior stabilization but with a lower complication rate.[42] The theoretical benefit of an anterior approach is the increased clearance of the spinal canal by removal of retropulsed bone fragments, as compared to a posterior approach, which does so indirectly.[37,43] The anterior approach selected depends on the surgeon's experience. Approaches described include a thoracotomy in the thoracic spine, a thoracoabdominal approach across the thoracolumbar junction, and retroperitoneal and transperitoneal approaches in the lumbar spine.[21] Lumbar endoscopic and thoracoscopic

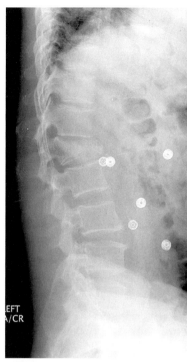

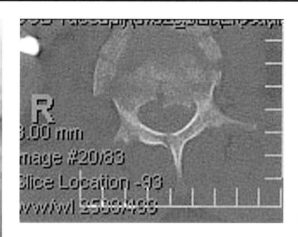

A

B

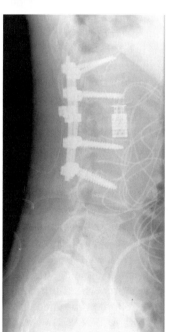

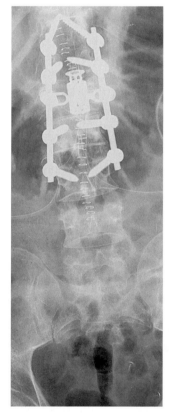

Fig. 10.5 (A,B) Plain radiographs and CT demonstrating an unstable burst fracture at L1 where evidence of PLC disruption was noted on MRI. **(C–E)** The patient was treated with transpedicular decompression, cage placement with autologous bone graft, pedicle screw fixation two levels above and below with onlay bone graft.

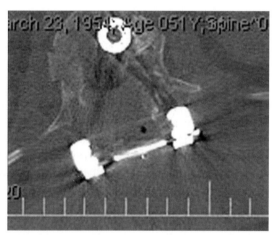

C

D

E

approaches have also been performed with good outcomes.[44–48] Anterior procedures allow direct decompression and reconstruction of the anterior and middle columns using bone strut grafting or metallic or synthetic cages. The construct can then be further reinforced with a screw-rod system or screw-plate system. Dual rods with a cross-link are effectively similar to rodding.[49] Although numerous systems are effective in restoring the stability of the spine in conjunction with an anterior bone strut, the Kaneda device has been known to be particularly strong in regard

to rotational stability.[50] Dynamized instrumented stabilization may also be useful, as it allows compression of the graft, thus promoting fusion while protecting the graft from shear and rotational stresses.[51]

If there is also a PLC injury in the setting of an anterior column injury, a posterior procedure is often required in addition to the anterior procedure. Circumferential fusion may also be useful in sparing additional segments of the fusion should a posterior procedure be done alone, and also may be useful in reducing the need for rigid anterior

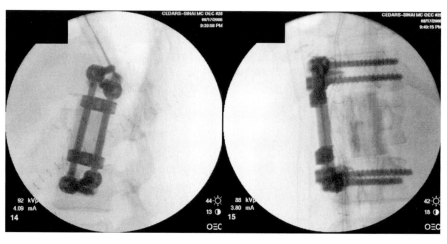

A   B

Fig. 10.6 (A) Unstable L1 burst fracture in a patient sustaining a motorcycle accident. This resulted in the patient being a T12 American Spinal Injury Association (ASIA) class A paraplegic. **(B)** The patient was initially treated with anterior vertebrectomy with femoral shaft allograft strut grafting with anterolateral rodding and cross-linking.

fixation (**Fig. 10.7**).[52] Alternatives to a combined anterior and posterior approach include the lateral extracavitary approach and the transpedicular approach for ventral decompression.[53,54] The lateral extracavitary approach may be associated with a relatively high morbidity in up to 55% of patients in the acute setting, with hemothorax and pleural effusions being among the more common complications. The morbidity of a lateral extracavitary approach or circumferential decompression and stabilization procedure must be weighed against the biomechanical advantages conferred by these procedures.[54]

Surgical management of flexion/distraction injuries is guided by the fulcrum axis of rotation of the injury.[20] If the axis of rotation of injury lies within the anterior vertebral body (i. e., compression failure), distraction may be applied to the anterior longitudinal segment via a posterior approach using a pedicle screw posterior cantilever construct. If this is done, great caution must be taken to avoid distracting the posterior vertebral body and posterior elements. The risk of this may be reduced by using temporary wires around the bony posterior elements of the segments bordering the fracture while the distraction maneuver is being performed. If the posterior vertebral body is intact, a posterior compression construct may be performed, extending one level above and below the injury.[55] If, however, the posterior vertebral body is disrupted, then due to the more posterior location of the axis of rotation, compression must be performed very carefully to avoid retropulsion of either disk or bone into the spinal canal.[56–58] In the situation of a flexion-distraction injury with posterior vertebral body disruption, it may be of benefit to extend the fusion segment two levels rostral and caudal to the injury or to consider an anterior procedure in addition to posterior stabilization.[21]

Fracture-dislocation injuries are highly unstable and usually require an initial posterior reduction and stabi-

lization, which would span at least two levels above and below the level of injury (**Fig. 10.8**). If there is a neurologically incomplete injury, CT scanning should be performed after posterior reduction and stabilization to assess the adequacy of the decompression of the spinal canal. If the spinal canal is insufficiently decompressed, a subsequent anterior decompression and stabilization can be performed. Patients sustaining complete injuries, however, can undergo an isolated posterior reduction and multisegment stabilization.[20,21]

Several authors have proposed techniques in an attempt to avoid long posterior fusions and thus reduce the morbidity from decreased mobility and theoretically higher rates of adjacent segment degeneration. Ebelke et al[59] advocated a supplemental anterior bone grafting via a transpedicular approach at the levels of fracture to theoretically supplement the anterior vertebral column and decrease bending moments on posterior instrumentation. Nevertheless, a prospective trial of bone grafting with short-segment instrumentation failed to find an increased benefit over short-segment fixation with only a posterior applied fusion mass. Both groups had unacceptably high failure rates of 40 to 50%.[60] Transpedicular injection of polymethylmethacrylate at levels of pedicle screw placement has also been performed to theoretically decrease the rate of screw failure in short-segment fusions.[61,62]

Recently, minimally invasive spine surgery techniques have been used for the treatment of thoracolumbar fractures.[63–66] Minimal invasive techniques may allow decompression and stabilization with reduced patient morbidity. One example of this is percutaneous posterior stabilization, which may be used to supplement anterior vertebrectomy and fusion (**Fig. 10.9**). As technologies evolve in this area, more widespread adaptation may be seen.

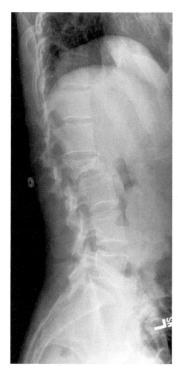

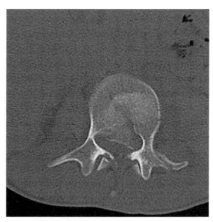

Fig. 10.7 **(A)** Lateral radiograph and **(B)** axial CT scan demonstrating an unstable burst fracture in a 22-year-old neurologically intact woman sustaining a fall. Postoperative **(C)** anteroposterior and **(D)** lateral plain radiographs, where an expandable cage with bone graft and anterolateral rodding/cross-linking followed by posterior pedicle screw fixation and onlay fusion were performed.

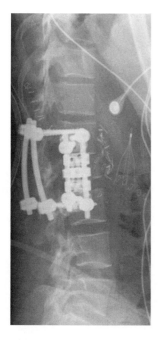

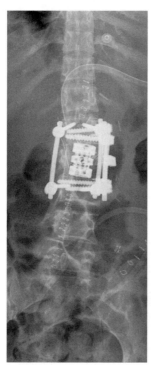

Complications

Surgery for thoracolumbar burst fractures has a defined complication rate ranging as high as 15% in one series. In a review of 682 patients, Knop et al[67] reported complications requiring surgical revision in 6% and a 9% rate of complications not requiring surgical revision in patients undergoing surgery for thoracolumbar fractures. Complications not requiring return to surgery included intraoperative bleeding, iatrogenic pedicle fracture, instrumentation misplacement, instability or subsequent malalignment, infection, healing problems at the bone graft site, iatrogenic rib fractures, pleural injury, spinal canal narrowing secondary to instrumentation, fracture at the iliac crest bone grafting harvesting site, and a dural tear. Complications requiring return to surgery included deep wound infections in 2.2% of patients, hematoma, persistent wound problems, instability or segmental malalignment, instrumentation misplacement, persistent spinal fluid leak, a sewn-in drain, and vascular thrombosis. Neurologic complications occurred in 2% of patients. Neurologic deterioration (cord) was seen in 0.4% of

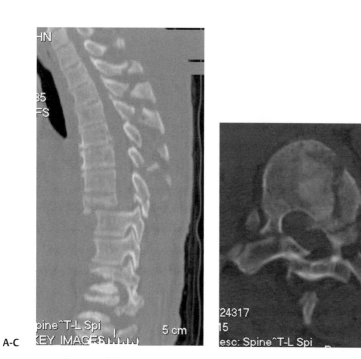
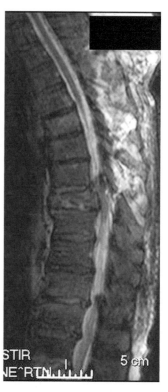

Fig. 10.8 T8 fracture dislocation demonstrated on CT scan on **(A)** sagittal reconstruction and on **(B)** axial imaging. **(C)** T2-weighted sagittal MRI through the region of injury.

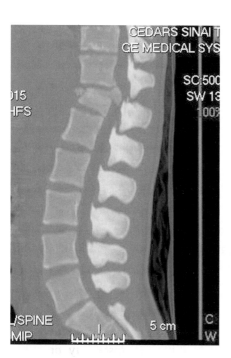
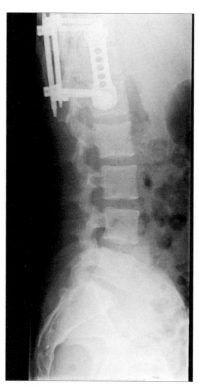
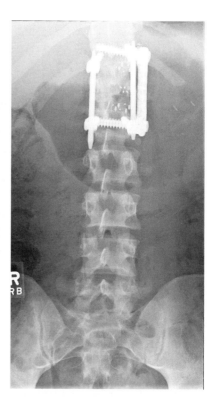

Fig. 10.9 (A) CT sagittal reconstruction of an unstable burst fracture at L1 in a 19-year-old man (with six lumbar vertebrae) sustaining a motor vehicle accident with a subsequent conus injury. **(B,C)** Plain radiographs following treatment demonstrating anterior corpectomy and placement of an expandable polyether-ether-ketone cage filled with local bone from the corpectomy followed by minimally invasive percutaneous pedicle screw stabilization.

patients, and nerve root injury was seen in 0.7% of patients. Nevertheless, given the fact that 42% of their patients had other injuries, the authors cautioned against generalizing the results to all patients undergoing surgery for thoracolumbar fractures.

Instrumentation failure has been reported at a rate of 15% in patients undergoing surgical treatment of thoracolumbar fractures followed for longer than 5 years. Nevertheless, only one third of the patients experiencing instrumentation failure required revision in one series.[68] Pseudarthrosis following surgical treatment of thoracolumbar fractures has been described as occurring in 2 to 8% of cases, with the highest incidence seen at the thoracolumbar junction.[20]

■ Conclusion

The majority of thoracolumbar fractures can be treated in a conservative fashion. A thorough physical examination and radiographic work-up are critical in determining the most appropriate treatment of these patients. The use of advanced imaging including three-dimensional reconstruction images is improving our understanding of these complex injuries. The introduction of MRI with higher strength magnetic fields and the use of more sophisticated software to interpret CT image data will potentially provide the clinician with more information that will become relevant to fracture care. It is critical to evaluate the patient in a systematic fashion, with emphasis being placed on the mechanism of injury, neurologic status of the patient, and the integrity of the PLC. These elements should define the mechanical and neurologic stability of patients and help stratify them into operative versus nonoperative treatment.

Surgical indications are based on whether neurologic compromise, deformity, and instability are present. The posterior approach effectively addresses injury to the PLC and may be used to achieve spinal alignment and decompression. An anterior approach may result in better neural element decompression, restoration of the anterior and middle columns, and possibly restoration of lordosis. Although a circumferential short-segment fusion may offer the best biomechanical solution, any theoretical benefit must be carefully weighed against the morbidity of additional surgical intervention. Complications seen with surgical management of thoracolumbar fractures are predictable and can be minimized through thorough operative planning, meticulous technique, and attentive postoperative care.

References

1. Gertzbein SD. Scoliosis Research Society. Multicenter spine fracture study. Spine 1992;17:528–540
2. Ball ST, Vaccaro AR, Albert TJ, Cotler JM. Injuries of the thoracolumbar spine associated with restraint use in head-on motor vehicle accidents. J Spinal Disord 2000;13:297–304
3. Holmes JF, Miller PQ, Panacek EA, Lin S, Horne NS, Mower WR. Epidemiology of thoracolumbar spine injury in blunt trauma. Acad Emerg Med 2001;8:866–872
4. Nicoll EA. Fractures of the dorso-lumbar spine. J Bone Joint Surg Br 1949;31:376–394
5. Holdsworth FW. Fractures, dislocations, and fracture-dislocations of the spine. J Bone Joint Surg Br 1963;45:6–20
6. Denis F. The three column spine and its significance in the classification of acute thoracolumbar spinal injuries. Spine 1983;8:817–831
7. McAfee PC, Yuan HA, Fredrickson BE, Lubicky JP. The value of computed tomography in thoracolumbar fractures: an analysis of one hundred consecutive cases and a new classification. J Bone Joint Surg Am 1983;65:461–473
8. McCormack T, Karaikovic E, Gaines RW. The load sharing classification of spine fractures. Spine 1994;19:1741–1744
9. Magerl F, Aebi M, Gertzbein SD, Harms J, Nazarian S. A comprehensive classification of thoracic and lumbar injuries. Eur Spine J 1994;3:184–201
10. Lee JY, Vaccaro AR, Lim MR, et al. Thoracolumbar Injury Classification and Severity Score: a new paradigm for the treatment of thoracolumbar spine trauma. J Orthop Sci 2005;10:671–675
11. Vaccaro AR, Zeiller SC, Hulbert RJ, et al. The Thoracolumbar Injury Severity Score: a proposed treatment algorithm. J Spinal Disord Tech 2005;18:209–215
12. Mehta JS, Reed MR, McVie JL, Sanderson PL. Weight-bearing radiographs in thoracolumbar fractures: do they influence management? Spine 2004;29:564–567
13. Hauser CJ, Visvikis G, Hinrichs C, et al. Prospective validation of computed tomographic screening of the thoracolumbar spine in trauma. J Trauma 2003;55:228–234 discussion 234–225
14. Brandt MM, Wahl WL, Yeom K, Kazerooni E, Wang SC. Computed tomographic scanning reduces cost and time of complete spine evaluation. J Trauma 2004;56:1022–1026 discussion 1026–1028
15. Lee HM, Kim HS, Kim DJ, Suk KS, Park JO, Kim NH. Reliability of magnetic resonance imaging in detecting posterior ligament complex injury in thoracolumbar spinal fractures. Spine 2000;25:2079–2084
16. Oner FC, van Gils AP, Faber JA, Dhert WJ, Verbout AJ. Some complications of common treatment schemes of thoracolumbar spine fractures can be predicted with magnetic resonance imaging: prospective study of 53 patients with 71 fractures. Spine 2002;27:629–636
17. Oner FC, van Gils AP, Dhert WJ, Verbout AJ. MRI findings of thoracolumbar spine fractures: a categorisation based on MRI examinations of 100 fractures. Skeletal Radiol 1999;28:433–443
18. Weinstein JN, Collalto P, Lehmann TR. Thoracolumbar "burst" fractures treated conservatively: a long-term follow-up. Spine 1988;13:33–38
19. Shen WJ, Shen YS. Nonsurgical treatment of three-column thoracolumbar junction burst fractures without neurologic deficit. Spine 1999;24:412–415
20. Singh K, Vaccaro AR, Eichenbaum MD, Fitzhenry LN. The surgical management of thoracolumbar injuries. J Spinal Cord Med 2004;27:95–101

21. Baron EM, Zeiller SC, Vaccaro AR, Hilibrand AS. Surgical management of thoracolumbar fractures. Contemporary Spine Surg. 2005;6:1–9

22. Wood K, Buttermann G, Mehbod A, et al. Operative compared with nonoperative treatment of a thoracolumbar burst fracture without neurological deficit: a prospective, randomized study. J Bone Joint Surg Am 2003;85-A:773–781

23. Vollmer DG, Gegg C. Classification and acute management of thoracolumbar fractures. Neurosurg Clin N Am 1997;8:499–507

24. Mikles MR, Stchur RP, Graziano GP. Posterior instrumentation for thoracolumbar fractures. J Am Acad Orthop Surg 2004;12:424–435

25. McDonough PW, Davis R, Tribus C, Zdeblick TA. The management of acute thoracolumbar burst fractures with anterior corpectomy and Z-plate fixation. Spine 2004;29:1901–1908, discussion 1909

26. Rechtine GR II, Cahill D, Chrin AM. Treatment of thoracolumbar trauma: comparison of complications of operative versus nonoperative treatment. J Spinal Disord 1999;12:406–409

27. Chipman JG, Deuser WE, Beilman GJ. Early surgery for thoracolumbar spine injuries decreases complications. J Trauma 2004;56:52–57

28. Yazici M, Gulman B, Sen S, Tilki K. Sagittal contour restoration and canal clearance in burst fractures of the thoracolumbar junction (T12–L1): the efficacy of timing of the surgery. J Orthop Trauma 1995;9:491–498

29. Vaccaro AR, Daugherty RJ, Sheehan TP, et al. Neurologic outcome of early versus late surgery for cervical spinal cord injury. Spine 1997;22:2609–2613

30. Peh WC, Gilula LA. Percutaneous vertebroplasty: indications, contraindications, and technique. Br J Radiol 2003;76:69–75

31. Feltes C, Fountas KN, Machinis T, et al. Immediate and early postoperative pain relief after kyphoplasty without significant restoration of vertebral body height in acute osteoporotic vertebral fractures. Neurosurg Focus 2005;18:e5

32. Singh K, Heller JG, Samartzis D, et al. Open vertebral cement augmentation combined with lumbar decompression for the operative management of thoracolumbar stenosis secondary to osteoporotic burst fractures. J Spinal Disord Tech 2005;18:413–419

33. Starr JK, Hanley EN Jr. Junctional burst fractures. Spine 1992;17:551–557

34. Leferink VJ, Nijboer JM, Zimmerman KW, Veldhuis EF, ten Vergert EM, ten Duis HJ. Burst fractures of the thoracolumbar spine: changes of the spinal canal during operative treatment and follow-up. Eur Spine J 2003;12:255–260

35. Kuner EH, Kuner A, Schlickewei W, Mullaji AB. Ligamentotaxis with an internal spinal fixator for thoracolumbar fractures. J Bone Joint Surg Br 1994;76:107–112

36. Aebi M, Etter C, Kehl T, Thalgott J. Stabilization of the lower thoracic and lumbar spine with the internal spinal skeletal fixation system: indications, techniques, and first results of treatment. Spine 1987;12:544–551

37. Schnee CL, Ansell LV. Selection criteria and outcome of operative approaches for thoracolumbar burst fractures with and without neurological deficit. J Neurosurg 1997;86:48–55

38. Cripton PA, Jain GM, Wittenberg RH, Nolte LP. Load-sharing characteristics of stabilized lumbar spine segments. Spine 2000; 25:170–179

39. Esses SI, Botsford DJ, Kostuik JP. Evaluation of surgical treatment for burst fractures. Spine 1990;15:667–673

40. Kaneda K, Abumi K, Fujiya M. Burst fractures with neurologic deficits of the thoracolumbar-lumbar spine: results of anterior decompression and stabilization with anterior instrumentation. Spine 1984;9:788–795

41. Kostuik JP. Anterior fixation for burst fractures of the thoracic and lumbar spine with or without neurological involvement. Spine 1988;13:286–293

42. Wood KB, Bohn D, Mehbod A. Anterior versus posterior treatment of stable thoracolumbar burst fractures without neurologic deficit: a prospective, randomized study. J Spinal Disord Tech 2005;18(suppl):S15–S23

43. McAfee PC, Bohlman HH, Yuan HA. Anterior decompression of traumatic thoracolumbar fractures with incomplete neurological deficit using a retroperitoneal approach. J Bone Joint Surg Am 1985;67:89–104

44. Beisse R, Muckley T, Schmidt MH, Hauschild M, Buhren V. Surgical technique and results of endoscopic anterior spinal canal decompression. J Neurosurg Spine 2005;2:128–136

45. Horn EM, Henn JS, Lemole GM Jr, Hott JS, Dickman CA. Thoracoscopic placement of dual-rod instrumentation in thoracic spinal trauma. Neurosurgery 2004;54:1150–1153, discussion 1153–1154

46. Kim DH, Jahng TA, Balabhadra RS, Potulski M, Beisse R. Thoracoscopic transdiaphragmatic approach to thoracolumbar junction fractures. Spine J 2004;4:317–328

47. McAfee PC, Regan JR, Fedder IL, Mack MJ, Geis WP. Anterior thoracic corpectomy for spinal cord decompression performed endoscopically. Surg Laparosc Endosc 1995;5:339–348

48. Schultheiss M, Hartwig E, Kinzl L, Claes L, Wilke HJ. Thoracolumbar fracture stabilization: comparative biomechanical evaluation of a new video-assisted implantable system. Eur Spine J 2004;13:93–100

49. Errico T. Point of view: anterior instrumentation of the spine in thoracic and thoracolumbar fractures: the single rod versus the double rod slot-Zielke device. Spine 1996;21:739–740

50. An HS, Lim TH, You JW, Hong JH, Eck J, McGrady L. Biomechanical evaluation of anterior thoracolumbar spinal instrumentation. Spine 1995;20:1979–1983

51. Carl AL, Tranmer BI, Sachs BL. Anterolateral dynamized instrumentation and fusion for unstable thoracolumbar and lumbar burst fractures. Spine 1997;22:686–690

52. Gertzbein SD, Court-Brown CM, Jacobs RR, et al. Decompression and circumferential stabilization of unstable spinal fractures. Spine 1988;13:892–895

53. Kaya RA, Aydin Y. Modified transpedicular approach for the surgical treatment of severe thoracolumbar or lumbar burst fractures. Spine J 2004;4:208–217

54. Resnick DK, Benzel EC. Lateral extracavitary approach for thoracic and thoracolumbar spine trauma: operative complications. Neurosurgery 1998;43:796–802, discussion 802–803

55. Hoshikawa T, Tanaka Y, Kokubun S, Lu WW, Luk KD, Leong JC. Flexion-distraction injuries in the thoracolumbar spine: an in vitro study of the relation between flexion angle and the motion axis of fracture. J Spinal Disord Tech 2002;15:139–143

56. Glantz SA. Primer of Biostatistics. 5th ed. New York: McGraw-Hill; 2002

57. Katonis PG, Kontakis GM, Loupasis GA, Aligizakis AC, Christoforakis JI, Velivassakis EG. Treatment of unstable thoracolumbar and lumbar spine injuries using Cotrel-Dubousset instrumentation. Spine 1999;24:2352–2357

58. Vaccaro AR. Combined anterior and posterior surgery for fractures of the thoracolumbar spine. Instr Course Lect 1999;48:443–449

59. Ebelke DK, Asher MA, Neff JR, Kraker DP. Survivorship analysis of VSP spine instrumentation in the treatment of thoracolumbar and lumbar burst fractures. Spine 1991;16(suppl):S428–S432

60. Alanay A, Acaroglu E, Yazici M, Oznur A, Surat A. Short-segment pedicle instrumentation of thoracolumbar burst fractures: does transpedicular intracorporeal grafting prevent early failure? Spine 2001;26:213–217

61. Acosta FL Jr, Aryan HE, Taylor WR, Ames CP. Kyphoplasty-augmented short-segment pedicle screw fixation of traumatic lumbar burst fractures: initial clinical experience and literature review. Neurosurg Focus 2005;18:e9

62. Cho DY, Lee WY, Sheu PC. Treatment of thoracolumbar burst fractures with polymethyl methacrylate vertebroplasty and short-segment pedicle screw fixation. Neurosurgery 2003;53:1354–1360, discussion 1360–1361

63. Muhlbauer M, Pfisterer W, Eyb R, Knosp E. Minimally invasive retroperitoneal approach for lumbar corpectomy and reconstruction: technical note. Neurosurg Focus 1999;7:e4

64. Rampersaud YR, Annand N, Dekutoski MB. Use of minimally invasive surgical techniques in the management of thoracolumbar trauma: current concepts. Spine 2006;31(suppl):S96–S102, discussion S104

65. Kossmann T, Jacobi D, Trentz O. The use of a retractor system (SynFrame) for open, minimal invasive reconstruction of the anterior column of the thoracic and lumbar spine. Eur Spine J 2001;10:396–402

66. Muhlbauer M, Pfisterer W, Eyb R, Knosp E. Minimally invasive retroperitoneal approach for lumbar corpectomy and anterior reconstruction: technical note. J Neurosurg 2000;93(suppl):161–167

67. Knop C, Bastian L, Lange U, Oeser M, Zdichavsky M, Blauth M. Complications in surgical treatment of thoracolumbar injuries. Eur Spine J 2002;11:214–226

68. McLain RF, Burkus JK, Benson DR. Segmental instrumentation for thoracic and thoracolumbar fractures: prospective analysis of construct survival and five-year follow-up. Spine J 2001;1:310–323

11 Spinal Cord Injuries in the Athlete

Brian Kwon, David H. Kim, and Alexander R. Vaccaro

Spinal cord injuries (SCIs) in athletes are uncommon and occur at an annual rate of 40 injuries per 1 million. These injuries are potentially devastating and particularly tragic when they occur in the setting of recreational or organized sports participation. SCIs occurring in sports typically involve the cervical spine during so-called collision sports, such as football and hockey (**Table 11.1**). The victims are characteristically young and healthy, and the injuries often result in permanent and significant disability or even death.[1]

The high-profile nature of organized sports in the United States has enhanced awareness of the potential for SCI, and many measures have been taken to reduce the risks of sustaining these injuries. Proper training and supervision of the athletes participating in high-risk sports have been shown to minimize the occurrence of injury to the head and neck during sports-related collisions. Due to such interventions and significant rule changes, the overall incidence of cervical SCI in both American football and North American hockey has significantly decreased over the past 30 years.[2–4]

Early injury recognition, appropriate stabilization of the injured athlete, and prompt treatment may improve the ultimate outcome following these injuries. SCIs that occur during sporting events are managed the same way as other traumatic cervical cord injuries. An organized system that includes personnel knowledgeable with the special requirements of protecting and mobilizing an athlete with potential SCI is essential.

■ Epidemiology (Table 11.2)

Over the past 30 years, sports participation has represented the fourth most common etiology of SCI and comprises between 10 and 15% of total SCIs. In the under-15-year age group, sports are the second most common etiology of SCIs. Males outnumber females 4:1, although this figure likely reflects the ratio of males to females involved in high-risk sports. For sports-related SCIs, the mean age at the time of injury is 24,[5] significantly younger than the average age of 33 years for SCIs in general.[1] Broken down by individual sporting events, diving accounts for the majority of SCIs, almost two thirds of the total sports-related injuries, followed by American football (**Table 11.3**). **Figure 11.1** shows the overall distribution of SCIs. **Figure 11.2** shows the distribution of SCIs by etiology in the under-15-year age group.

Football (Table 11.4)

Historically, American football has been associated with a significant number of injuries in general and a relatively larger number of SCIs. However, there has been a dramatic decrease in the incidence of football-related SCIs in the past 30 years. The risk of neck injuries was noted during the initial organization of the sport. A further increase in the rate of injury was observed with the advent of the football helmet. First worn during the traditional Army-Navy

Table 11.1 Spinal Cord Injuries in Sports

Etiology	• Typically involve the cervical spine in collision sports
	• Victims are often young and healthy
	• Injuries result in severe disability and even death
Preventative measures	• Proper training
	• Increased supervision
	• Rule changes
Improving outcomes	• Early recognition of injury
	• Appropriate stabilization
	• Prompt treatment
	• Organized system with knowledgeable personnel

Table 11.2 Epidemiology of Spinal Cord Injuries in Sports

Incidence rates	• Fourth most common etiology of SCIs
	• Second most common etiology of SCIs in age group under 15
	• 10 to 15% of total SCIs
Gender differences	Male to female ratio 4:1
Age	Mean age at time of injury = 24
Sports	• Diving accounts for approximately two thirds of SCIs
	• Football has next highest incidence

Table 11.3 Number and Percentages of Sports and Sports-Related Injuries in the National Spinal Cord Injury Statistical Center Database

Etiology	Number	Percentage
Diving	1601	65.4
Football	124	5.1
Snow skiing	118	4.8
Horseback riding	106	4.3
Winter sports	95	3.9
Other sports	80	3.3
Surfing	80	3.3
Wrestling	76	3.1
Gymnastics	47	1.9
Field sports	37	1.5
Water skiing	28	1.1
Baseball	19	0.8
Rodeo	18	0.7
Basketball	10	0.4
Track and field	5	0.2
Skateboard	4	0.2
Total	2448	

Source: From the National Spinal Cord Injury Statistical Center, University of Alabama at Birmingham, Annual Statistical Report, July 2005.

game in 1893, the helmet was designed and implemented to protect players from head injuries. By 1940 both the National Collegiate Athletic Association (NCAA) and the National Football League (NFL) made its use mandatory. Despite this rule, serious head and neck injuries continued to plague the sport at all levels of play. In the 1950s, face masks were added to the helmet. Interestingly, the rate of head and neck injuries increased,[6] as players may have felt more protected by face masks and became more apt to use their helmets and heads during high-risk blocking and tackling.

Dr. Joseph Torg et al[7] developed a registry to record and monitor serious cervical spine injuries occurring during football games. The ensuing observations and reports led to significant rule changes that prohibited players from using their helmets as blocking and tackling mechanisms or as projectiles. The NCAA and the National Federation of

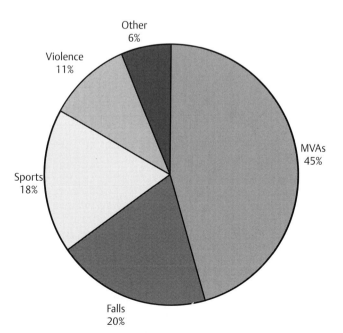

Fig. 11.1 Overall distribution of spinal cord injuries over a 30-year study period. MVAs, motor vehicle accidents.

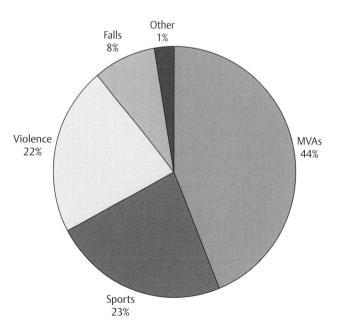

Fig. 11.2 In the under-15-year age group, sports injuries are the second most common etiology of spinal cord injuries.

Table 11.4 Football-Related Spinal Cord Injuries

Evolution	• Neck injuries noted during initial organization of the sport
	• Introduction of helmet wear led to an increase in rate of injury
	• Many feel these increases are a result of players feeling more protected, so are more apt to use helmets during blocking and tackling
Torg et al[7]	• Developed sports registry to record cervical spine injuries
	• National Center for Catastrophic Sports Injury Research
	• "Spearing" (tackling by leading with one's head) made illegal by NCAA and high school sports associations
Cantu and Mueller[3]	• Observations from 1977 to 2001
	• Total 223 SCIs
	• Incidence of SCIs increased with increased speed, forces, and level of play
	• SCIs observed (per 100,000):
	• 0.52 = high school
	• 1.55 = college
	• 14.0 = professional
Boden et al[9]	• Observations from 1989 to 2002
	• Showed significant increase in football-associated SCIs
	• Overall incidence spine injuries (per 100,000):
	• 1.10 = high school
	• 4.72 = college
	• Incidence of quadriplegia (per 100,000):
	• 0.50 = high school
	• 0.82 = college
	• Approximately six quadriplegic injuries per year
	• Most injuries occur while playing defense (57.5%) and making tackles (79.7%)
	• 43 cases of cervical cord neurapraxia (CCN)
	• None suffered SCI
	• Incidence of CCN (per 100,000):
	• 0.17 = high school
	• 2.05 = college
Efforts to reduce incidence of SCI	• Coaches urged to enforce illegal nature and danger of spearing
	• Concentrate on teaching proper tackling technique
	• Physical conditioning (pericervical musculature)

State High School Associations disallowed so-called spearing maneuvers in which the crown of the head is used during blocking and tackling.[8]

Cantu and Mueller[3] reported on catastrophic cervical spine injuries from 1977 to 2001, the 25 years following implementation of the aforementioned rule changes. They studied data from the National Center for Catastrophic Sports Injury Research at the University of North Carolina at Chapel Hill, which collects reports from physicians treating injured athletes on the high school, collegiate, and professional levels. The study reported a total of 223 cervical spine injuries in which no or incomplete neurologic recovery was documented. There were 183 injuries in high school players, 29 in college athletes, and 7 in professional athletes. When factoring in the number of participants at risk, the incidence of catastrophic SCIs appeared to increase in direct association with the increased speed, forces, and level of play. SCIs observed, per 100,000 participants, were 0.52 at the high school level, 1.55 in college athletes, and 14.0 at the professional level.

Subsequently, Boden et al[9] published an updated report from the National Center for Catastrophic Sports Injury Research on data collected between 1989 and 2002. These figures suggest that there has again been a significant increase in the rate of football-associated SCIs. During the time period of the study, the overall incidence of cervical spine injuries was 1.10 per 100,000 high school athletes and 4.72 injuries per 100,000 college participants. The incidence of quadriplegia in high school and college was 0.50 and 0.82 injuries per 100,000 athletes, respectively. There were 76 quadriplegic injuries sustained, leading to an overall incidence of approximately 6 per year in scholastic football. The mean age of the players at the time of injury was 17 years. Most injuries occurred while playing on defense (57.5%) and making a tackle (79.7%). The expert opinion in most cases, including four cases documented on videotape, was that the mechanism of injury involved spear tackling.

In the same study,[9] there were also 43 reported episodes of cervical cord neurapraxia (CCN). The calculated mean incidence of CCN in college players was 2.05 per 100,000 participants and 0.17 per 100,000 high school participants. Two players reported a previous episode of CCN, and none of the 43 players suffered permanent quadriplegia during the study period. It is likely that these figures represent an underestimate of the true incidence of CCN in organized football and that cases are not reported at the same rate as more significant SCIs.

Despite widespread belief that the number of SCIs has decreased over time, as seen by most recent data, there has been an apparent increase in the rate of these injuries. Coaches have been urged to enforce the illegal nature of

and dangers involved in spear tackling. Proper tackling technique and physical conditioning, particularly of the pericervical musculature, have been strongly encouraged. The NCAA, effective for the 2005–2006 academic year, removed the term *intentional* from the spearing rule in efforts to strengthen the wording. This may give referees freedom to call the penalty more often as they would not have to judge intent.[3,9,10] Of note, there were 18 lawsuits or insurance settlements associated with the injuries included in the most recent study by Boden et al.[9]

Ice Hockey (Table 11.5)

Ice hockey in North America has undergone increased scrutiny because of the regular occurrence of high-profile cases of quadriplegia. In 1981 a registry to document and track SCIs due to ice hockey was created. Following the creation of the Committee on Prevention of Spinal Cord Injuries Due to Hockey, an abrupt increase in SCIs was noted in the late 1980s. It was not known at the time whether this was due to better reporting and awareness or to a true increase in the rate of SCIs. A report following evaluation of the initial data did not provide much in the way of conclusions other than the suggestion that SCIs occurring during ice hockey were multifactorial and worthy of study.[11,12]

Tator et al[4] reviewed reports of 271 SCIs documented between 1943 and 1999 in Canada. The 16- to 20-year-old age group was most frequently affected and comprised 49% of the total. The overall mean age at the time of injury was 20.6 years. The injury mechanism in the majority of cases involved a player striking the boards with his head (67%), and the most frequent cause was being pushed or checked from behind by another player (37%) and being

Table 11.5 Ice Hockey–Related Spinal Cord Injuries

Committee on Prevention of SCIs Due to Hockey	• Created in 1981
	• Abrupt increase in SCIs seen in the late 1980s; could be from better reporting and awareness or actual increase
Tator et al[4]	• 271 reported SCIs between 1943 and 1999 in Canada
	• 49% between ages 16 and 20 years
	• Mean age at time of injury = 20.6 years
	• Injury mechanisms:
	• Striking boards with head = 67%
	• Checked from behind = 37%
	• Checked (not from behind) = 24%
	• 83.0% involved cervical spine, 47.3% sustained permanent neurologic loss
Increased incidence	• Increased speed and size of players
	• More aggressive risk-taking behavior (based on psychosocial profile)
	• False sense of security with helmet wear

checked but not from behind (24%). The cervical spine was involved in 83.0% of injuries, and 47.3% of players sustained permanent neurologic losses. The overwhelming majority of injuries (91%) occurred during supervised games.

An increase in the speed and physical size of players may account to some degree for observed increases in the rate of spinal injuries. Recommendations have been made to change the rules and enforce penalties for illegal techniques, such as checking a player from behind. Possible changes in equipment have been proposed, such as rounding the helmet tops. More importantly, changing attitudes about smart play have begun. As previously suggested, the use of helmets has lowered rates of head injury but may also give athletes a false sense of security and lead to more aggressive, less protected behavior.[4,11] A study of the psychosocial profiles of hockey players has also suggested that aggressive, risk-taking behaviors contribute directly to a higher incidence of spinal injury.[12]

Rugby (Table 11.6)

Another popular sport with relatively high rates of SCI is rugby. Although there are several rule variations, all versions of the sport involve high-velocity collisions between players who wear relatively little or no protective gear. Several authors have studied SCIs that occur in the Rugby Union and Rugby League in Australia, New Zealand, and Ireland.[8,13–15] In each study, a relatively constant high rate of SCI was identified spanning several years.

Overall, the Rugby Union had the highest incidence of SCIs. Between 1986 and 1991 there were 9.2 reported cases of SCI per 100,000 players. Between 1995 and 2003 the rate decreased somewhat to 6.8 injuries per 100,000. This decrease, however, was not significant. During the same time periods the rate of SCI per 100,000 players in the Rugby League, which has several rule differences with the Rugby Union, were 2.3 and 1.7, respectively. The difference was significant. The majority of injuries in union players occurred during the scrum, whereas in league players they tended to occur during tackling. This difference is felt to be due to major rule differences governing the scrum between union play and league play. Among 31 injuries in the Rugby Union reported by Berry et al,[14] 11 were caused by scrums, and 9 were caused by tackling, with both representing 64% of the total injuries observed. In the Rugby League, Berry et al reported 1 SCI during the scrum and 18 during tackling, with both mechanisms making up 82% of the injuries in league play.

In the Rugby Union a scrum involves eight players lined up in a 3–4–1 formation. The scrum occurs after specific events, such as accidental offsides, rucks (group tackles), and mauls (group tackles where the player stays standing and the referee whistles the ball dead). In the Rugby League the scrum is reduced in power by involving fewer players (six in a 3–2–1 pattern) and does not allow for any pushing or contesting. Although likely reducing the risk of injury during the scrum, this form of scrummage has been criticized as not embodying the true nature of the scrum. Efforts to enforce stricter scrummage regulations have been resisted, as teams continue to attempt to gain tactical advantage in recovering the ball during this phase of the game by thrusting and engaging opponents as forcefully as possible. One of the goals of the scrum quoted on a Web site was explicitly stated as follows: "to push the other side off the ball or at least break the opposing hooker/prop's neck/spine."

In a cadaver study modeling scrums, the horizontal force during initial contact was measured at 4.4 kilonewton (kN) to 8 kN,[16] which exceeds the upper limit of the axial load required to cause compression failure of the cervical spine.[11] Not surprisingly, several health care officials

Table 11.6 Rugby-Related Spinal Cord Injuries

Incidence rates	• Highest rates of SCI were seen in Rugby Union (as opposed to Rugby League)
	Rugby Union (per 100,000):
	• 1986–1991 = 9.2 cases
	• 1995–2003 = 6.8 cases
	Rugby League (per 100,000):
	• 1986–1991 = 2.3 cases
	• 1995–2003 = 1.7 cases
Rugby League vs Rugby Union	• Rule differences between the two specifically regarding the scrum
	• Scrummage injuries:
	• Rugby Union = 11/31 cases
	• Rugby League = 1/19 cases (18/19 during tackling)
	• Efforts to enforce stricter regulations have been resisted

Table 11.7 Water Sports–Related Spinal Cord Injuries

Incidence and causes	Diving is leading cause of SCIs; represents two thirds of all such injuries
Demographic and temporal pattern[17]	• Average age of 23
	• Occurred between May and September
	• Reckless behavior, ignorance, and alcohol were all factors

have called for governmental-level changes in the rules of rugby, stating that to allow players, particularly schoolboys, to continue with the current rules "constitutes culpable negligence."[15]

Water Sports (Table 11.7)

Diving is the leading cause of SCIs related to sports and leisure activities and represents the cause of nearly two thirds of all such injuries.[1,17] SCIs from diving accidents occur to a distinct demographic and in a specific temporal pattern. A recent review by Korres and colleagues[17] retrospectively reviewed SCIs due to diving accidents. They found 20 patients (19 males and 1 female) whose average age was 23 years at the time of injury. All injuries occurred between May and September. They found reckless behavior, ignorance, and alcohol use in young males to be the typical factors in those injured. Poor judgment and diving head first into shallow pools were the most frequently reported injury mechanisms.

Tumbling Sports (Table 11.8)

Cheerleading has developed into a competitive sport and as such has experienced progressive increase in the apparent rate of injuries resulting from more acrobatic high-energy maneuvers. Over a 17-year period from 1983 to 2000, cheerleading accounted for almost half of the serious cervical spine injuries in women. The rate of these injuries over that time period was 1.03 per 100,000 participants. New rules have changed the methods and height at which the cheerleaders can be catapulted into the air, and it is hoped these rules will lead to fewer catastrophic injuries.[18]

Skiing/Snowboarding (Table 11.8)

Skiing and snowboarding accidents are a major concern due to the very high volume of participants, estimated at 14 million in the United States and over 200 million worldwide.[18] Although most serious injuries are head injuries, spine injuries also occur at a reported incidence of 1 per 100,000 skier days and 4 per 100,000 snowboarder days. In contrast to other sports activities, most spine injuries occurring in association with skiing and snowboarding are thoracolumbar injuries.[18] Specific data regarding the rates of cervical spine and SCI are unavailable.

■ Injury Syndromes (Table 11.9)

Cervical SCIs occur when the athlete's head is rapidly decelerated against an immobile object. The head is fixed in position, and the cervical spine becomes an intervening mobile segment between the head and the body. The momentum of the body contributes a significant axial load during its deceleration. The resulting injury pattern depends in part on the position of the neck at the time the axial load is applied. When the neck is in a neutral or lordotic position, axial loads can be dissipated by paraspinal musculature and ligamentous structures. However, when the neck is flexed, lordosis is eliminated, and the cervical spine then behaves biomechanically like a rigid column (**Fig. 11.3**). Axial loads are dissipated through the bony structures, resulting in significant force transfer.[2]

Torg et al[19] have also examined the mechanism by which football players suffer cervical SCIs. As previously noted, a majority of such injuries occur during tackling,

Table 11.8 Tumbling Sports– and Skiing/Snowboarding–Related Spinal Cord Injuries

Tumbling sports	• 1983–2000: cheerleading was almost one half of cervical spine injuries in women
	• Rule changes, including height at which cheerleaders can be catapulted, may reduce incidence
Skiing/snowboarding	• Major concern due to high volume of participants
	• 14 million in United States, > 200 million worldwide
	• Spine injury incidence (per 100,000 skier days):
	• Skiers = 1
	• Snowboarders = 4
	• Most injuries are thoracolumbar injuries

Table 11.9 Injury Syndromes

Cervical SCI mechanisms	• Occur when head is rapidly decelerated against immobile object
	• Cervical spine becomes intervening mobile segment between head and body
	• Injury pattern depends on neck position at time axial load is applied
	• Neutral, lordotic position: axial loads dissipated by paraspinal musculature and ligaments
	• Flexed position: cervical spine becomes rigid column, with axial loads dissipated through bony structures
Transient neurapraxia	• "Burners" (stingers): benign events from stretch injury to upper roots and trunks of brachial plexus or foraminal compression of nerve roots
	• Radiating pain down one extremity (if bilateral, could be more serious)
	• Return to play if symptoms quickly resolve with no strength deficits or limitations in range of motion
	• MRI or EMG if symptoms persist after 2 to 4 weeks
	• "Burning hands syndrome": variant of central cord syndrome and implies actual SCI
Cervical cord neurapraxia (CCN)	• Definition: temporary paralysis lasting for 15 minutes and up to 48 hours, followed by full recovery
	• Torg ratio: sagittal diameter of spinal canal/sagittal diameter of vertebral body
	• Smaller Torg ratio (< 0.8, normal $= 1.0$) does not predict catastrophic SCI and should not prevent a player from participating
Spear-tackler's spine	• Constellation of radiographic findings:
	• Developmental cervical stenosis
	• Persistent straightening or loss of normal cervical lordosis
	• Persistent radiographic evidence of previous injury
	• Clinical history of previous use of spear tackling
	• Absolute contraindication to participation in collision sports

particularly with the head in the down position. This observation gave rise to the "nose-to-the-numbers" technique of tackling that is currently being taught. Many authors have urged coaches and trainers to emphasize the importance of these principles during play.[3,9]

Transient Neurapraxias

"Burners" (also known as "stingers") are relatively benign events that are thought to arise from a stretch injury to the upper roots and trunks of the brachial plexus or foraminal compression of the existing nerve roots. Players often experience radiating pain down one extremity. Bilateral stingers are less benign and may represent a potentially more significant injury involving the cervical spinal cord. Associated weakness, especially of the deltoid, biceps, and spinatus muscles, can occur and should be specifically tested for on the sidelines. Athletes can return to play if symptoms quickly resolve and there are no strength deficits and sensory changes and no limitation to neck range of motion.

Persistent symptoms from a stinger should warrant advanced imaging with magnetic resonance imaging (MRI) to look for possible cervical disk herniation, cervical stenosis, cord compression, or signs of actual cord injury. Electromyography (EMG) performed 2 to 4 weeks after injury can be helpful. Typical findings include a mild conduction block, but sharp waves and fibrillation potentials can also be seen. Even with abnormal EMG findings, athletes can return to play if symptoms resolve. However, persistent sensory symptoms or muscle-specific weakness with concordant EMG changes should preclude a player from returning to play in contact sports.[11,20]

"Burning hands" syndrome is an entirely different diagnosis. It is considered a variant of central cord syndrome and implies actual SCI. Radiographic evidence of cervical spine injury can be seen in up to 50% of cases.

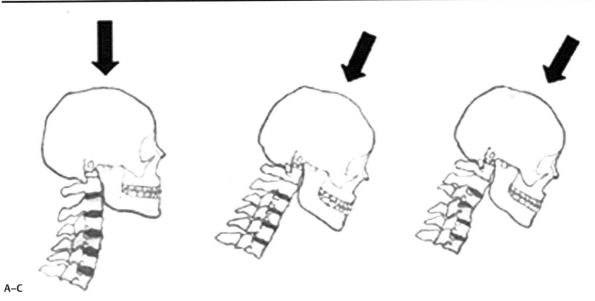

A–C

Fig. 11.3 Influence of neck position and injury at time of axial impact to head. **(A)** With the neck in neutral alignment, the vertebral column is extended. The compressive force can be dissipated by the spinal musculature and ligaments. **(B)** With the neck in a flexed posture, the spine straightens out and becomes collinear with the axial force. **(C)** At the time of impact, the straightened cervical spine undergoes a rapid deformation and buckles under the compressive load. (From Banerjee R, Palumbo MA, Fadale PD. Catastrophic cervical spine injuries in the collision sport athlete: 1. Epidemiology, functional anatomy, and diagnosis. Am J Sports Med 2004;32(4):1077–1087, with permission.)

Cervical Cord Neurapraxia

Cervical cord neurapraxia is defined as temporary paralysis that lasts for 15 minutes and up to 48 hours followed by full recovery and a completely normal physical examination. The term is taken from the nomenclature of peripheral nerve injuries where "neurapraxia" implies return to normal function. Its relationship to congenital stenosis of the cervical canal and cervical SCI has been well studied.

Torg et al[21] described a radiographic measurement comparing the anteroposterior diameter of the cervical canal to the anteroposterior diameter of the corresponding vertebral body (**Fig. 11.4**). This ratio was devised because of the significant interindividual variation in measured values for spinal canal diameter by routine radiographic techniques. Torg et al found the ratio of normal individuals to be around 1.0, and this value was in contrast to the ratio found in a majority of athletes experiencing CCN in whom the ratio was found to be below 0.8. On the basis of this finding, it was concluded that congenitally narrow spinal canals may predispose an athlete to episodes of CCN and SCI. In a follow-up study, the Torg ratios in high school and professional football players, in athletes with permanent SCI as well as CCN, and in nonathlete control groups were studied. The group with permanent SCIs had smaller absolute canal diameter measurements but did not have significantly lower Torg ratios. It was observed that none of the SCI group reported prior episodes of CCN. In the athlete groups, the vertebral body diameters were significantly

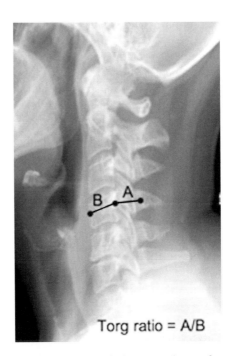

Torg ratio = A/B

Fig. 11.4 Radiograph showing technique for measuring Torg ratio. The anteroposterior diameter of the canal is measured with a perpendicular line from the cephalocaudal midpoint of the posterior vertebral body wall to the spinolaminar line. The anteroposterior diameter of the vertebral body is measured at the midpoint of the body from the anterior wall to the posterior wall.

larger on average than those in the nonathletes. The interpretation for this finding was that those with larger bony anatomy are better suited for competitive football. Because of this anatomical difference, the prevalence of congenital cervical stenosis as defined by the Torg ratio may be artificially high in this population. Overall, the positive predictive value of a Torg ratio less than 0.8 was 0.2%, indicating that it cannot be reasonably used as a screening tool. The conclusion of the study was that a smaller Torg ratio does not predict catastrophic SCI and should not prevent a player from being allowed to participate in collision sports. It does, however, appear to predict an increased susceptibility to episodes of CCN.[22]

Spear-Tackler's Spine

In 1993 Torg et al reported on a small subset of injured patients who presented with cervical spine complaints or catastrophic SCIs.[23] They demonstrated a constellation of radiographic findings, including (1) developmental cervical stenosis, (2) persistent straightening or loss of the normal cervical lordosis, (3) persistent radiographic evidence of previous injury, and (4) a clinical history of previous use of the spear-tackling technique (**Fig. 11.5**). Torg et al considered spear-tackler's spine an absolute contraindication to participation in collision sports that may expose the athlete to high-energy, axial cervical spinal loads.[23,24]

■ Evaluation and Management

The events that occur immediately after a potential sports-related SCI are pivotal in determining the ultimate outcome. Because these injuries are rare, trainers and medical staff may not be accustomed to the specific steps necessary to care for an athlete with a possible SCI. Preparation for such events is vital. This includes availability of trained and knowledgeable staff and the availability of appropriate

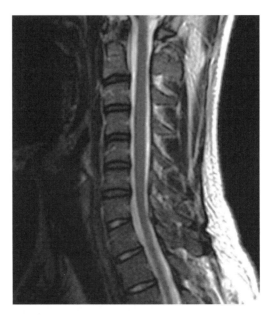

Fig. 11.5 Magnetic resonance image of a spear-tackler's cervical spine. This is an 18-year-old high school football player who in the preceding season had had two episodes of spear tackling. Prior to beginning his next season, he complained of axial neck pain but had no neurologic symptoms.

stabilization and mobilization equipment (**Table 11.10**). Backboards with attachments for immobilization of the head and neck as well as emergency airway devices should be available and in good working condition. Appropriate transportation to an emergency room prepared to manage and stabilize an athlete with SCI is important.

Initial management begins with establishing the basics of trauma resuscitation: airway, breathing, and circulation. Cervical spine immobilization must be maintained along with a patent airway. A cervical spine injury should be assumed until proven otherwise, particularly if an axial loading injury was witnessed or the athlete complains of neck pain, altered sensation, or extremity weakness.

Table 11.10 Evaluation and Management of Spinal Cord Injuries in Sports

Initial management	• Crucial to patient outcome; important to have knowledgeable personnel on staff and available
	• Initial management:
	• Begin with establishing basics of trauma resuscitation: airway, breathing, and circulation
	• Maintenance of cervical spine immobilization
	• Assume cervical spine injury until proven otherwise
Presence of concomitant head injury	• In unconscious patient, emergent airway control is necessary
	• Removal of both helmet and shoulder pads necessary if airway cannot be secured
	• Conscious and responsive patient: *leave helmet and shoulder pads on*
	• Logroll onto backboard and transport to trauma center
	• Thorough neurologic exam repeated often during transportation

A concomitant closed head injury may be present. If the patient is unconscious, emergent airway control is necessary, and the face mask may need to be removed to perform bag mask techniques or intubation. If the helmet or shoulder pads do not allow for proper immobilization or access to the patient's airway, both pieces need to be removed. This should be done carefully and preferably with a team of medically trained personnel performing the task in unison. Failure to remove both helmet and shoulder pads could lead to excessive flexion or extension of the injured cervical spine and exacerbation of any underlying SCI. Again, if the patient begins having cardiopulmonary distress, the shoulder pads may need to be removed for resuscitation, and the helmet will need to be removed with the pads.

If the patient is conscious and responsive and medically stable, then both helmet and pads should remain in place. The patient should be logrolled onto a backboard and immobilized for transport to the nearest trauma center. If feasible, the face mask should be removed before transport regardless of mental status. A thorough neurologic exam should be performed and documented as soon as possible.[25,26]

In the emergency room, care of the patient becomes the responsibility of the emergency room staff. The on-field medical staff and trainers should provide relevant information regarding mechanism of injury and findings on initial evaluation. Additionally, the emergency staff may not be familiar with helmet and shoulder pad removal and may require assistance. Any protective equipment that may potentially interfere with radiographs should be removed.[27] The use of methylprednisolone in SCI has engendered considerable debate.[28] The decision to use it should be considered, but it may not be essential to improving the overall neurologic outcome.

■ Return to Play

The issue of returning an injured athlete to participation in sports at his or her previous level of play carries psychological, emotional, and financial implications. Physician responsibility is to promote the athlete's safety and well-being. A study by Morganti et al[29] showed considerable variation in the criteria used by medical professionals to determine whether a player should be returned to play. Surprisingly, they found few significant correlations between return-to-play recommendations and the risk of the sport, physician years in practice, or subspecialty interest. Torg and Ramsey-Emrheim[24] published their opinions regarding congenital, developmental, and posttraumatic conditions that confer absolute, relative, and no contraindications to play in collision sports. Despite a paucity of objective supporting data to back up their recommendations, they presented a starting point from which to debate and develop future more evidence-based guidelines. Vaccaro and colleagues[30] reviewed the literature on return-to-play criteria and have summarized their own recommendations. They added contraindications that include a category of postoperative conditions. Although there is little high-quality data upon which to formulate absolute guidelines, these expert opinions are useful to aid the responsible physician in making reasoned decisions in individual situations.

Based on expert opinion, the proposed absolute contraindications to participation in collision sports are shown in **Table 11.11**, as are relative contraindications and those conditions that present no contraindication.

Table 11.11 Return to Play

Proposed absolute contraindications	
	1. Odontoid anomalies
	2. Klippel-Feil anomalies that involve multilevel fusion
	3. MRI evidence for cervical spinal cord abnormality
	4. Subaxial instability (lateral x-rays that show more than 3.5 mm of displacement and 11 degrees of angulation)
	5. Atlanto-occipital fusion, instability, rotatory fixation, or hypermobility
	6. Spear-tackler's spine
	7. More than two episodes of CCN
	8. Cervical myelopathy
	9. Ankylosing spondylitis or diffuse idiopathic skeletal hyperostosis (DISH)
	10. Acute fracture of vertebral body or posterior elements with or without ligamentous instability
	11. Posttraumatic vertebral body fracture with kyphosis
	12. Radiographic evidence for distraction/extension injury

(Continued on page 168)

Table 11.11 *(Continued)* **Return to Play**

	13. Radiographic evidence of posttraumatic cervical canal stenosis
	14. Persistent neck pain, pain with range of motion, or focal neurologic deficit
	15. Symptomatic disk herniation
	16. Rheumatoid arthritis
	17. Cervical laminectomy
	18. Three-level cervical spine fusion
Proposed relative contraindications	1. The absence of any absolute contraindications to play; recurrent injury may occur, and the severity of injury may be uncertain but potentially catastrophic
	2. Previous episode of CCN; athlete must have a complete recovery
	3. Three or more stingers in one season
	4. Healed single-level posterior fusion with instrumentation
	5. Healed two-level anterior fusion
	6. Occipital-cervical fusion
No contraindications to play	1. Klippel-Feil abnormality with single-level fusion
	2. Spina bifida occulta
	3. Torg ratio less than 0.8 with no history of CCN
	4. One or two stingers in one season
	5. Cervical spondylosis without need for interventional care (i.e., athlete previously sought treatment for neck pain or stiffness)
	6. Stable, healed C1 or C2 fracture that did not require operative intervention
	7. Healed subaxial spine fracture without kyphotic deformity
	8. Asymptomatic clay-shoveler's fracture
	9. Single-level anterior cervical fusion, healed
	10. Single- or multilevel posterior cervical foraminotomy

■ Special Considerations (Table 11.12)

Os Odontoideum

Os odontoideum refers to a smoothly corticated ossicle replacing the odontoid process and without osseous continuity with the body of C2.[31] Acquired and congenital etiologies have been supported, with a majority of experts favoring a traumatic etiology. The natural history of an asymptomatic os odontoideum is unknown. Predictions for instability and neurologic deterioration have been based on small retrospective reports. Although stable asymptomatic patients can be observed without surgical treatment, most authors believe that the diagnosis of os odontoideum is an absolute contraindication to participation in contact/collision sports.[24]

Down Syndrome

Down syndrome caused by trisomy 21 is considered the most commonly observed chromosomal abnormality

and is seen in 1 in 660 live births. It is characterized by low intelligence, facial abnormalities, and ligamentous laxity. Orthopedic manifestations include cervical (occipitocervical and atlantoaxial) hypermobility, hip and patellofemoral instability, and foot deformities. Atlantoaxial instability occurs in 10 to 30% of Down syndrome patients. Approximately 15% of those with instability develop neurologic sequelae.[31,32]

In 1995, the Committee on Sports Medicine and Fitness of the American Association of Pediatrics published a statement on use of screening radiographs for Down syndrome patients prior to participation in sports.[33] It argued that the low incidence of symptomatic instability and difficulty in obtaining and interpreting appropriate images precluded the use of cervical radiographs as a screening tool. Nevertheless, the Special Olympics continues to require that all Down syndrome participants obtain screening lateral flexion-extension cervical spine radiographs. The athlete is not allowed to participate in certain events such as diving, soccer, and gymnastics if there is evidence of instability defined as an anterior atlanto-dens interval greater than 4 mm.

Table 11.12 Special Considerations

Os odontoideum	• Definition: smooth corticated ossicle replacing odontoid process without osseous continuity with body of C2
	• Can be congenital or acquired; natural history is unknown
	• Diagnosis is absolute contraindication to play in collision sports
Down syndrome (trisomy 21)	• Most common chromosomal abnormality (1 in 660 births)
	• Characterized by intelligence and developmental abnormalities
	• Special Olympics requires Down syndrome participants to obtain screening lateral flexion-extension cervical spine radiographs
	• If evidence of instability (anterior atlanto-dens interval > 4 mm), athlete is not allowed to participate

■ Conclusion

Cervical SCI is a potentially devastating injury in general and is potentially even more tragic when it occurs in the course of organized, supervised athletic participation. Over the past several decades, significant changes in equipment, techniques, conditioning, and coaching in several at-risk sports have led to a notable decrease in the incidence of SCIs. Unfortunately, in recent years, there is evidence that this trend has reversed, possibly related to the steady increase in speed and energy of the play involved.

The management of sports-related SCIs requires the immediate availability of personnel with appropriate train-ing and experience in managing such injuries. Appropriate early management of the athlete with an acute SCI can positively influence the overall outcome by minimizing the risk of reinjury during initial evaluation and transport. Following proper evaluation and treatment, return-to-play criteria for these athletes have not been well established, and the vast majority of current recommendations are based on expert opinion only and unsupported by high-quality data. In many cases, expert opinion regarding a specific condition or situation is contradictory and is best considered an aid to the treating specialist in making an informed recommendation for a given athlete. Absolute guidelines are largely unavailable.

References

1. Jackson AB, Dijkers M, DeVivo MJ, Poczatek RB. A demographic profile of new traumatic spinal cord injuries: change and stability over 30 years. Arch Phys Med Rehabil 2004;85:1740–1748
2. Banerjee R, Palumbo MA, Fadale PD. Catastrophic cervical spine injuries in the collision sport athlete: 1. Epidemiology, functional anatomy, and diagnosis. Am J Sports Med 2004;32:1077–1087
3. Cantu RC, Mueller FO. Catastrophic spine injuries in American football, 1977–2001. Neurosurgery 2003;53:358–363
4. Tator CH, Provvidenza CF, Lapczak L, Carson J, Raymond D. Spine injuries in Canadian ice hockey: documentation of injuries sustained from 1943–1999. Can J Neurol Sci 2004;31:460–466
5. DeVivo MJ. Causes and costs of spinal cord injury in the United States. Spinal Cord 1997;35:809–813
6. Levy ML, Ozgur BM, Berry C, Aryan HE, Apuzzo MLJ. Birth and evolution of the football helmet. Neurosurgery 2004;55:656–662
7. Torg JS, Quedenfeld TC, Burstein A, Spealman A, Nichols C. National football head and neck injury register: report on cervical quadriplegia. Am J Sports Med 1979;7:127–132
8. McIntosh AS, McCrory P. Preventing head and neck injury. Br J Sports Med 2005;39:314–318
9. Boden BP, Robin L, Tacchetti RL, Cantu RC, Knowles SB, Mueller FO. Catastrophic cervical spine injuries in high school and college football players. Am J Sports Med 2006;34:1223–1232

10. Heck JF, Clarke KS, Peterson TR, Torg JS, Weis MP. National Athletic Trainers' Association position statement: head-down contact and spearing in tackle football. J Athl Train 2004;39:101–111
11. Kim DH, Vaccaro AR, Berta SC. Acute sports related spinal cord injury: contemporary management principles. Clin Sports Med 2003;22:501–522
12. Tator CH, Carson JD, Edmonds VE. Spinal injuries in ice hockey. Clin Sports Med 1998;17:183–194
13. Shelly MJ, Butler JS, Timlin M, Walsh MG, Poynton AR, O'Byrne JM. Spinal injuries in Irish rugby: a ten-year review. J Bone Joint Surg Br 2006;88:771–775
14. Berry JG, Harrison JE, Yeo JD, Cripps RA, Stephenson SCR. Cervical spinal cord injury in Rugby Union and Rugby League: are incidence rates declining in NSW? Aust N Z J Public Health 2006;30:268–274
15. Carmody DJ, Taylor TKF, Parker DA, Coolican MRJ, Cumming RG. Spinal cord injuries in Australian footballers 1997–2002. Med J Aust 2005;182:561–564
16. Milburn PD. The Biomechanics of Rugby Scrummaging. Wollongong: University of Wollongong; 1990
17. Korres DS, Benetos IS, Themistocleous GS, Mavrogenis AF, Nikolakakos L, Liantis PT. Diving injuries of the cervical spine in amateur divers. Spine J 2006;6:44–49

18. Cooper MT, McGee KM, Anderson DG. Epidemiology of athletic head and neck injuries. Clin Sports Med 2003;22:427–443

19. Torg JS, Vegso JJ, O'Neill MJ. The epidemiologic, pathologic, biomechanical, and cinematographic analysis of football induced cervical spine trauma. Am J Sports Med 1990;18:50–57

20. Weinstein SM. Assessment and management of the athlete with a "stinger." Clin Sports Med 1998;17:127–135

21. Torg JS, Pavlov H, Gennario SE, et al. Neurapraxia of the cervical spinal cord with transient quadriplegia. J Bone Joint Surg Am 1986;68:1354–1370

22. Torg JS, Naranja RJ Jr, Pavlov H, et al. The relationship of developmental narrowing of the cervical spinal canal to reversible and irreversible injury of the cervical spinal cord in football players. J Bone Joint Surg Am 1996;78:1308–1314

23. Torg JS, Sennett B, Pavlov H, Leventhal M, Glasgow S. Spear tackler's spine: an entity precluding participation in tackle football and collision activities that expose the cervical spine to axial energy inputs. Am J Sports Med 1993;21:640–649

24. Torg JS, Ramsey-Emrheim JA. Suggested management guidelines for participation in collision activities with congenital, developmental, or postinjury lesions involving the cervical spine. Med Sci Sports Exerc 1997;29:S256–S272

25. Banerjee R, Palumbo MA, Fadale PD. Catastrophic cervical spine injuries in the collision sport athlete: 2. Principles of emergency care. Am J Sports Med 2004;32:1760–1764

26. Kleiner DM, Almquist JL, Bailes J, et al. Prehospital Care of the Spine-Injured Athlete: A Document from the Inter-Association Task Force for Appropriate Care of the Spine-Injured Athlete. Dallas, TX: National Athletic Trainers' Association; 2001

27. Davidson RM, Burton JH, Snowise M, Owens WB. Football protective gear and cervical spine imaging. Ann Emerg Med 2001;38:26–30

28. Hurlbert RJ. Methylprednisolone for acute spinal cord injury: an inappropriate standard of care. J Neurosurg 2000;93(suppl):1–7

29. Morganti C, Sweeney CA, Albanese SA, Burak C, Hosea T, Connolly PJ. Return to play after cervical spine injury. Spine 2001;26:1131–1136

30. Vaccaro AR, Klein GR, Ciccoti M, et al. Return to play criteria for the athlete with cervical spine injuries resulting in stinger and transient quadriplegia/paresis. Spine J 2002;2:351–356

31. Hadley MN. Os odontoideum. Neurosurgery 2002;50:S148–S155

32. Pueschel SM. Should children with Down syndrome be screened for atlantoaxial instability? Arch Pediatr Adolesc Med 1998;152:123–125

33. Committee on Sports Medicine and Fitness. Atlantoaxial instability in Down syndrome: subject review. Pediatrics 1995;96:151–154

34. White AA III, Panjabi MM: The problem of clinical instability in the human spine: a systematic approach, in Clinical Biomechanics of the Spine, ed 2. Philadelphia: JB Lippincott, 1990, pp 278–378

12 Critical Care of Acute Spinal Cord Injuries

Melissa Y. Macias and Dennis J. Maiman

In the United States, 160,000 new traumatic vertebral column injuries occur annually, 10 to 30% with concomitant spinal cord injury (SCI), yielding an average of 10,000 new cases of SCI per year.[1] Currently, an estimated 225,000 to 288,000 individuals live with paralysis. In order of decreasing frequency, the most common level of neurologic injury is cervical (51.0%), thoracic (34.3%), and lumbosacral (10.7%). The most frequently injured regions are cervical C4-C6 (39.4%) and thoracolumbar T12-L1 (11.6%).[1]

The majority of spine and spinal cord traumas are caused by motor vehicle accidents (MVAs), followed by falls, acts of violence (most commonly gunshot wounds), and recreational sports activities (e.g., diving and contact sports). Interestingly, the proportion of sports-related and violence-related spinal cord injuries has decreased since 2000, whereas those due to falls have increased. The average age at injury is 37.6 years, an increase likely reflecting the rise in the median age of the general population since the mid-1970s.[1] Accordingly, SCI in the elderly population (> 60 years of age) is most commonly caused by falls and has doubled since the 1980s. More common causes of SCI in younger populations remain MVAs, violence, and sports.[1]

Initial management of SCI is focused on basic emergency and trauma management protocols that institute immediate immobilization, stabilization, and safe transport to a high-level care facility. Improved medical management of SCI has facilitated a 60 to 90% reduction in the high mortality associated with SCI[2] and remains crucial for the improvement in quality of life for SCI patients.[2-4] Management of acute SCI patients requires knowledge of the postinjury pathophysiologic changes specific to this patient population and is optimized in an intensive care unit (ICU) setting, as both morbidity and mortality after acute SCI have been shown to be improved with continuous monitoring in the ICU.[5] Though the evidence is at best anecdotal, some authors believe that timely surgical stabilization of an unstable spinal column injury with associated SCI appears clinically beneficial, facilitating more rapid mobilization and treatment of associated traumatic injuries, potentially reducing medical complications and reducing the duration of the stay in the ICU and the duration of the overall hospitalization.[6-8] However, instability due to undiagnosed associated trauma is increased.[9,10]

This chapter identifies key medical considerations for management of acute SCI patients in the posttraumatic phase of care. The preeminent goals of ICU management are anticipation of acute complications and the prevention of intermediate and long-term complications of SCI. A systems approach is recommended, with specific attention to respiratory, cardiovascular, gastrointestinal, urologic, and integument systems with utilization of pharmacologic agents where appropriate.

■ Pharmacologic Considerations

Methylprednisolone

High-dose steroid infusion, primarily with methylprednisolone (MP), is the main pharmacologic treatment that is widely utilized following SCI, and the decision to initiate treatment is made during the initial resuscitation phase, but treatment remains rather controversial. When treatment is started within 8 hours of injury, beneficial effects at 6 weeks, 6 months, and 1 year were reported in the National Acute Spinal Cord Injury Study (NASCIS II) in 1990.[11] The protocol included a bolus dose of 30 mg/kg intravenous (IV) over 15 minutes followed by 5.4 mg/kg/h IV for 23 hours if administered within 3 hours and for 47 hours if administered after 3 hours but before 8 hours of injury (**Table 12.1**). Though the mechanism of action remains incompletely understood, the beneficial effects are potentially mediated by their ability to reduce postinjury vasogenic edema and inflammation. Once considered the standard of care, more recent studies advocate not using methylprednisolone, primarily due to a critique of several shortcomings of the initial NASCIS II study, including lack of reproducibility.[12-17] In other studies, including NASCIS

Table 12.1 Methylprednisolone Protocol

Dosage	
Bolus	30 mg/kg over 15 minutes
Maintenance	5.4 mg/kg/h
Duration of treatment 45 minutes after bolus	
23 hours	Initiation < 3 hours from injury
47 hours	Initiation > 3 but < 8 hours from injury

Source: Bracken, et al. N Engl J Med 1990;322:1405–1411

III, high-dose MP failed to provide clinical benefit but rather demonstrated significant morbidity, which included prolonged ventilator dependency, hyperglycemia, pneumonia, gastrointestinal (GI) hemorrhage, acute corticosteroid myopathy, infection, and sepsis.[12,18,19] The subsequent medical evidence fails to support high-dose MP treatment following SCI; however, the possibility of some clinical benefit following a catastrophic SCI injury has led to its continued use by some clinicians. Generally, treatment that commences during the resuscitation phase should be continued to completion in the ICU setting, with awareness and attention to its potential adverse systemic effects. Contraindications to high-dose MP usage include cauda equina syndrome, gunshot wounds to the spine, pregnancy, pediatric population ($<$ 13 years of age), prior use of maintenance steroids, and narcotics addiction.[20]

■ Respiratory Considerations

Ventilation

Respiratory sufficiency and pulmonary function may be profoundly altered following neurologic dysfunction, especially following SCI at the cervical or thoracic levels.[3,21] After ensuring airway protection during initial resuscitation following acute SCI, the adequacy of ventilation must be maintained. The key muscles of respiration are the intercostal, diaphragm, abdominal, and cervical accessory muscles.[3,22,23] Intercostal muscles (T1-T12) stabilize the chest during expiration, and paralysis leads to a functional flail chest phenomenon that contributes to loss of adequate tidal volume (Vt). The diaphragm (C3-C5) generates approximately 50 to 60% of the inspiratory force of respiration or forced vital capacity (FVC). Diaphragmatic dysfunction may occur either by high cervical SCI or from fatigue following low cervical or high thoracic SCI where the diaphragm has assumed 100% of the workload of respiration. In either situation, lung volumes become diminished.[3,23,24] As the primary muscles of expiration, loss of abdominal muscle function (T7-L1) may lead to increased end-tidal volumes and compromised lung capacity.[3,25] Cervical accessory muscles, the scalene muscles (C3-C8), and the clavicular portion of the pectoralis major muscle (C5-C7) may be lost in patients with high quadriplegia. More often, however, these muscles augment respiratory mechanics following acute SCI.

Marked reductions in tidal volume, FVC, and expiratory volumes may lead to the development of hypercarbia, hypoxemia, atelectasis, and inability to mobilize secretions. Generally accepted parameters for positive pressure ventilation include hypoxemia ($PaO_2 <$ 80 mm Hg), hypercarbia ($PaCO_2 >$ 50 mm Hg), or elevated respiratory rate ($>$ 35 breaths per minute).[3,22] In the awake, cooperative patient, ventilation-perfusion abnormalities may be assessed with serial measurements of FVC, which is the

maximal volume that may be exhaled after maximal inhalation. FVC incorporates tidal volume and inspiratory and expiratory reserve volumes, and is normally 65 to 75 mL/kg of ideal body weight. A drop to less than 15 mL/kg is indicative of impending respiratory failure.[26]

Continuous pulse oximetry monitoring, supplemental oxygen, and frequent arterial blood gas measurements are the mainstays in respiratory management of the SCI patient. Caution must be used, however, when interpreting arterial blood gas values, as they may be poor indicators of adequate ventilation, changing only after pulmonary and cardiovascular reserves are depleted.[3] Early hypocapnia may reflect activation of primary pulmonary receptors innervated by vagal afferents producing dyspnea and an increased ventilatory drive rather than a carotid chemoreceptor response to hypoxemia.[27] Subsequently, normal to low $PaCO_2$ may be misinterpreted to reflect adequate respiratory reserve in the face of respiratory distress. Treatment of supplemental oxygen may mask ensuing hypoxemia, further exacerbating altered pulmonary pathophysiology. Thus, as fatigue inevitably ensues with progressive tachypnea, exacerbation of profound ventilation-perfusion abnormalities may lead to acute respiratory arrest. Consequently, close attention to the respiratory rate is essential in the SCI patient as it may reflect impending respiratory failure.[3,28]

High cervical cord injuries often result in respiratory mechanical insufficiency requiring intubation. Even so, lower cervical, thoracic, or lumbar cord injured patients may require intubation in the setting of trauma to the chest or respiratory complications secondary to impaired cough or mobilization of respiratory secretions. The form of mechanical ventilation varies according to the level of alertness and respiratory effort. Altered pulmonary physiology in the SCI patient results in inadequate lung expansion. Therefore, positive pressure ventilation is preferred and can be provided with volume-cycled mechanical ventilation using either synchronized intermittent mandatory ventilation (SIMV) or assist control ventilation (ACV).[28] The former allows spontaneous and unassisted breathing between mechanical breaths. With SIMV, pressure support is advised to minimize fatigue that may result from an increased work of breathing through the high resistance of the ventilatory circuit. Extrinsic positive end-expiratory pressure (PEEP), which ceases expiratory flow at a preselected pressure, may be added to IMV settings. By preventing alveolar collapse, PEEP improves lung compliance and overall gas exchange, allowing inspired oxygen (FIO_2) to be reduced to less toxic levels ($<$ 60%). The latter, ACV, fully assists all spontaneous breaths through a full cycle and provides breaths at a pre-selected rate and by the ventilator. Hyperinflation is an undesirable feature of ACV, resulting from a decreased time for exhalation, and is accompanied by intrinsic or auto-PEEP, leading potentially to hypercarbia, alkalosis, and tachypnea. Patients with sufficient respiratory effort but at risk of fatigue benefit most from SIMV, whereas

ACV is appropriate in those with minimal respiratory effort.[3,28]

No single protocol for weaning a SCI patient off ventilator support appears to have a greater advantage over another. General criteria indicative that a patient may be successfully weaned include a vital capacity > 10 mL/kg, tidal volume > 5 mL/kg, peak inspiratory pressure > 20 cm H_2O, and a respiratory rate < 30 breaths per minute.[22,26] A gradual wean may be accomplished by slowly decreasing the rate of intermittent mandatory ventilation, continuous positive airway pressure support, or extending periods off ventilator support by using a T-piece trial for increasing periods of time. The latter is commonly used in our institution; there is clinical evidence that the diaphragm can be "trained."[3,21] Quadriplegic patients from high cervical cord injury are least likely to be weaned off ventilator support and may require a tracheostomy,[29] the timing of which should be coordinated with the possible necessity of surgical stabilization. Yet any patient requiring prolonged mechanical ventilation, usually more than 14 days, with inability to be successfully weaned off the ventilator should be considered for tracheostomy.

Pneumonia

Although postural changes, sterile nasotracheal suctioning, and aggressive chest physiotherapy remain important in the armamentarium for minimizing atelectasis and bronchial secretions, pulmonary complications are the most common cause of morbidity and mortality following SCI, with the majority of them due to pneumonia.[2,26,30] Pneumonia occurs in 5 to 20% of cervical-level SCI patients.[2,30,31] Even so, the use of prophylactic antibiotics is not recommended owing to the increased risk of antibiotic-resistant infection.[25,30] Early placement of a nasogastric tube for removal of stomach contents is indicated to minimize the risk of aspiration pneumonia in the right lower lobe resulting from gastric atony with SCI.[32] Nonetheless, the vicious cycle of poor secretion clearance, progressive bronchiole obstruction, ventilation-perfusion abnormalities, and atelectasis is the more common cause of pneumonia in SCI patients.[3,22,31] Combined with these factors and the acute angle of the left bronchus compared with the right bronchus, pneumonia is more frequently observed in the left lower lobe following SCI.[29] The microorganisms involved are likely similar to those found in most nosocomial pneumonias, which are polymicrobial and derived from the flora of the oropharynx.[28,31] The most common isolates are gram-negative aerobic pathogens.[28] In mechanically ventilated patients, development of ventilator-associated pneumonia (VAP) is usually caused by *Streptococcus pneumoniae* or *Haemophilus influenzae* if within the first 4 days of ventilation or *Pseudomonas aeruginosa* or *Staphylococcus aureus* after 4 days.[28]

The clinical signs of pneumonia in SCI patients include fever, leukocytosis, hypoxia, and purulent sputum associated with infiltrates evident on chest radiographs.[31] Chest radiographic diagnosis remains challenging owing to the likely presence of atelectasis that predisposes patients to pneumonia.[3,31] Further caution is noted in interpretation of these clinical signs as fever and leukocytosis may accompany atelectasis alone. Tracheal suctioning or bronchoscopy may be used to obtain a sampling of tracheal secretions for Gram stain and culture analysis. Antibiotic therapy should be directed at the most likely organisms until final culture results are available, but it should not be withheld during progressive infection while awaiting culture results. Alternatively, antibiotic treatment should not be changed if the patient shows improvement concomitant with radiographic evidence of clearance based solely on a culture report suggesting different or additional organisms.[3]

Thromboembolic Disease

Following SCI, venous stasis secondary to decreased vascular resistance and the loss of muscle contraction potentiates thromboembolic disease. The incidence of thromboembolic complications in the acutely SCI patient population may be as high as 100% based on radiolabeled fibrinogen scanning.[3,20,33,34] The risk for deep vein thrombosis (DVT) may be nearly ninefold greater in SCI patients compared with the generalized trauma population.[34,35] Likewise, the risk for catastrophic pulmonary embolism (PE) following DVT is elevated in the SCI population, 2 to 10%, compared with the general surgical population, 0.1% to 0.8%.[36] Yet the incidence of clinically recognizable DVT in the SCI patient has been reported at 15% and for PE only 5%.[37] The risk of either DVT or PE appears greatest in the acute phase of injury and up to at least 3 months following injury.[22,33,38] Not surprisingly, substantial morbidity and mortality is associated with the development of thromboembolism.[2,33,35] Consequently, a high index of clinical suspicion and aggressive prophylactic measures are recommended for 3 months' duration.

Choices for prophylactic treatment in patients with SCI and severe motor deficits include mechanical devices, such as external pneumatic compression devices, compression stockings, rotating beds or electrical stimulation, and anticoagulants, such as low-dose heparin, low molecular weight heparin (LMWH), and Coumadin.[3,20,33,39] Clearly, mechanical devices carry little if any risk; however, they do not appear to provide sufficient prophylaxis in isolation. Similarly, anticoagulation modalities, while potentially increasing the risk of hemorrhage within the injured spinal cord, particularly within the first 72 hours of injury, do not provide optimal thromboembolic prophylaxis when used alone.[3,20,33] Instead, combined therapy appears to provide the greatest protection against thromboembolism employing the use of LMWH or adjusted-dose or low-dose heparin in conjunction with pneumatic compression

Table 12.2 Thromboembolic Disease

Prophylaxis	
Mechanical devices*	
External pneumatic compression devices	
Compression stockings	
Rotating beds	
Electrical stimulation	
Anticoagulation*	
Low molecular weight heparin	1 mg/kg SC q12h
Low-dose heparin	5000 units SQ q8h
Adjusted-dose heparin	Titration of SQ heparin to partial thromboplastin time (PTT) 1.5 × normal
Deep vein thrombosis (DVT) diagnosis	
Clinical	
Unexplained fever	
Leg swelling or redness	
Diagnostic	
Duplex Doppler ultrasound (most common)	

devices, electrical stimulation, or rotational beds.[3,20,33,40,41] Neither low-dose heparin nor oral anticoagulation alone is recommended for prophylactic treatment of thromboembolic disease.[20,33] Thus, a reasonable ICU management strategy would be to employ mechanical devices in the acute phase followed by the addition of low-dose heparin (5000 units subcutaneously every 8 hours), adjusted-dose heparin (titration of subcutaneous heparin every 12 hours to a partial thromboplastin time [PTT] of 1.5 times control), or LMWH once primary hemostasis is evident and the risk of hemorrhage is significantly reduced, approximately 72 hours after SCI.[3,33,35,40] At our institution, we routinely employ Lovenox (LMWH) as our anticoagulation agent of choice, concomitant with pneumatic compression devices.

In the SCI patient, the diagnosis of DVT should be suspected with the development of an unexplained fever, leg edema, or redness, or an increase in leg circumference or skin temperature.[22,39] Mortality from DVT in SCI patients is 9%.[20] Diagnostic tests for DVT include duplex Doppler ultrasound, venous occlusion plethysmography (VOP), fibrinogen scanning, D-dimer analysis, and venography.[20,33] Once the "gold standard," venography is invasive and costly; therefore, it is reserved in the setting of high clinical suspicion with a negative ultrasound study.[33] Duplex Doppler ultrasonography is the mainstay test because of its availability, low cost, and accuracy in detecting DVT with a sensitivity of approximately 90%.[3,33] D-dimer measurement is highly sensitive but not specific,[42] and fibrinogen scanning is not widely employed.[3,20,21,33]

Upon confirmatory diagnosis of DVT, full anticoagulation with heparin followed by oral warfarin for 3 to 6 months with international normalized ratio (INR) levels of 1.5 to 2.5 is recommended.[40,43] In patients with confirmed DVT but in whom anticoagulation therapy is contraindicated or ineffective, a vena cava filter should be placed.[3,40,43–45] Subsequently, the PE must be attentively monitored, as the typical symptoms of tachypnea, tachycardia, or pleuritic pain may be obfuscated from the underlying respiratory pathophysiology observed following SCI. Although pulmonary angiography remains the gold standard in diagnosis of PE, more often chest radiography, ventilation-perfusion scans, or, more commonly, spiral computed tomography[46] with acute changes in arterial blood gases and electrocardiogram may be useful in establishing the presence of PE.[3,21,22,40] The arterial blood gas changes may be difficult to interpret with the pretext of underlying pulmonary compromise, yet decreases in oxygen saturation or arterial oxygen with a concomitant increase in arterial carbon dioxide should raise the suspicion of pulmonary emboli. The electrocardiogram may demonstrate signs of acute cor pulmonale, especially with a large PE. The classic triad on the electrocardiogram, though seldom observed, includes a large S wave in lead I, a large Q wave in lead III, and an inverted T wave in lead III ("S1Q3T3"). More commonly observed is sinus tachycardia. In addition to full anticoagulation as with DVT treatment described above, the placement of a vena cava filter is recommended to prevent further emboli[44] (**Table 12.2**).

Table 12.2 *(Continued)* **Thromboembolic Disease**

Venous occlusion plethysmography	
Fibrinogen scanning	
D-dimer analysis	
Venography (gold standard but rarely used)	
Treatment of DVT	
Anticoagulation	
First phase:	24 to 48 hours with full anticoagulation with heparin
Second phase:	> 48 hours, warfarin for 3 to 6 months with goal international normalized ratio (INR) of 1.5 to 2.5
Pulmonary emboli diagnosis:	
Clinical findings	
Tachypnea	
Tachycardia	
Pleuritic pain	
Diaphoresis/anxiety	
Diagnostic findings	
Acute changes in arterial blood gases and ECG with confirmatory study:	
Spiral computed tomography (most common)	
Ventilation-perfusion scan	
Pulmonary angiography (gold standard)	
Treatment	
Full anticoagulation usually for 3 to 6 months (as above for DVT but INR goal of 2–3)	
Anticoagulation with vena cava filter	

* Combination therapy recommended, neither proven effective in isolation; initiate anticoagulation once risk of hemorrhage is decreased, approximately 72 hours postinjury.[6,16,22,27]

Some centers advocate placement of vena cava filters in all SCI patients as a principal prophylactic measure.[2,47] Others, however, have demonstrated significant complications particular to SCI patients with compromised abdominal muscle tone that include distal migration, intraperitoneal erosion, and symptomatic IVC occlusion.[48–50] Therefore, current recommendations for caval filters are for patients with thromboembolic events despite anticoagulation or for those in whom anticoagulation or pneumatic compression devices are contraindicated.[2]

■ Cardiac/Hemodynamic Considerations

Hemodynamic complications frequently accompany acute SCI and may include hypotension, dysrhythmias, reduced peripheral vascular resistance, and reduced cardiac output.[51–53]

This compilation of symptoms manifests as neurogenic shock and are principally the result of interrupted sympathetic pathways with unopposed vagal activity.[3,53] Loss of sympathetic outflow causes vasodilation (leading to the pooling of blood in the periphery and third spacing of fluids) and the inability to generate tachycardia to increase cardiac output, subsequently relying mostly on increased stroke volume, which may or may not be obtained. The inevitable outcome is relative hypovolemia and hypotension.[3,45,52] Hypotension with systolic blood pressure < 90 mm Hg and a decreased heart rate of < 90 beats per minute are observed in approximately 25% of patients following acute SCI,[52] and may persist even after 4 to 6 L of fluid resuscitation.[3] Clearly, volume depletion is not the cause of hypotension. Thus, in the absence of hemorrhagic hypovolemia from associated injuries, judicious administration of fluids is advised secondary to the risk of iatrogenic congestive heart failure, pulmonary edema, and hyponatremia.[3,21,45,51]

Table 12.3 Vasopressors in Spinal Cord Injury

Drug	Dose	Effects
Epinephrine	1–8 μg/min	α- and β-agonist: prominent vasoconstriction but also activates B_2-receptors causing vasodilatation and ↓ diastolic blood pressure; + chronotropic and inotropic cardiac effects
Norepinephrine	1–20 μg/min	α- and $β_2$-agonist minimal effect on B_2-receptors; prominent increase in peripheral resistance with increases in systolic and diastolic blood pressure but may get reflex bradycardia; + chronotropic and inotropic effects
Phenylephrine	40–100 μg/min	Purely α-sympathomimetic; noninotropic; use in SCI is highly cautioned due to reflex bradycardia
Dopamine	0.5–2.0 μg/kg/min	Dopaminergic with renal, mesenteric, coronary, and cerebral vasodilatation; + inotropic cardiac effect
	2–10 μg/kg/min	α- and $β_1$-agonist; vasoconstriction with ↑ systolic and diastolic blood pressure; + inotropic cardiac effect
	> 10 μg/kg/min	α-, β-agonist and dopaminergic effects
Dobutamine	2.5–10.0 μg/kg/min	Primarily $β_1$- selective increasing cardiac output; + inotropic cardiac effect

Continuous electrocardiographic monitoring of hemodynamic parameters is essential in the ICU setting. Once the diagnosis of hemorrhagic hypovolemia is excluded or adequately addressed, the placement of a pulmonary artery catheter is useful to monitor peripheral resistance, which may be < 50% normal, and cardiac output.[3,21,52] Treatment with vasopressors is often required. Optimally, a vasopressor with both α- and β-adrenergic components is used because of the desired vasoconstrictive effect to the peripheral vasculature and chronotropic/inotropic effects to the heart (**Table 12.3**). Either norepinephrine (0.05 to 0.20 μg/kg/min) or dopamine (1 to 10 μg/kg/min) is commonly used as a single agent. The former has prominent $α_1$-/$β_1$- with mild $β_2$-adrenergic effects, resulting in prominent increases in peripheral resistance and both chronotropic and inotropic support to the heart, but may also be associated with undesired reflex bradycardia. The latter, on the other hand, is the pressor of choice. Dopamine, in a dose-dependent manner, primarily activates $α_1$- and $β_1$-adrenergic receptors, resulting in optimal chronotropic cardiac and peripheral vascular improvement. Dobutamine (5–15 μg/kg/min), selective for $β_1$-receptors, augments cardiac function but may reduce systemic blood pressure and is not widely used for patients with SCI. Although peripheral vascular resistance increases effectively with pure α-adrenergic agonists, such as phenylephrine, they are seldom used independently secondary to ensuing reflex bradycardia that is detrimental to cardiac function.[3,21]

The preeminent goal of therapy is the maintenance of adequate organ perfusion, which may be demonstrated by urine output of ≥ 0.5 ml/kg/h, prevention of acid/base abnormalities, and appropriate mentation.[3,21,52] The optimal mean arterial pressure (MAP) to achieve this goal is unknown and may vary among patients. In the acute phase of injury, disrupted perfusion to the injured spinal cord may be further compromised by systemic hypotension, thereby potentially exacerbating secondary ischemic cord injury. Maintenance of a MAP at high to normal levels, > 85 to 90 mm Hg for a minimum of 7 days, has been suggested to enhance neurologic outcome and reduce morbidity and mortality following acute SCI.[51,52,54]

■ Gastrointestinal Considerations

The spectrum of GI dysfunction following disruption of sympathetic innervation following SCI includes gastric atony, stress ulcerations, bowel obstruction, constipation, abdominal bloating, and fecal incontinence. Nutritional requirements and timing of enteral feeding are additional management considerations in the SCI patient population.[3,22,55] Early placement of a nasogastric tube for decompression of stomach contents and secretions reduces the risk of vomiting and acute gastric dilatation, either of which may compromise pulmonary function through aspiration or decreased lung capacity, respectively.[3] A decrease in nasogastric output typically occurs 2 to 3 days after admission and usually indicates a return of gastric motility.[22,56] Additionally, the return of flatus and bowel movements provides more direct evidence of regained GI motility. Once gastric motility has returned, enteral nutrition should be slowly introduced and may play a key role in the prevention of stress ulceration.[41] The key complication of early enteral feedings is high gastric residuals with an associated risk of aspiration.[56] Additional concerns with premature feeding include exacerbation or recurrence of GI ileus, especially when vomiting is observed after prior tolerance of enteral feeding.[3]

Nutritional Support

Nutritional support is a key consideration for the hypermetabolic and hypercatabolic state of SCI patients. The resting energy expenditure calculated by the Harris-Benedict equation overestimates the caloric needs of patients with isolated SCI, likely attributed to the flaccidity of denervated musculature.[57,58] The loss of muscle tone and activity also contributes significant nitrogen losses, resulting in prolonged overall negative nitrogen balance. Nutritional goals are to meet the caloric and nitrogen needs of the patient but not to restore nitrogen balance. Consequently, indirect calorimetry is the energy expenditure assessment method of choice, especially in the early postinjury period.[55,57,58] Providing nutritional support in this early period of injury, within 7 days, is essential to minimize hormonal alterations manifest as increased plasma cortisol and adrenocorticotropic levels, nutritional deficiencies, and immune dysfunction, all of which may lead to increased susceptibility to infection and delayed wound healing.[3,55,59] Enteral feedings are the preferred route, providing maintenance of GI integrity and function. Parenteral nutrition should be reserved for patients with GI injury, prolonged ileus, or mechanical obstruction.[3,55]

Many commercial solutions are available for enteral feedings. Initially, continual rather than bolus feeding is better tolerated in the critically ill patient, with starting rates of 20 to 30 mL/h, incrementally increased to deliver the final goal amount as tolerated by the patient, approximately 30 to 40 kcal/kg/d in the acute postinjury setting.[45,60,61] Enteral nutrition may be provided by nasogastric, orogastric, or, in the presence of high gastric retention volumes, small-bore nasoduodenal or nasojejunal tubes.[28,31,60]

Stress Ulceration/Gastrointestinal Hemorrhage

Stress ulcerations may occur in the GI tract due to an unopposed, persistent vagal tone accompanying the sympathectomy effect of SCI; they peak at 4 to 10 days postinjury.[3,22,62] Patients with cervical injuries are the most prone to stress ulceration. High-dose steroid treatment may[18] or may not[63] increase the risk. Prophylactic treatment with antacids, H_2-receptor antagonists, or sucralfate has been proven effective against stress-related mucosal damage.[62,64] Maintenance of gastric pH > 4 is associated with decreased incidence of GI hemorrhage.[63] Antacids, such as magnesium hydroxide, aluminum, and aluminum-magnesium combinations, quickly neutralize gastric pH but have untoward side effects with the required dosing regimens, such as diarrhea, constipation, hypophosphatemia, and metabolic alkalosis.[22,62] Intravenous H_2-antagonists (cimetidine, ranitidine, famotidine) may be administered instead; for example, ranitidine, 50 mg IV q6h, reduced the risk of GI hemorrhage from 43 to 17%.[64] Possible side effects of H_2-antagonists include hypotension, thrombocytopenia, and inhibition of cytochrome P-450 enzyme system with subsequent interference with the hepatic metabolism of other drugs, including phenytoin, antibiotics, and warfarin.[62,65] A third potential agent to consider is sucralfate, a mixture of sucrose, sulfates, and aluminum hydroxide that binds to gastric mucosa, increasing its viscosity, mucin content, and hydrophobicity.[22,62,66] Beneficial effects of sucralfate, including stimulation of prostaglandin, protection of the mucosal proliferative zone, with facilitation of mucosal regeneration and healing, combined with no major adverse effects, make this agent an attractive choice for the prevention of stress ulceration.[62] Indeed, sucralfate, 1 g PO/NG q6h, was found to be more effective that IV ranitidine, 50 mg IV q6h, in preventing GI ulceration or hemorrhage.[67] Further, a meta-analysis study reports sucralfate to be as effective as antacids, absent the deleterious side effects, and slightly more protective than IV H_2-antagonists administered in the prevention of clinical bleeding[68] (**Table 12.4**).

Declining hematocrit and platelet levels on serial cell blood counts should raise the suspicion of GI hemorrhage, especially when no other etiology may account for blood loss. Elevations in blood urea nitrogen (BUN) with adequate urine output and stable creatinine may indicate a hemorrhage within the GI tract.[63] In patients in whom a GI ulceration/hemorrhage is highly suspected, endoscopic

Table 12.4 Stress Ulceration Prophylactic Agents

Category	Example Agents	Effects
Antacids	Magnesium hydroxide	Maintain gastric pH > 4.5 and inactivates pepsin
	Aluminum hydroxide	
	Aluminum-magnesium combinations	
H_2-antagonists	Cimetidine	Inhibit parietal cell, histamine type 2, receptors; ↓ acid production
	Famotidine	
	Ranitidine	
Other	Sucralfate	Protects GI mucosa

evaluation is diagnostic and may provide hemostatic intervention. In recurrent or refractory GI bleeding, urgent surgical intervention is warranted.[3,62]

Abdominal and Bowel Dysfunction

The spectrum of bowel disorders in SCI patients ranges from acute life-threatening complications such as splenic rupture or liver laceration to more insidious issues such as bloating, bowel obstruction, constipation, fecal incontinence, and abdominal pain.[60,61,69] Acute intra-abdominal problems should be identified by computed tomography of the abdomen and pelvis during the early assessment phase following SCI and managed accordingly.

Although vagal efferent innervation remains intact, loss of sympathetic outflow from the bowel often results in impaired colonic transit. Progression to ileus with concomitant constipation is not uncommon. If untreated, resultant fecal impaction may precipitate a more severe bowel obstruction with an associated distention and risk of perforation. Initiating a daily bowel regimen is paramount in the early phase of SCI. A standard regimen consists of a combination of stool softeners, rectal suppositories, and enemas.[3] Paradoxically, although these agents improve colonic motility, looser and more frequent bowel movements may exacerbate the incidence of fecal incontinence, already manifest secondary to loss of sphincter control. Subsequently, supplying a source of fiber and maintaining adequate hydration are important considerations in the bowel regimen following SCI.[69] Functional bowel disorders persist outside the window of ICU management, and have been found to be an unfortunate yet understandable source of anxiety and psychological distress.[61,69] Therefore, early bowel retraining must be incorporated into the early management of SCI patients.

In injuries below C5, diaphragmatic irritation from abdominal distention may manifest as referred pain to the shoulder regions.[3] Yet visceral pain may be perceived below the sensory level of injury, possibly secondary to an imbalance of sensory channels, loss of spinal inhibitory tone, or the presence of a central pain generator.[70] Irrespective of the mechanism, elevated anxiety has been associated with SCI patients experiencing visceral pain symptoms.[60]

■ Urologic Considerations

Bladder hypotonia or flaccidity accompanies acute SCI during the period of spinal shock, lasting, on average, 3 weeks postinjury. Initial management involves the placement of an indwelling Foley catheter for accurate volume monitoring during hemodynamic stabilization and bladder decompression. A direct correlation between length of catheterization and risk of urinary tract infection (UTI) has been shown;[71] however, evidence is lacking for support of prophylactic antibiotic treatment as catheter bacteriuria is common.[71,72] The diagnosis of a UTI in SCI patients remains difficult as signs and symptoms may be occult due to loss of sensation. Clinical features may include fever, discomfort over the back or abdomen, increased urinary incontinence or spasticity, autonomic dysreflexia, malaise, and urine cloudiness or odor.[31,71,72] Gram-negative bacilli (*Escherichia coli, Pseudomonas, Klebsiella*) and commensal organisms of the bowel (*Enterococcus*) are the predominating causative microorganisms of UTIs in SCI patients.[31,71] Diagnosis should be confirmed with a urine culture. Empiric treatment may be started with broad-spectrum antibiotics and then tailored once the microorganism is identified and susceptibilities are known.

Once medically stable, consideration of removing the indwelling catheter and initiating a bladder regimen may commence; usually this occurs beyond the time of initial ICU management and is done after transfer to SCI rehabilitation. Return of bladder function after spinal shock has resolved is dependent on the level of SCI. Most commonly observed in SCI patients, hypertonic bladder dysfunction occurs with injury above the sacral spinal cord and is categorized as upper motor neuron dysfunction. Resultant bladder-sphincter dyssynergia may lead to incomplete bladder emptying and progressively increasing urinary volumes and distention.[22,73] Stimulated by excessive bladder distention, autonomic dysreflexia, a condition of massive sympathetic overdrive, may have life-threatening consequences. Symptoms of autonomic dysreflexia include sweating, headache, hypertension, and bradycardia.[22] Detrussor areflexia, or hypocontractility, occurs following injuries that interrupt the local reflex arc and is the hallmark of lower motor neuron bladder dysfunction.[73] Associated symptoms include saddle anesthesia, absent bulbocavernous reflex, and loss of both anal sphincter tone and control[73] (**Table 12.5**).

Urodynamic studies may guide appropriate management regimens. Overall, intermittent, clean, straight catheterization is the treatment of choice because of lower risk for UTI.[71–73] In a hypertonic bladder dysfunction regimen, goals include adequate drainage with low postvoid residuals, low-pressure storage, and low-pressure voiding. This can be accomplished numerous ways, including intermittent straight catheterization, external condom catheterization, functional electrical stimulation via an implanted device, volitional voiding, and anticholinergic pharmacologic agents such as oxybutynin and tolterodine tartrate.[3,73] In detrussor areflexia, the goal is the prevention of overdistention, which may be accomplished with scheduled bladder emptying using abdominal pressure, the Credé maneuver, or intermittent straight catheterization.[22,73] In either upper or lower motor neuron bladder dysfunction, long-term indwelling catheters are the choice of last resort, as they are associated with increased abnormal intravenous pyelograms, calculi, urethral lesions, leakage, and previously mentioned UTIs.[3,31,71,73]

Table 12.5 Bladder Dysfunction Categories and Treatments

Category	Manifestation/Treatment
Upper motor neuron dysfunction	
Complications	Ureteral reflux, hydronephrosis pyelonephritis, renal dysfunction
Detrussor-sphincter dyssynergia (elevated bladder pressures)	Anticholinergics, α-antagonists, antihypertonics, transurethral sphincterotomy, urethral stent placement, functional electrical stimulation
Detrussor hyperreflexia (urge incontinence)	Anticholinergics, afferent desensitization agents, functional electrical stimulation
Lower motor neuron dysfunction	
Complications	Saddle anesthesia, reduced anal sphincter tone, loss of sphincter control and bulbocavernous reflex
Detrussor areflexia (overdistention)	Intermittent straight catheterization, chronic, indwelling catheter (treatment of last resort)

Nonetheless, if necessary, indwelling catheters may be implemented through either transurethral or suprapubic placement.[71,73]

Priapism following acute SCI in men is nonischemic but rather appears to be in consequence of the sympathectomy effects following cord interruption. Conservative management by means of observation may be preferred over intracorporeal phenylephrine irrigation without interference of long-term erectile function in patients who regain erectile function after SCI.[74]

■ Integument Considerations

Decubitus ulcers are an unfortunate yet frequent problem in SCI patients. Immobility, insensate integument, low blood pressure, and resultant decreased skin perfusion predispose the skin to necrosis and breakdown.[3,22] For example, an SCI patient may develop decubiti even if left on a spine board for less than 6 hours.[3] The level and completeness of the injury appear to be proportional to the risk of decubiti formation. The most common sites for decubiti include the ischial tuberosities, sacrum, lateral malleoli, greater trochanter, heels, and coccyx.[3,22,31] Vigilant attentiveness to susceptible areas with frequent inspection and hygienic care is paramount in prevention, which remains the primary goal of treatment. Padding of pressure points, positioning, frequent turning with spine precautions as necessary, and utilizing air flotation beds constitute the mainstay of preventative measures currently employed.[3,8,22] Management of pressure ulcers once formed involves immediate relief of pressure and wound débridement. Antibiotic therapy is indicated in the presence of infection or bacteremia. *Bacteroides, E. coli, Proteus, Enterococcus,* and anaerobic streptococci are most prevalent in decubiti associated with necrotic tissue; *P. aeruginosa* and *S. aureus* are more frequent isolates from healing ulcerations.[31] Once formed, infection may result in cellulites, abscess formation, or osteomyelitis, with potentially catastrophic progression to bacteremia and sepsis.

References

1. The National SCI Statistical Center. Spinal Cord Injury: Facts and Figures at a Glance. University of Alabama at Birmingham National Spinal Cord Injury Center, June 2005
2. DeVivo MJ, Krause JS, Lammertse DP. Recent trends in mortality and causes of death among persons with spinal cord injury. Arch Phys Med Rehabil 1999;80:1411–1419
3. Benzel EC. Spine Surgery. 2nd ed. Philadelphia: Elsevier Churchill Livingstone; 2005:512–571
4. DeVivo MJ, Kartus PL, Stover SL, Rutt RD, Fine PR. Cause of death for patients with spinal cord injuries. Arch Intern Med 1989;149: 1761–1766
5. Management of acute spinal cord injuries in an intensive care unit or other monitored setting. Neurosurgery 2002;50(suppl): 63–72
6. Albert TJ, Kim DH. Timing of surgical stabilization after cervical and thoracic trauma. J Neurosurg Spine 2005;3:182–190
7. Fehlings MF, Perrin RG. The role and timing of early decompression for cervical spinal cord injury: update with a review of recent clinical evidence. Injury 2005;36:B13–B26
8. Management of acute central spinal cord injuries. Neurosurgery 2002;50:S166–S172
9. Larson SJ, Holst RA, Hemmy DC, et al. Lateral extracavitary approach to traumatic lesions of the thoracic-level spinal cord injury. Spine 1993;45:628–637
10. Marshall LF, Knowlton S, Garfin SR, et al. Deterioration following spinal cord injury: a multicenter study. J Neurosurg 1987;66:400–404
11. Bracken MB, Shepard MJ, Collins WF, et al. A randomized, controlled trial of methylprednisolone or naloxone in the treatment of acute spinal cord injury: results of the Second National Acute Spinal Cord Injury Study. N Engl J Med 1990;322:1405–1411
12. Fehlings MG, Baptiste DC. Current status of clinical trials for acute spinal cord injury. Injury 2005;36:B113–B122

13. George ER, Scholten DJ. Failure of methylprednisolone to improve the outcome of spinal cord injuries. Am Surg 1995;61:659–665

14. Hurlbert RJ. Methylprednisolone for acute spinal cord injury: an inappropriate standard of care. J Neurosurg 2000;93:1–7

15. Hurlbert RJ. The role of steroids in acute spinal cord injury: an evidence based analysis. Spine 2001;26(suppl):S39–S46

16. Hugenholtz H, Cass DE, Dvorak MF, et al. High-dose methylprednisolone for acute spinal cord injury: only a treatment option. Can J Neurol Sci 2002;29:227–235

17. Pharmacological therpy after acute cervical spinal cord injury. Neurosurgery 2002;50(suppl):S63–S72

18. Bracken MB, Shepard MJ, Holford TR, et al. Administration of methylprednisolone for 24 or 48 hours or tirilazad mesylate for 48 hours in the treatment of acute spinal cord injury: results of the Third National Acute Spinal Cord Injury Randomized Controlled Trial. JAMA 1997;277: 1597–1604

19. Qian T, Guo X, Levi AD, et al. High-dose methylprednisolone may cause myopathy in acute spinal cord injury patients. Spinal Cord 2005;43:199–203

20. Greenberg MS. Handbook of Neurosurgery. 6th ed. New York: Thieme; 2006:702–707

21. Ball PA. Critical care in spinal cord injury. Spine 2001;26:S27–S30

22. Andrews BT. Intensive Care in Neurosurgery. New York: Thieme; 2003:137–141

23. Estenne M, Detroyer A. Respiratory muscle involvement in tetraplegia. Prob Respir Care 1990;3:360–374

24. Bluechardt MH, Wiens M, Thomas SG, et al. Repeated measurements of pulmonary function following spinal cord injury. Paraplegia 1992;30:768–774

25. Kocan MJ. Pulmonary considerations in the critical care phase. Crit Care Nurs Clin North Am 1990;2:369–374

26. Schmitt J, Midha M, McKenzie N. Medical complications of spinal cord disease. Neurol Clin 1991;9:779–795

27. St John WM, Ahou D. Reduction of neural activities to upper airway muscles after elevations in static lung volume. J Appl Physiol 1992;73:701–707

28. Marino PL. The ICU Book. 2nd ed. Philadelphia: Lippincott Williams & Wilkins; 1998:421–448

29. Suderman VS, Crosby ET, Lui A. Elective oral tracheal intubation in the cervical spine-injured adult. Can J Anaesth 1991;38: 785–789

30. Fishburn MJ, Marino RJ, Ditunno JF. Jr. Atelectasis and pneumonia in acute spinal cord injury. Arch Phys Med Rehabil 1990;71: 197–200

31. Montgomerie JZ. Infections in patients with spinal cord injuries. Clin Infect Dis 1997;25:1285–1290

32. Gore RM, Mintzer RA, Calenoff L. Gastrointestinal complications of spinal cord injury. Spine 1981;6:538–544

33. Deep venous thrombosis and thromboembolism in patients with cervical spinal cord injuries. Neurosurgery 2002;50(suppl):S73–S80

34. Merli GJ, Crabbe S, Paluzzi RG, et al. Etiology, incidence, and prevention of deep vein thrombosis in acute spinal cord injury. Arch Phys Med Rehabil 1993;74:1199–1205

35. Green D, Sullivan S, Simpson J, Soltysik RC, Yarnold PR. Evolving risk for thromboembolism in spinal cord injury (SPIRATE study). Am J Phys Med Rehabil 2005;84:420–422

36. Green D, Twardowski P, Wei R, et al. Fatal pulmonary embolism in spinal cord injury. Chest 1994;105:853–855

37. Waring WP, Karuna RS. Acute spinal cord injuries and the incidence of clinically occurring thromboembolic disease. Paraplegia 1991;29:8–16

38. Lamb GC, Tomski MA, Kaufman J, Maiman DJ. Is chronic spinal cord injury associated with increased risk of venous thromboembolism? J Am Paraplegia Soc 1993;16:153–156

39. Kurtoglu M, Yanar H, Bilsel Y, et al. Venous thromboembolism prophylaxis after head and spinal trauma: intermittent pneumatic compression devices versus low molecular weight heparin. World J Surg 2004;28:807–811

40. Geerts WH, Pineo GF, Heit JA, et al. Prevention of venous thromboembolism. Chest 2004;126(suppl 1):338S–400S

41. Kuric J, Lucas CE, Ledgerwood AM, et al. Nutritional support: a prophylaxis against stress bleeding after spinal cord injury. Paraplegia 1989;27:140–145

42. Roussi J, Bentolila S, Boudaoud L, et al. Contribution of D-dimer determination in the exclusion of deep vein thrombosis in spinal cord injury patients. Spinal Cord 1999;37:548–552

43. Hamilton MG, Hull RD, Pineo GF. Venous thromboembolism in neurosurgery and neurology patients: a review. Neurosurgery 1994;34:280–296

44. Johns JS, Nguyen C, Sing RF. Vena cava filters in spinal cord injuries: evolving technology. J Spinal Cord Med 2006;29:183–190

45. Licina P, Nowitzke AM. Approach and considerations regarding the patient with spinal injury. Injury 2005;36:B2–B12

46. van Rossum AB, Pattynama PM, Ton ER, et al. Pulmonary embolism: validation of spiral CT angiography in 149 patients. Radiology 1996; 201:467–470

47. Wilson JT, Rogers FB, Wald SL, et al. Prophylactic vena cava filter insertion in patients with traumatic spinal cord injury: preliminary results. Neurosurgery 1994;35:234–239

48. Balshi JD, Cantelmo NL, Menzoian JO. Complications of caval interruption by Greenfield filter in quadriplegics. J Vasc Surg 1989; 9:558–562

49. Greenfield LJ. Does cervical spinal cord injury induce a higher incidence of complications after prophylactic after Greenfield usage? J Vasc Interv Radiol 1997;8:719–720

50. Kinney TB, Rose SC, Valji K, et al. Does cervical spinal cord injury induce a higher incidence of complications after prophylactic Greenfield inferior vena cava filter usage? J Vasc Interv Radiol 1996;7:907–915

51. Blood pressure management after acute spinal cord injury. Neurosurgery 2002;50(suppl):S58–S62

52. Levi L, Wolf A, Belzberg H. Hemodynamic parameters in patients with acute cervical cord trauma: description, intervention, and prediction of outcome. Neurosurgery 1993;33:1007–1017

53. Piepmeier JM, Lehmann KB, Lane JG. Cardiovascular instability following acute spinal cord trauma. Cent Nerv Syst Trauma 1985;2:153–160

54. Vale FL, Burns J, Jackson AB, et al. Combined medical and surgical treatment after acute spinal cord injury: results of a prospective pilot study to assess the merits of aggressive medical resuscitation and blood pressure measurement. J Neurosurg 1997;87: 239–246

55. Nutritional support following spinal cord injury. Neurosurgery 2002;50(suppl):S81–S84

56. Rowan CJ, Gillanders LK, Paice RL, Judson JA. Is early enteral feeding safe in patients who have suffered spinal cord injury? Injury 2004;35:238–242

57. Kearns PJ, Thompson JD, Werner PC, et al. Nutritional and metabolic response to acute spinal cord injury. JPEN J Parenter Enteral Nutr 1992;16:11–15

58. Rodriguez DJ, Benzel EC, Clevenger FW. The metabolic response to spinal cord injury. Spinal Cord 1997;35:599–604

59. Cruse JM, Lewis RE, Dilioglu S, et al. Review of immune function, healing of pressure ulcers, and nutritional status in patients with spinal cord injury. J Spinal Cord Med 2000;23:129–135

60. Barrett H, McClelland JM, Ritkowski S, Siddall P. Pain characteristics in patients admitted to hospital with complications after spinal cord injury. Arch Phys Med Rehabil 2003;84:789–795

61. Ng C, Prott G, Rutkowski S, et al. Gastrointestinal symptoms in spinal cord injury: relationships with level of injury and psychologic factors. Dis Colon Rectum 2005;48:1562–1568

62. Schmitt J, Midha M, McKenzie N. Medical complications of spinal cord disease. Neurol Clin 1991;9:779–795

63. Albert TJ, Levine MJ, Balderston RA, et al. Gastrointestinal complications in spinal cord injury. Spine 1991;16:S522–S525

64. Chan KH, Lai ECS, Tuen H, et al. Prospective double-blind placebo-controlled randomized trial on the use of ranitidine in preventing postoperative gastroduodenal complications in high-risk neurosurgical patients. J Neurosurg 1995;82:413–417

65. Tryba M. Side effects of stress bleeding prophylaxis. Am J Med 1989;86:85–93

66. Slomiany BL, Piotrowski J, Okazaki E, et al. Nature of the enhancement of the protective qualities of gastric mucus by sucralfate. Digestion 1989;44:222–231

67. Eddleston JM, Vohra A, Scott P, et al. A comparison of the frequency of stress ulceration and secondary pneumonia in sucralfate or ranitidine treated intensive care unit patients. Crit Care Med 1991;19:1491–1496

68. Tryba M. Sucralfate versus antacids or H2-antagonists for stress ulcer prophylaxis: a meta-analysis on efficacy and pneumonia rate. Crit Care Med 1991;19:942–949

69. Lynch AC, Wong C, Anthony A, et al. Bowel dysfunction following spinal cord injury: a description of bowel function in a spinal cord-injured population and comparison with age and gender matched controls. Spinal Cord 2000;38:717–723

70. Yezierski RP. Pain following spinal cord injury: the clinical problem and experimental studies. Pain 1996;68:185–194

71. Garcia Leoni ME, Esclarin De Ruz A. Management of urinary tract infection in patients with spinal cord injuries. Clin Microbiol Infect 2003;9:780–785

72. National Institute on Disability and Rehabilitation Research. Consensus statement: the prevention and management of urinary tract infections among people with spinal cord injuries. J Am Paraplegia Soc 1992;15:194–204

73. Burns AS, Rivas DA, Ditunno JF. The management of neurogenic bladder and sexual dysfunction after spinal cord injury. Spine 2001;26(suppl):S129–S136

74. Gordon SA, Stage KH, Tansey KE, Lotan Y. Conservative management of priapism in acute spinal cord injury. Urology 2005;65:1195–1197

IV Outcome

13 Pediatric Spinal Injuries

William S. Anderson and George I. Jallo

■ Pediatric Spine Development and Anatomy

Cervical Spine Development

Understanding the differences in pediatric versus adult spinal trauma can begin with the development and growth of the spine in general (**Table 13.1**). The healthy development of the spine is governed by the proper segmentation and specialization of the different spinal elements under genetic control.[1,2] Of interest in the cervical spine is the complexity of formation of the C1 and C2 elements. Most cases of os odontoideum are clearly linked with traumatic events (**Fig. 13.1**), but there are also well-described twin studies of patients with similar upper cervical defects resulting in congenital dens malformations.[3] It has been hypothesized

Table 13.1 Cervical Spine Development

Healthy development	Proper segmentation and specialization of different spinal elements under genetic control	
Os odontoideum	Dens malformations commonly linked to trauma, but can be congenital as well (weakness at synchondrosis)	
C1 and C2 formation	Atlas (C1)	Forms from three ossification centers:
		• 1 single center in anterior body
		• 2 paired centers forming posterior ring (unfused posterior ring commonly seen in dissection)
	Axis (C2)	Forms from four ossification centers:
		• 1 for the dens
		• 1 for the body
		• 2 for the posterior arch
	Atlanto-dens interval	Larger in children; can be as high as 4.5 mm on radiograph
Klippel-Feil syndrome	• Developmental anomaly showing incomplete spinal segmentation	
	• Three major subtypes:	
	• Type I: multilevel cervical and thoracic vertebral fusion	
	• Type II: 1 or 2 interspace fusions, hemivertebrae, occipitoatlantal fusion	
	• Type III: cervical and lower thoracic or lumbar level fusions	
Normal findings in child subaxial spine	• Pseudosubluxation of C2 on C3 by up to 3 mm	
	• Wedge-shaped vertebral bodies during ossification	
Additional factors affecting spinal injury in children	• Orientation of cervical facet joints:	
	• Child: fairly horizontal (30 degree angle relative to sagittal plane)	
	• Teenager: 60 to 70 degree angle	
	• Intersegmental instability until 7 years due to delay in ossification of uncinate processes	
	• Lymph drainage of upper cervical spine into deep cervical and nasopharyngeal nodes; can lead to Grisel syndrome and C1-C2 rotary subluxation	

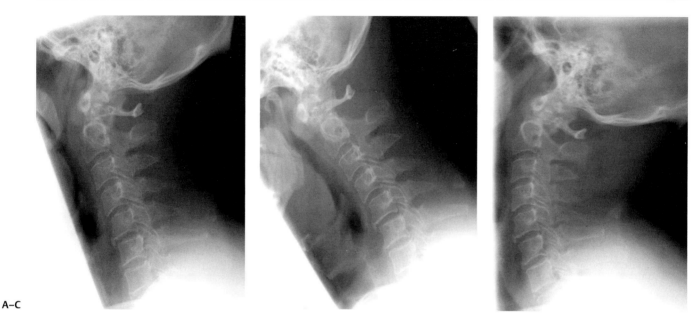

A–C

Fig. 13.1 Plain x-ray views of a young patient with os odontoideum. **(A)** Neutral view of the os odontoideum. **(B)** Flexion view of patient demonstrating the dens. **(C)** Extension view of the same patient.

that a congenital weakness at the synchondrosis might also predispose certain patients to os formation caused by mild trauma.[3] The axis itself is formed from four separate ossification centers: one for the dens, one for the body, and two for the posterior arch.[4] The atlas is complex as well and forms from three ossification centers: one single center in the anterior body, and two paired centers forming the posterior ring. An unfused posterior ring between the two latter centers is frequently encountered during dissection around C1.[4] The atlanto-dens interval is larger in children than in adults and can be as high as 4.5 mm on a normal radiograph.[5]

One particular development anomaly affecting the cervical spine and occipitocervical junction is the Klippel-Feil syndrome,[6] which illustrates many features of incomplete spinal segmentation. There are three major subtypes of the malformation per the classification scheme of Nagib et al:[6] type I involves multilevel cervical and thoracic vertebral fusion; type II affects patients with one or two interspace fusions, hemivertebrae, and occipitoatlantal fusion; and type III consists of patients with cervical and lower thoracic or lumbar level fusions. Several authors have identified specific fusion patterns that result in unstable cervical spine configurations, including a fused C2-C3 level with occipitalization of the axis, multilevel cervical fusion with a malformed occipitocervical level, and an unfused space between two long fused segments.[7,8] Normal findings in the subaxial spine in children include pseudosubluxation of C2 on C3 by up to 3 mm,[9] as well as in general more wedge-shaped vertebral bodies during ossification.

An additional factor affecting spinal injury patterns in children is the orientation of the cervical facet joints, especially in the young child.[10] The upper cervical spine facet joints start at a fairly horizontal angle of 30 degrees relative to the sagittal plane at birth, which increases to 60 to 70 degrees by the teenage years.[10] Intersegmental stability is also not mature until after the ossification of the uncinate processes, which occurs after 7 years of age.[10,11] Additionally, in the young child, the upper cervical spine segments drain via the lymphatic system into the deep cervical and nasopharyngeal lymph node chains, the same drainage as the nasopharynx itself, which can lead to Grisel syndrome and C1-C2 rotatory subluxation.[12] It is conceivable that this form of instability can occur after surgical procedures performed in the pharynx as well.[13]

Thoracic Spine Development

During the growth period between infancy and adolescence, the thoracic spine changes morphology enormously (**Table 13.2**). In a large longitudinal study of thoracic spine curvature following healthy children, the thoracic kyphosis increased by 6 degrees between the ages of 5–6 and 15–16 years. In the same time period, lumbar lordosis increased by 6 degrees.[14] The thoracic spine mobility decreases a great deal during this time period, by as much as 27 degrees.[14] The increase in magnitude of the thoracic kyphosis during growth is not linear, but seems to take off very quickly between the ages of 13 and 15.[15] Just prior to this age range, during the

Table 13.2 Thoracic Spine Development

Morphology	Changes drastically between infancy and adolescence:
	• Thoracic kyphosis increases 6 degrees between 5–6 and 15–16 years of age
	• Lumbar kyphosis increases 6 degrees
Mobility	Decreases by as much as 27 degrees during this period
Kyphotic changes	• Not linear; most change between ages 13 and 15
	• Actually decrease between ages 10 and 12
	• Slight difference in timing of these changes between sexes

time of the adolescent growth spurt, the amount of kyphosis actually decreases somewhat, with the anterior vertebral growth exceeding the posterior growth during the 10- to 12-year age range.[15,16] There are also slightly different timings of these kyphotic changes as a function of sex.

Lumbar Spine Development

Similarly, developmental disorders of the lumbar spine can predispose the pediatric population to further risk from trauma (**Table 13.3**). Spondylolysis and slippage are not uncommon in the pediatric population and seem to be more prevalent during the growth spurt.[17,18] The slippage itself, which occurs in association with spondy-lolysis, appears to be a problem of epiphyseal separation or epiphyseal plate injury due to the defect in the isthmus[19,20] (**Fig. 13.2**). The growth plate of the vertebral body is exposed to enormous stresses due to the bilateral pars defects and can frequently shear apart, leading to the listhesis. This does not appear to be a degeneration of the disk itself.[19]

Additionally, there is a spectrum of caudal agenesis disorders that can affect growth of the sacral vertebral segments, as well as neural structures, and the spinal dysraphism disorders affecting the posterior bony elements.[21] In severe cases of caudal agenesis, spinopelvic

instability can be an issue requiring operative intervention, and frequently these children have scoliosis problems as well.[21] Although not necessarily predisposing these children to additional traumatic injury, they are commonly

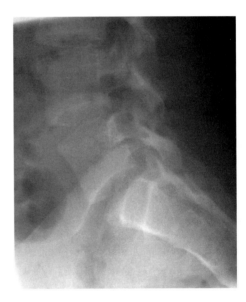

Fig. 13.2 A 13-year-old athletic boy with low back pain without radiation. The cone-down lateral x-ray clearly demonstrates the defect in the pars of the L4 vertebrae.

Table 13.3 Lumbar Spine Development

Spondylolysis and slippage	• Most prevalent during growth spurt
	• Slippage: problem of epiphyseal separation or epiphyseal injury due to isthmus defect
	• Listhesis: may occur due to shearing effects of bilateral pars defects on growth plate of vertebral bodies
Caudal agenesis disorders	• Affects growth of sacrum and neural structures
	• Spinal dysraphism affecting posterior bony elements
	• Spinopelvic instability requires operative treatment

enough encountered to complicate the surgical treatment of trauma in this group.

■ Pediatric Spinal Injury Characteristics

Overview

In general, cervical spine injury patterns in children (**Table 13.4**) are different from those in adults because of the pediatric disproportionate head size, looser cervical spinal biomechanics, and immaturity of bone formation.[22,23] Anthropometric growth data for children demonstrate vastly different growth rates for head circumference versus the more linearly related growth of other body structures, with this growth rate difference persisting to an age of 6 to 7 years.[24] Children do seem to be safer than adults in falls from great heights (> 15 feet); they survive in higher percentages, and have fewer internal organ injuries and fewer spinal fractures.[25] Younger children who do sustain spine trauma tend to exhibit cord injury more frequently than older children and die more frequently,[26,27] although as a group, the younger patients (< 11 years) present less frequently.[27] In one large series from the Mayo Clinic, the age- and sex-adjusted annual incidence rate for trauma-induced fracture and dislocation of the cervical spine was 7.41 per 100,000 population.[27]

Characteristic Injury Patterns in the Cervical Spine

Pediatric cervical spine injuries frequently occur in association with motor vehicle accidents (60% in the Rancho Los Amigos series).[28] Of interest, if the injured victim was a pedestrian, the victim's age was most likely less than 11 years old. Another age division occurs in sports-derived cervical spine injuries, with most patients ranging from 12 to 16 years of age.[28] Because of the large pediatric head size, the levels of greatest movement in the cervical spine are different from those in an adult (**Table 13.5**). In infants, it occurs at C2-C3, at 5 to 6 years it moves downward to C3-C4, and in adolescents and young adults it occurs at the C5-C6 level, as in maturity.[29] This categorization also correlates with the predominant level of injury in the pediatric population. These patients are subject to the gross patterns of injury demonstrated in the adult population as well, including atlantoaxial subluxation via transverse ligament disruption, Jefferson-type fractures, hangman's fractures, odontoid fractures, and atlantoaxial rotatory subluxation, as well as subaxial spine fractures (**Fig. 13.3**).[4] Additionally, the phenomenon of spinal cord injury without radiographic abnormality (SCIWORA) is present in perhaps 10 to 20% of spine-injured children and may represent various forms of ischemic injury or cartilaginous failure.[4,30]

The criteria of Panjabi and White need to be relaxed somewhat when evaluating the pediatric spine due to the higher mobility and elasticity in the pediatric population.[29,31] One set of criteria marking instability under the age of 8 years includes more than 4.5 mm of subluxation at the C2-C3 or C3-C4 levels, and more than 3.5 mm of subluxation at any level for patients older than 8 years. Furthermore, angulation of a deformity greater than 7 degrees can also be a sign of ligamentous injury.[29] The younger population frequently suffers from trauma-induced rotatory atlantoaxial subluxation as well (**Fig. 13.4**), and very rarely may have a pure component of strict atlantoaxial subluxation after tearing the transverse ligament.[32] In children, this is much more likely due to Grisel inflammatory syndrome or from congenital problems. Other causes of atlantoaxial stability leading to problems after trauma include Down syndrome, juvenile rheumatoid arthritis, and the skeletal dysplasias.[4] Birth injury as a

Table 13.4 Pediatric Cervical Spine Injury

Patterns of injury differ compared with adults due to	• Disproportionate head size
	• Loose cervical spine biomechanics
	• Immature bone formation
Falls from heights > 15 feet	Children actually safer than adults:
	• Higher survival percentage
	• Fewer internal organ injuries
	• Fewer fractures
Mayo Clinic study[27]	Age- and sex-adjusted incidence of cervical spine fracture and dislocation due to trauma = 7.41 per 100,000

Table 13.5 Imaging Patterns in Pediatric Cervical Spine

Associations	Motor vehicle accidents, sports injuries (12–16 years)
Levels of greatest movement	Correlate with predominant level of injury in pediatric population:
	• Infants: C2-C3
	• 5 to 6 years: C3-C4
	• Adolescent/young adult: C5-C6
Gross injury patterns	• Atlantoaxial subluxation via transverse ligament disruption
	• Jefferson-type fractures
	• Hangman's fractures
	• Odontoid fractures
	• Atlantoaxial rotatory subluxation
	• Subaxial spine fractures
SCIWORA	Spinal cord injury without radiographic abnormality:
	• Present in 10 to 20%
	• May represent ischemic injury or cartilaginous failure
Cervical spine instability	• Criteria:
	• > 4.5 mm subluxation at C2-C3 or C3-C4 under age of 8
	• > 3.5 mm subluxation at any level over age 8
	• Angulation of deformity > 7 degrees: sign of ligamentous injury
	• Trauma-induced rotatory atlantoaxial subluxation common
	• Strict atlantoaxial subluxation following transverse ligament tear is rare; more likely due to Grisel syndrome or congenital
	• Other causes of atlantoaxial instability: Down syndrome, juvenile rheumatoid arthritis, skeletal dysplasias
	• Birth injury rare but needs consideration, especially in diagnosis of neonatal hypotonia

cause of cervical spine fracture-dislocation is rare but does occur and needs to be included in the differential diagnosis of neonatal hypotonia. Many of these cases involve cervical hyperextension of the neck with the child in breech position.[33]

Characteristic Injury Patterns of the Thoracolumbar Spine

Thoracolumbar fractures (**Table 13.6**) in the pediatric population in the United States are most frequently caused by motor vehicle accidents, followed by falls, and pedestrian versus vehicle accidents.[34] Simple physical exam of these patients has a relatively high sensitivity (87%) for diagnosing a fracture and can be used as a filter before imaging.[34] Physical exam findings correlated with injury include midline spinal tenderness and ecchymosis.

The most common type of thoracic and thoracolumbar fracture in children is the compression fracture, and these fractures frequently are multiple.[35] Fortunately, because of continued bone growth, these types of fractures are remodeled quickly, and persistent kyphotic deformities are unusual in children after compression fractures.[35] Besides thoracic compression fractures occurring after motor vehicle accidents or falls, this age range also exhibits Chance-type multicolumnar fractures (**Fig. 13.5**), more often in the upper lumbar region. They have been reported in both restrained and unrestrained passengers.[26] Burst-type fractures are more common in older children.[26]

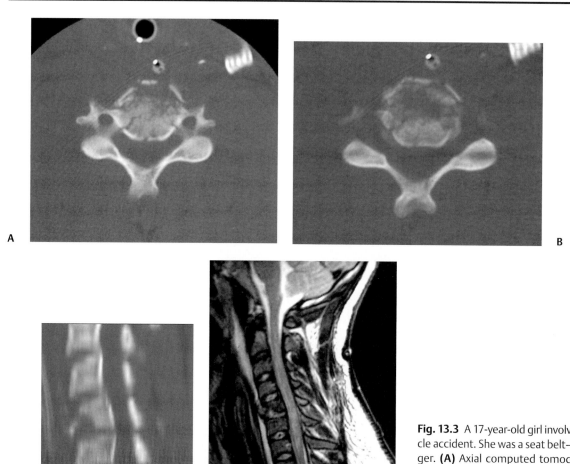

Fig. 13.3 A 17-year-old girl involved in a motor vehicle accident. She was a seat belt–restrained passenger. **(A)** Axial computed tomography (CT) image demonstrates a C5 burst fracture. **(B)** Another axial slice inferior to the previous image. **(C)** Sagittal CT reconstruction demonstrates the fracture. **(D)** T2-weighted sagittal magnetic resonance imaging (MRI) scan demonstrates the soft tissue swelling and compression on the thecal sac.

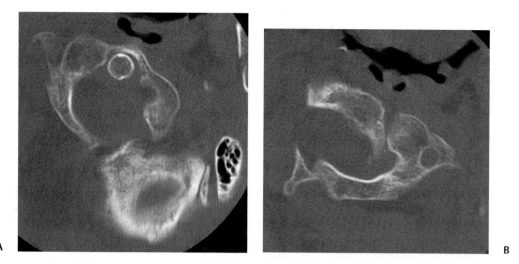

Fig. 13.4 **(A)** Axial CT scan of a 5-year-old boy with rotatory subluxation of C1 on C2 following an upper respiratory infection. **(B)** This is a purely rotatory component with no canal compromise.

Table 13.6 Injury Patterns in the Thoracolumbar Spine

Associations	Motor vehicle accidents, falls, pedestrian vs vehicle accidents
Physical exam	High sensitivity for diagnosis of fracture (87%)
Most common fracture type in children	Compression fracture
	• Remodeled quickly due to continued bone growth
	• Rare persistent kyphotic deformity
Chance-type multicolumnar fractures	• Common in upper lumbar region
	• Reported in restrained and unrestrained children
Burst fractures	More common in older children

■ Management of Pediatric Cervical Spine Trauma (Table 13.7)

Initial Assessment

Clearance of the pediatric cervical spine after trauma can be based on the National Emergency X-Radiography Utilization Study (NEXUS) criteria if the child is communicative and older than 3 years.[36–38] Upon examination, the patient is cleared if there is an absence of midline tenderness, there is no intoxication, the patient is alert, there is no distracting injury, and the patient has a normal neurologic exam. Any deviation from these normal findings requires imaging the patient, which can include flexion/ extension cervical spine radiography as well as computed tomography (CT) or magnetic resonance imaging (MRI) scanning.[36–38] Preverbal patients require a more extensive work-up as well. Patients younger than age 5 probably do not need transoral radiographs to view the odontoid, given the low sensitivity of this test in this age group.[31] Because of the relatively large heads in this age group, the emergency department staff must be careful when placing the child on a firm backboard because there is a tendency to induce additional kyphosis in the spine.[24,29] Many authors advocate torso elevation with pads or sheets to bring the neck into neutral position during the trauma evaluation or before.[29,39] As many as 18% of these patients have multilevel fractures or dislocations, mandating evaluation of the whole spine.[40]

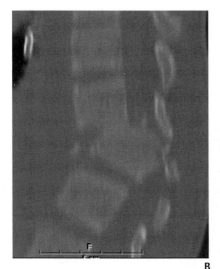
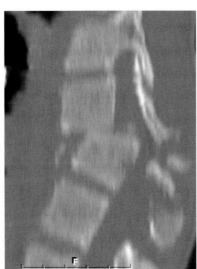
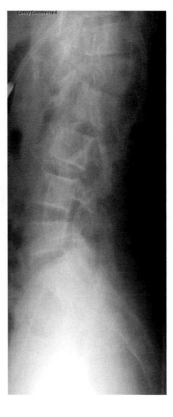

Fig. 13.5 (A) Sagittal reconstruction CT of a young boy with a traumatic L1 multicolumnar Chance-type fracture. **(B)** Sagittal view demonstrates the deformity and compression of the spinal cord. **(C)** Lateral x-ray of the same child with displacement of the vertebral bodies.

Table 13.7 Pediatric Cervical Spine Trauma Management

Initial assessment	Clearance via NEXUS criteria if child is communicative and over 3 years:
	• Midline tenderness absent
	• No intoxication
	• Patient alert
	• No distracting injury
	• Neurologic exam normal
	Any deviation from these requires imaging (radiography, CT, MRI)
Brace utility	• Nonoperative treatment, including use of halo vest (treatment of choice)
	• In halo ring fixation, skull thickness of child needs to be considered
	• Criteria for skipping halo and proceeding directly to surgical intervention:
	• No reduction achieved
	• Persistent instability
	• Ligamentous injury with facet instability
	• Kyphosis > 15 degrees
	• Compression fracture of involved vertebral body
	• Spinal cord compression resulting in neurologic deficit
	• Halo use in type II odontoid fractures; reduction and fusion achieved in 80%, with time to fusion between 10 and 18 weeks (13-week average)
Surgical management	• Posterior approach: common in upper cervical spine injuries
	• Anterior approach: in cases of disk herniations, severe fracture/dislocation injuries of both posterior and anterior elements, corpectomy in vertebral body fractures, and misalignment causing cord compression
	• In C1-C2 transarticular screw study, virtually a 100% fusion rate (preoperative CT required)

Brace Utility

In many large series of pediatric cervical spine injuries, most patients are treated nonoperatively,[40] with the halo vest proving to be of use even in very young patients. For instance, immobilization can be achieved in patients ranging in age from 7 to 24 months for periods of 2.0 to 3.5 months.[41] Of note with halo ring fixation, the skull thickness of children ages 2 to 5 years averages 4.8 mm, and great care must be taken to keep the pin torque at an acceptable level yet maintain a stable ring system.[42] Reasons for proceeding to surgical intervention with or without attempting halo fixation include no reduction achieved, persistent instability, ligamentous injury with facet instability, spinal kyphosis > 15 degrees, a significant compression fracture of an involved vertebral body, and spinal cord compression resulting in neurologic deficit.[40]

In a small series of predominantly type II odontoid fractures, which in children are frequently avulsions of the synchondrosis in the dens (**Fig. 13.6**), 8 of 10 children younger than 6 years of age achieved reduction and fusion using halo fixation alone, with the other 2 requiring

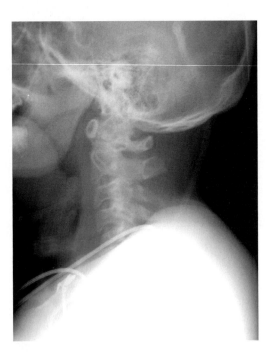

Fig. 13.6 A lateral x-ray of a type II odontoid fracture in a child, just under the ring of C1.

operative management.[43] The time to fusion in these patients was reported as 13 weeks (range 10–18 weeks).[43] A few authors have investigated the use of Minerva-type cervicothoracic orthoses, which include an upper thoracic brace, a cervical collar with an occipital flare, and a forehead strap for cervical immobilization.[44] Data indicate that this type of device limits motion adequately below C2 and might be useful for reducing motion at the C1-C2 level. However, halo ring fixation remains the treatment of choice for high cervical injuries.[44]

Surgical Management

Surgical management of spine injuries in the pediatric population is complicated by the growing needs of the child. As discussed above, injuries in the younger pediatric population (younger than 6 or 7 years) frequently involve the upper cervical spine, including the axis and atlas. Most of these injuries are treated via a posterior approach. However, it is not uncommon to encounter traumatic disk herniations in children, which become more common in the older child, when the spine assumes more adult proportions. An anterior approach in this situation is warranted. Some authors also consider anterior approaches in children for severe fracture/dislocation injuries involving both posterior and anterior elements, severe vertebral body fractures to perform a corpectomy, and major misalignment problems causing cord compression.[45] Long anterior constructs typically require posterior fusion as well, and in children the newer bioabsorbable plates and spacer systems may prove to be more appropriate in the long run than metal hardware.[45]

Sixty-seven patients with an average age of 9 years underwent C1-C2 transarticular screw placement in a large series of pediatric spine trauma and cervical anomaly patients (24 patients had trauma-induced C1-C2 instability) at the University of Utah over an 11-year period.[46] This was combined with occipitocervical fixation in 23 of the patients. The youngest patient was 18 months of age. These authors reported two vertebral artery injuries in this series and virtually a 100% fusion rate, which befits the age of the patients. Preoperative CT planning with reconstructed images is necessary for these cases, and when only one side is amenable to screw placement, reinforcement of the construct with one of the cable fusion techniques is advised.[46]

■ Management of Pediatric Thoracolumbar Spine Trauma (Table 13.8)

Additional Complications

Children suffering spine fractures secondary to trauma at the sites of great curvature in the lumbar and thoracic spine typically do develop deformity (scoliotic or kyphotic) during the period of a year after the injury. It is not clear that these early resultant deformities remain stable into adulthood for most patients or whether any increase in deformity is clinically important viewing the population as a whole.[47] Growth plate injuries are significant in this population as well and, depending on their locations, may produce progressive kyphosis (anterior injury) or scoliosis (posterior injury).[36] Thoracolumbar injuries in the pediatric population are also frequently associated with abdominal organ injuries, including splenic and liver lacerations, intestinal damage, and injury to the genitourinary system. Many of these patients require urgent laparotomy exploration on presentation.[35] This age group also presents with multiple thoracolumbar fractures that can skip levels.[35] One interesting unexplained feature of pediatric thoracolumbar injuries is that boys tend to develop abdominal

Table 13.8 Pediatric Thoracolumbar Spine Trauma Management

Additional complications	• Deformities (scoliosis or kyphosis) develop during period of 1 year following fracture at site of great curvature
	• Growth plate injuries
	• Abdominal organ injuries, including splenic and liver lacerations, intestinal damage, genitourinary damage
	• Boys tend to develop abdominal injuries more easily and have worse outcomes
Surgical management	• Decompression of affected neurologic tissue
	• Reduction of fracture
	• Fixation or fusion in unstable fractures
	• Pedicle screw fixation (decreases kyphotic deformity and spondylolisthesis)
	• Nonoperative vs operative study: those treated operatively showed stable to improved kyphosis, whereas those treated with bracing showed progressive kyphosis and anterior vertebral compression

injuries more easily than girls, and they also tend to have a worse outcome.[48]

Surgical Management

The goals of treatment of thoracolumbar fractures are similar to adult cases, namely, decompression of affected neurologic tissue, fracture reduction, and fixation or fusion in the case of unstable fractures.[36] Pedicle screw fixation in the pediatric population is useful for correcting, a kyphotic deformity, reducing spondylolisthesis, or, later down the road, correcting postlaminectomy-induced kyphosis.[49] There is a great deal of literature and experience in hardware applications in the correction of scoliotic deformity in this age group, so concomitantly many surgeons have become facile at posttraumatic instrumentation as well in the thoracic spine.[49] There are very few series of pediatric patients who have been followed long term after fracturing their thoracic spine. Lalonde et al[50] published a series of 11 patients with thoracolumbar burst fractures, with 5 being treated non-operatively, and 6 undergoing treatment with posterior fixation and fusion. These latter six were described as having the worst fractures. On average the operative cases demonstrated stable to improved fracture kyphosis, which differed considerably from the cases treated with bracing, which over time demonstrated progressive kyphosis and anterior vertebral compression. Other studies of thoracolumbar region fractures have further risk stratified the development of later kyphotic deformity for conservatively treated patients.[51]

■ Management of Pediatric Lumbosacral Spine Trauma (Table 13.9)

Additional Complications

Lumbosacral fractures are rarer than the thoracolumbar region fractures in the pediatric population and tend to occur in older children.[48] As described earlier, the seatbelt-type fractures in children can be devastating. These are flexion-distraction injuries, with the most frequent level involved being L2. These injuries can result in Chance-type fractures, producing a horizontal fracture line extending through the lamina, pedicles, and vertebral body, and are frequently associated with lap-belt injuries.[52] This is why shoulder restraints are also advocated for this age group. A form of lumbosacral fracture that can mimic a herniated disk is a fracture involving the posterior rim apophysis of the vertebral body.[53] If these fractures are symptomatic, they may require removal of the offending bone fragment.[35]

Surgical Management

Conservative management including bracing can result in improvements in vertebral body height in pediatric thoracolumbar compression fractures. Some authors have used plaster body casts with the patient placed in hyperextension, specifically for anterior vertebral body angulation > 10 degrees and Risser sign (skeletal maturity index) ≤ 2 at the time of injury.[51] One worry involving instrumentation that parents and pediatricians may have is the effect of pedicle screw placement on further vertebral column growth in a child. A series of 19 patients (ages 1 to 2 years) was published by Ruf and Harms,[54] which followed these children after thoracolumbar pedicle screw placement (91 total screws). Measurements of the subsequent vertebral body growth appear to demonstrate continued age-appropriate growth in both the vertical and horizontal dimensions of the vertebral body. These authors also note the rarity of development of spinal stenosis in these patients.[54] The correction of high-grade spondylolisthesis at L5-S1 has also been described in children ages 8, 11, and 12 years with partial reduction of the slip.[55]

■ Rehabilitation in the Pediatric Patient (Table 13.10)

Motor Issues

Rehabilitation issues for children are somewhat different from those for adults, especially in the cervical spine, where children can suffer severe injuries yet regain a considerable

Table 13.9 Pediatric Lumbosacral Spine Trauma Management

Additional complications	• Rarer than thoracolumbar trauma; more common in older children
	• Associated with flexion-distraction (seatbelt) injuries; most frequently involved level is L2
	• Can produce Chance-type fractures
	• Posterior rim apophysis fracture mimics herniated disk
Surgical management	• Concern: effect of pedicle screw on continued vertebral column growth
	• Ruf and Harms[54] study showed no such evidence; continued age-appropriate growth seen

Table 13.10 Pediatric Rehabilitation for Spinal Cord Injury

Motor issues	• Unlike adults, children with cervical spine injury can regain considerable function
	• Case study showed:
	• 17 of 23 patients demonstrate independent communication at end of rehab
	• 14 of 23 patients demonstrate independent feeding
	• 12 of 23 patients demonstrate independent locomotion
	• Mortality rate of 13%
	• Functional improvements show stability over time
Bowel/bladder issues	• Neurogenic bladder and bowel are frequent complications
	• Involves loss of sensation of bladder fullness and inability to urinate, leading to hydronephrosis and urinary tract infections
	• Important to teach children by age of 5 to 7 how to perform scheduled catheterizations
	• Scheduled bowel program may be necessary as well

amount of function. There are frequently reports of children surviving atlanto-occipital dislocation.[56] In a small case series that had a mortality rate of cervical spine injuries of 13%, 17 of 23 injured patients demonstrated independent communication at the time of rehabilitation discharge, 14 of 23 had independent feeding, and 12 of 23 demonstrated independent locomotion.[56] Improvements in functional outcome in the pediatric population suffering spinal cord injury is stable over time as well, with one large series of patients followed into adulthood demonstrating relatively high levels of employment, independence, and life satisfaction.[57] Occasionally, spinal cord injuries in the acute phase have no radiologic manifestations as in SCIWORA. It is sometimes necessary to carry out thorough evoked potential studies in these patients as an aid to accurate identification of the affected levels, which can help in rehabilitation planning.

Bowel/Bladder Issues

Neurogenic bladder and bowel are frequent complications of spinal cord injuries in children.[58] This can involve the loss of sensation of fullness in the bladder and the inability to urinate at desired times. Many of these patients go on to develop hydronephrosis and frequent urinary tract infections, so it is thought best to teach children at least by the age of 5 to 7 how to perform scheduled intermittent catheterizations.[58] A scheduled bowel program may also be necessary, with young children placed on the potty for brief regular periods.[58] The transition to self-care in these two areas is frequently a source of frustration for parents and highlights the enormous challenges the families of injured children need to overcome.

■ Surgical Failures (Table 13.11)

Kyphotic Deformities

In a small series of patients that included predominantly pediatrics patients (age range 2 to 35 years) studied by Otsuka et al,[59] it was noted that patients undergoing previous multilevel laminectomies frequently require structural stabilization or fusion for progressive kyphotic deformity

Table 13.11 Surgical Failures

Kyphotic deformities	• Otsuka et al[59] study: showed patients undergoing previous multilevel laminectomies often require stabilization or fusion for progressive kyphotic deformity close to operative level
	• Prophylactic bracing following laminectomy does not prevent this long term
	• Meyer et al[60] study: showed 5 of 31 patients develop persistent kyphotic deformity at surgical level
Hardware failure	• May be more significant in pediatrics due to longer cycle duty of pedicle screws and growth stresses
	• Brown et al[49] study: 17 of 759 screws needed to be removed in perioperative period
	• Ruf and Harms[54] study: showed two screw breakages and two screw connection losses in 91 total screws

close to the operative level. This can become an issue in trauma patients when initial emergent decompressions are performed without immediate fusion. Unfortunately, prophylactic bracing after performing laminectomies in a child probably does not prevent the formation of any kyphotic deformity in the long term.[59] As a comparison, in a small series of 31 patients followed on average for 7 years, Meyer et al[60] studied children who had undergone laminoplasties for a variety of cord pathologies. These involved cervical, thoracic, and lumbar cases; 5 of 31 of these patients developed a persistent kyphotic deformity at the level of surgery, 2 of which eventually required fusion.

Hardware Failure

Hardware failure occurs in the pediatrics population just as in adults and may be more significant in the younger group due to the longer duty cycles the pedicle screws are exposed to, as well as the growth stresses of the child. In Brown et al's[49] series of 759 pedicle screws placed in pediatrics patients (ages < 18 years), 2.2% (17/759) screws had to be removed in the perioperative period (< 2 years) for a variety of failure modes. These included cases of instrument failure, such as screw breakage, pseudarthrosis, and chronic draining infections eventually requiring hardware removal. In Ruf and Harms's[54] series of very young children (1 to 2 years of age) undergoing pedicle screw placement, out of 91 total thoracolumbar screws, there were 2 screw breakages and 2 cases of loss of screw connection. As described previously, in long-term follow-up with this series, there were no adverse effects due to the instrumentation on vertebral body growth or eventual spinal length or curvature.

References

1. Müller F, O'Rahilly R. Occipitocervical segmentation in staged human embryos. J Anat 1994;185:251–258
2. O'Rahilly R, Müller F, Meyer DB. The human vertebral column at the end of the embryonic period proper: 2. The occipitocervical region. J Anat 1983;136:181–195
3. Kirlew KA, Hathout GM, Reiter SD, et al. Os odontoideum in identical twins: perspectives on etiology. Skeletal Radiol 1993;22: 525–527
4. Sponseller PD. Cervical spine injuries in children. In: Clark CR, ed. The Cervical Spine. Philadelphia: Lippincott Williams & Wilkins; 2005:508–524
5. deBeer J, Hoffman EB, Kieck CF. Traumatic atlantoaxial subluxation in children. J Pediatr Orthop 1990;10:397–400
6. Nagib MG, Maxwell RE, Chou SN. Identification and management of high-risk patients with Klippel-Feil syndrome. J Neurosurg 1984;61:523–530
7. McRae DL. Bony abnormalities in the region of the foramen magnum: correlation of the anatomic and neurologic findings. Acta Radiol 1953;40:335–354
8. Hensinger RN, Lang JE, MacEwen GD. Klippel-Feil syndrome: a constellation of associated anomalies. J Bone Joint Surg Am 1974;56:1246–1253
9. Cattell HS, Filtzer DL. Pseudosubluxation and other normal variations in the cervical spine in children. J Bone Joint Surg Am 1965;47:1295–1309
10. d'Amato C. Pediatric spinal trauma: injuries in very young children. Clin Orthop Relat Res 2005;432:34–40
11. Ogden JA, Hensinger RN, McCollough N. Skeletal Injury in the Child. 3d ed. New York: Springer; 2000:708–789
12. Mezue WC, Taha ZM, Bashir EM. Fever and acquired torticollis in hospitalized children. J Laryngol Otol 2002;116:280–284
13. Samuel D, Thomas DM, Tierney PA, Patel KS. Atlanto-axial subluxation (Grisel's syndrome) following otolaryngological diseases and procedures. J Laryngol Otol 1995;109:1005–1009
14. Widhe T. Spine: posture, mobility and pain. A longitudinal study from childhood to adolescence. Eur Spine J 2001;10:118–123
15. Cil A, Yazici M, Uzumcugil A, et al. The evolution of sagittal segmental alignment of the spine during childhood. Spine 2005;30:93–100

16. Murray DW, Bulstrode CJ. The development of adolescent idiopathic scoliosis. Eur Spine J 1996;5:251–257
17. Laurent LE, Einola S. Spondylolisthesis in children and adolescents. Acta Orthop Scand 1961;31:45–64
18. Seitsalo S, Osterman K, Hyvarinen H, Tallroth K, Schlenzka D, Poussa M. Progression of spondylolisthesis in children and adolescents: a long-term follow-up of 272 patients. Spine 1991;16: 417–421
19. Sairyo K, Katoh S, Sakamaki T, et al. Vertebral forward slippage in immature lumbar spine occurs following epiphyseal separation and its occurrence is unrelated to disc degeneration: is the pediatric spondylolisthesis a physis stress fracture of vertebral body? Spine 2004;29:524–527
20. Farfan HF, Osteria V, Lamy C. The mechanical etiology of spondylolysis and spondylolisthesis. Clin Orthop Relat Res 1976;117: 40–55
21. Estin D, Cohen AR. Caudal agenesis and associated caudal spinal cord malformations. Neurosurg Clin N Am 1995;6:377–391
22. Birney TJ, Hanley EN. Traumatic cervical spine injuries in childhood and adolescence. Spine 1989;14:1277–1282
23. Fuchs S, Barthel MJ, Flannery AM, Christoffel KK. Cervical spine fractures sustained by young children in forward facing car seats. Pediatrics 1989;84:348–354
24. Herzenberg JE, Hensinger RN, Dedrick DK, Phillips WA. Emergency transport and positioning of young children who have an injury of the cervical spine. J Bone Joint Surg Am 1989;71: 15–22
25. Demetriades D, Murray J, Brown C, et al. High-level falls: type and severity of injuries and survival outcome according to age. J Trauma 2005;58:342–345
26. Carreon LY, Glassman SD, Campbell MJ. Pediatric spine fractures: a review of 137 hospital admissions. J Spinal Disord Tech 2004;17: 477–482
27. McGrory BJ, Klassen RA, Chao EYS, et al. Acute fractures and dislocations of the cervical spine fractures in children and adolescents. J Bone Joint Surg Am 1993;75:988–995
28. Haffner DL, Hoffer MM, Wiedebusch R. Etiology of children's spinal injuries at Rancho Los Amigos. Spine 1993;18:679–684
29. McCall T, Fassett D, Brockmeyer D. Cervical spine trauma in children: a review. Neurosurg Focus 2006;20:E5

30. Hamilton MG, Myles ST. Pediatric spinal injury: review of 61 deaths. J Neurosurg 1992;77:705–708

31. White AA, Johnson RM, Panjabi MM, Southwick WO. Biomechanical analysis of clinical stability in the cervical spine. Clin Orthop Relat Res 1975;109:85–96

32. deBeer JD, Hoffman EB, Kieck CF. Traumatic atlantoaxial subluxation in children. J Pediatr Orthop 1990;10:397–400

33. Caird MS, Reddy S, Ganley TJ, Drummond DS. Cervical spine fracture-dislocation birth injury: prevention, recognition, and implications for the orthopaedic surgeon. J Pediatr Orthop 2005; 25:484–486

34. Santiago R, Guenther E, Carroll K, Junkins EP. The clinical presentation of pediatric thoracolumbar fractures. J Trauma 2006; 60: 187–192

35. Price AE. Unique aspects of pediatric spine injuries. In: Errico TJ, Bauer RD, Waugh T, eds. Spinal Trauma. Philadelphia: JB Lippincott; 2005:581–625

36. Anderson RC, Kan P, Hansen KW, Brockmeyer DL. Cervical spine clearance after trauma in children. Neurosurg Focus 2006;20:E3

37. Anderson RC, Scaife ER, Fenton SJ, Kan P, Hansen KW, Brockmeyer DL. Cervical spine clearance after trauma in children. J Neurosurg 2006;105(suppl):361–364

38. Viccellio P, Simon H, Pressman BD, Shah MN, Mower WR, Hoffman JR. A prospective multicenter study of cervical spine injury in children. Pediatrics 2001;108:E20

39. Nypaver M, Treloar D. Neutral cervical spine positioning in children. Ann Emerg Med 1994;23:208–211

40. Dogan S, Safavi-Abbasi S, Theodore N, Horn E, Rekate HL, Sonntag VK. Pediatric subaxial cervical spine injuries: origins, management, and outcome in 51 patients. Neurosurg Focus 2006;20:E1

41. Mubarak SJ, Camp JF, Vuletich W, Wenger DR, Garfin SR. Halo application in the infant. J Pediatr Orthop 1989;9:612–614

42. Loder RT. Skull thickness and halo-pin placement in children: the effects of race, gender and laterality. J Pediatr Orthop 1996;16: 340–343

43. Mandabach M, Ruge JR, Hahn YS, et al. Pediatric axis fractures: early halo immobilization, management and outcome. Pediatr Neurosurg 1993;19:225–232

44. Sharpe KP, Rao S, Ziogas A. Evaluation of the effectiveness of the Minerva cervicothoracic orthosis. Spine 1995;20: 1475–1479

45. Baron EM, Loftus CM, Vaccaro AR, Dominique DA. Anterior approach to the subaxial cervical spine in children: a brief review. Neurosurg Focus 2006;20:E4

46. Gluf WM, Brockmeyer DL. Atlantoaxial transarticular screw fixation: a review of surgical indications, fusion rate, complications, and lessons learned in 67 pediatric patients. J Neurosurg Spine 2005;2:164–169

47. Bergstrom EM, Henderson NH, Short DJ, Frankel HL, Jones PR. The relation of thoracic and lumbar fracture configuration to the development of late deformity in childhood spinal cord injury. Spine 2003;28:171–176

48. Cirak B, Ziegfeld S, Knight VM, Chang D, Avellino AM, Paidas CN. Spinal injuries in children. J Pediatr Surg 2004;39:607–612

49. Brown CA, Lenke LG, Bridwell KH, Geideman WM, Hasan SA, Blanke K. Complications of pediatric thoracolumbar and lumbar pedicle screws. Spine 1998;23:1566–1571

50. Lalonde F, Letts M, Yang JP, Thomas K. An analysis of burst fractures of the spine in adolescents. Am J Orthop 2001;30:115–120

51. Pouliquen JC, Kassis B, Glorion C, Langlais J. Vertebral growth after thoracic or lumbar fracture of the spine in children. J Pediatr Orthop 1997;17:115–120

52. Santschi M, Echave V, Laflamme S, McFadden N, Cyr C. Seat-belt injuries in children involved in motor vehicle crashes. Can J Surg 2005;48:373–376

53. Takata K, Inoue S, Takahashi K, Ohtsuka Y. Fracture of the posterior margin of a lumbar vertebral body. J Bone Joint Surg Am 1988;70:589–594

54. Ruf M, Harms J. Pedicle screws in 1- and 2-year-old children: technique, complications, and effect on further growth. Spine 2002;27:E460–E466

55. Smith JA, Deviren V, Berven S, Kleinstueck F, Bradford DS. Clinical outcome of trans-sacral interbody fusion after partial reduction for high-grade L5–S1 spondylolisthesis. Spine 2001;26: 2227–2234

56. Partrick DA, Bensard DD, Moore EE, Calkins CM, Karrer FM. Cervical spine trauma in the injured child: a tragic injury with potential for salvageable functional outcome. J Pediatr Surg 2000;35: 1571–1575

57. Anderson CJ, Vogel LC, Willis KM, Betz RR. Stability of transition to adulthood among individuals with pediatric-onset spinal cord injuries. J Spinal Cord Med 2006;29:46–56

58. Vogel LC, Anderson CJ. Spinal cord injuries in children and adolescents: a review. J Spinal Cord Med 2003;26:193–203

59. Otsuka NY, Hey L, Hall JE. Postlaminectomy and postirradiation kyphosis in children and adolescents. Clin Orthop Relat Res 1998;354:189–194

60. Meyer NJ, Flatley TJ, Dunn DD. Superiorly based laminoplasty in children: average 6.8-year follow-up of 21 patients. J Spinal Disord Tech 2003;16:156–162

14 Rehabilitation and Recovery from Spinal Injuries

Tom Stanley, Bart Wojewnik, Alexander R. Vaccaro, and Kern Singh

Rehabilitating spinal cord injury (SCI) patients requires a multidisciplinary approach that goes far beyond restoration of physical function and medical management. SCI is a life-changing event, and the ultimate goals of postinjury rehabilitation are independence and reintegration into society. This chapter focuses on the physiologic complications of SCI and their management as well as current trends in physical rehabilitation.

■ Epidemiology

The National Spinal Cord Injury Database is the largest SCI registry, yet it captures only 13% of all SCIs in the United States.[1] There are 11,000 new SCI cases each year, with 250,000 SCI patients currently living in the United States. Eighty percent of injuries occur in males primarily between the ages of 16 and 30. Motor vehicle accidents account for the majority of injuries, followed by falls, acts of violence, and sports.

■ Medical Complications (Table 14.1)

Respiratory Function

Respiratory complications are the number one cause of death in patients with spinal cord injury.[2] Any injury above the level of T12 results in impaired respiratory function. Patients with injuries at functional levels below T12 are also prone to pulmonary complications from inactivity. Diminished vital capacity leads to atelectasis and pneumonia.[3]

Table 14.1 Medical Complications of Spinal Cord Injury

Respiratory function	• Respiratory complications are the primary cause of death in those with SCI
	• Results from any injury above T12 level
	• A decrease in vital capacity leads to atelectasis and pneumonia
	• Areas for improving pulmonary function:
	1. Improved cough generation
	2. Endurance training
Cardiovascular effects	• Cardiovascular compromise is the cause of death for two specific groups:
	1. Those surviving for over 30 years following an SCI
	2. Those who are over 60 years of age
	• Both acute and chronic effects on cardiovascular system are seen
	• SCI above T6 affects sympathetic outflow, causing autonomic dysfunction and resulting in hypotension or hypertension
	• Autonomic dysreflexia is the loss of sympathetic inhibition, causing vasoconstriction, hypertension, and headache
	• Decreased venous return results in a decrease in stroke volume and an increase in heart rate, which then cause left ventricular hypertrophy and cardiovascular collapse
Deep vein thrombosis (DVT)/pulmonary embolism	• Develops due to immobility and venous stasis
	• Prophylaxis should be mechanical and pharmacologic
	• Duration of treatment remains controversial

Table 14.1 *(Continued)* **Medical Complications of Spinal Cord Injury**

Heterotopic ossification		• Incidence in SCI is 10 to 53%
		• Risk factors include prolonged immobilization, autonomic deregulation, and neuroimmunologic changes
		• Typically found around joints below injury level and results in decreased range of motion
		• Radiation therapy or indomethacin can be used postoperatively to prevent reformation
Neurogenic bladder/bowel	Bladder	• Result of upper motor and lower motor neuron injury at S2-S4 level (areflexic bladder and sphincter)
		• Overdistention can lead to renal injury and urinary tract infections
		• Treatment methods include medications, intermittent catheterization, indwelling catheters, timed voiding, and urinary diversion
	Bowel	• Uncoordinated peristalsis and bowel dysmotility due to loss of autonomic regulation
		• Treatment includes planned bowel regimen, stool softeners, laxatives, suppositories, and enemas
Osteoporosis		• Multifactorial pathogenesis (loss of mechanical loading, poor nutrition, hypercortisolism, etc.)
		• Current treatment focuses on exercise and pharmacologic agents to improve bone density
		• Loss of mechanical loading is primary risk factor
		• Spasticity protects against osteoporosis in low extremities
		• Functional electrical stimulation can re-create mechanical stresses
Pressure ulcers		• Most common long-term complication of SCI
		• Development and healing are multifactorial (movement, immune conditions, nutrition)
		• Areas of high risk of ulcer development: trochanter, sacrum, ischium, and calcaneal tuberosities
		• National Pressure Ulcer Advisory Panel guidelines:
		• Turning schedule with no single position held for > 2 hours
		• Examine high-risk areas on daily basis
		• Specialty beds to decrease focal compression
		• Rotating beds change patient position more frequently
Spasticity		• Incidence following SCI is 25 to 67%
		• Frequent cause of pain leading to joint contractures, decreased range of motion, and sleep impairment
		• Treatment:
		• Passive range of motion and stretching
		• Pharmacologic adjuvant (baclofen)

Two primary areas for improving pulmonary function are cough generation and endurance training. In a prospective analysis of 187 patients, Haisma et al[4] demonstrated an increase in respiratory function after rehabilitation. Alternatively, Brooks et al[5] did not find any clear evidence that rehabilitation improved respiratory function. Some authors believe that focusing on cough generation helps prevent the majority of respiratory complications.[6] Future research needs to address the use of epidural spinal cord stimulators to induce coughing; however, these devices are still being fully developed.[7]

Cardiovascular Effects

Although pulmonary complications represent the number one cause of death in all SCI patients, patients surviving longer than 30 years and those older than 60 years of age die primarily from cardiac complications.[2,8,9] SCI has both acute and chronic effects on the cardiovascular system.

Spinal cord injuries above the T6 level affect sympathetic outflow and cause autonomic dysfunction, leading to episodes of profound hypotension or hypertension.[10,11] A specific condition termed autonomic dysreflexia results in a loss of sympathetic inhibition to noxious stimuli, leading to vasoconstriction, hypertension, and headache. Urgent treatment is required to reduce intracranial pressure and prevent stroke.

Decreased venous return from the nonfunctional lower extremities results in decreased stroke volume and increased resting heart rate. Long-term effects include left ventricular hypertrophy and cardiovascular collapse.

Deep Vein Thrombosis/Pulmonary Embolism

Spinal cord injury patients are prone to developing DVT and pulmonary embolism secondary to immobility and venous stasis. The incidence of venous thromboembolism (VTE) varies widely in the literature from 7 to 100% without the use of prophylaxis. In one of the largest series to date, Jones et al[12] reviewed over 16,000 SCI patients in the state of California over an 11-year period to determine thromboembolic risk factors. The authors noted that the incidence of VTE did not change with varying methods of prophylaxis.

The diagnosis of DVT begins with a daily physical examination. The use of ultrasound has become widely accepted, but venography still remains the gold standard. Screening ultrasounds prior to surgical procedures can prevent perioperative morbidity.

Various authors have published recommendations for VTE prophylaxis in SCI patients.[13–15] Current recommendations include a combination of mechanical and pharmacologic treatments (**Table 14.2**). The goal with newer

Table 14.2 Recommendations for Deep Vein Thrombosis Prophylaxis[15]

- Compression hose and mechanical compression devices should be applied for the first 2 weeks following injury.
  - In patients whose prophylaxis has been delayed by 72 hours after injury, a screening lower extremity ultrasound should be performed prior to mechanical prophylaxis.
- Vena cava filter placement is indicated in SCI patients who have failed anticoagulant prophylaxis or who have a contraindication to anticoagulation (active or potential bleeding sites not amenable to local control (e.g., the central nervous system, gastrointestinal tract, or lungs).
  - Filters should also be considered in patients with complete motor paralysis due to lesions in the high cervical cord (C2, C3), with poor cardiopulmonary reserve, or with a thrombus in the inferior vena cava despite anticoagulant prophylaxis.
  - Filter placement is not a substitute for thromboprophylaxis, which should be commenced as soon as feasible.
- Anticoagulant prophylaxis with either low molecular weight heparin (LMWH) or adjusted dose unfractionated heparin should be initiated within 72 hours after spinal cord injury provided there is no active bleeding or coagulopathy.
  - Anticoagulants should be continued for 8 weeks in patients with uncomplicated complete motor injury and for 12 weeks in patients with complete motor injury and other risk factors (e.g., lower limb fractures, a history of thrombosis, cancer, heart failure, obesity, or age over 70).
- Reinstitution of prophylactic measures should be considered in chronic SCI patients if they are immobilized with bed rest for a prolonged period of time, are readmitted for medical illnesses, or undergo surgical procedures.
- Early mobilization and passive exercise should be initiated as soon as the patient is medically and surgically stable.
  - With documented deep vein thrombosis, mobilization and exercise of the lower extremities should be delayed 48 to 72 hours until appropriate medical therapy is implemented.
- In symptomatic patients, perform ultrasound of the lower extremities or ventilation/perfusion lung scanning.
  - If clinical suspicion is strong but the tests are negative or indeterminate, obtain venography of the legs, spiral computed tomography of the lungs, or pulmonary angiography.

pharmacologic agents is to reduce the risk of complications associated with anticoagulation. Recent literature has looked at various pharmaceuticals, but no study has shown improved efficacy over traditional agents.[16–18]

The duration of prophylaxis remains controversial. Anecdotally, many physicians continue prophylaxis until the patient regains mobility. Some physicians stop prophylaxis in the setting of spastic paralysis. Multiple studies have shown a significant decrease in the incidence of VTE after the first 3 months irrespective of the level of mobility.[14] Analysis of other patient groups suggests that chronic immobility does not predict VTE.[19]

Heterotopic Ossification

Heterotopic ossification (HO) is a known complication of SCI, with an incidence ranging from 10 to 53%.[20] The exact mechanism by which HO occurs is unknown; however, risk factors include prolonged immobilization, autonomic deregulation, and neuroimmunologic changes. HO is typically observed around joints below the level of injury and usually manifests as a decreased range of motion.

Diagnosis is most easily accomplished with plain radiographs, although triple-phase bone scanning is positive earlier and is more sensitive. Serum levels of alkaline phosphatase are elevated in HO and can be used to monitor the effectiveness of treatment.

Surgical excision of HO may be considered in severe cases with the primary goal of increasing the range of motion of the affected joint. Radiation therapy or indomethacin can be used postoperatively to prevent reformation. Early passive motion is effective at reducing joint contractures and may reduce HO formation; however, excessive exercises should be avoided to prevent microtrauma-inducing HO.

Pharmacologic HO prophylaxis is the mainstay of treatment. Bisphosphonates have been shown to decrease the formation of HO, but rebound ossification after cessation of therapy has been reported.[21,22] Current research is evaluating the use of nonsteroidal antiinflammatory drugs in the immediate postinjury period to prevent HO formation. In a prospective, randomized, double-blind placebo-controlled study, researchers analyzed the use of a selective cyclooxygenase-2 (COX-2) inhibitor in the prevention of HO after SCI.[23] Patients who received the COX-2 inhibitor were 2.5 times less likely to develop HO. Similar results with indomethacin were also noted by the same group of authors.[24]

Neurogenic Bladder

Injury to upper and lower motor neurons at the S2-S4 level result in an areflexic bladder and sphincter, causing overflow incontinence. Chronic bladder overdistention causes renal injury and predisposes patients to acquiring urinary tract infections (UTIs). The goal of treatment is to prevent urinary incontinence, avoid renal injury from excessive bladder pressures, and minimize the likelihood of infection. Treatment involves medications, intermittent catheterization, indwelling catheters, timed voiding, and urinary diversion. Cholinergic agonists such as bethanecol may promote bladder contraction, whereas antimuscarinic agents (oxybutynin) are effective for treating bladder spasm.

Current research regarding neurogenic bladders after SCI is limited. Laboratory studies of dietary glycine supplementation have shown reduced bladder and urethral activity, but human studies have not been performed.[25] The use of stents to treat detrusor sphincter dyssynergia is currently recommended only as a temporary option.[26] Future treatment options may include the use of an artificial sphincter, and initial studies appear promising.[27]

Neurogenic Bowel

Spinal cord injury has two major effects on bowel function. First, loss of autonomic regulation leads to uncoordinated peristalsis and bowel dysmotility, causing both constipation and diarrhea.[28] Consensus guidelines were developed in 1998 for the treatment of neurogenic bowel and are up to date as of 2005.[29] Patients should be placed on a planned bowel regimen that incorporates the use of stool softeners, laxatives, suppositories, and enemas.[29,30] Prokinetic agents are being added to bowel programs to help induce gastric emptying.[28,31]

The second effect of SCI is loss of anal sphincter control. Diagnostic testing includes anal manometry and electromyography of the external anal sphincter. Medications to increase resting tone are under investigation, as are methods for electrodefecation.[31,32] Biofeedback may prove to be an effective method for improving sphincter function in partial injuries, but thus far the literature is inconsistent as to its efficacy.[33]

Osteoporosis

The pathogenesis of osteoporosis is multifactorial, with contributions from the lack of mechanical loading, poor nutritional status, hypercortisolism, and alterations in gonadal function.[34] Osteoporosis predisposes patients to fragility fractures, particularly of the lower extremities. Current treatment regimens focus on both functional exercise and pharmacologic therapies to improve bone density.

Loss of mechanical loading is the primary risk factor for developing osteoporosis.[35–42] Studies have demonstrated that spasticity protects against osteoporosis in the lower extremities, further suggesting the importance of mechanical loading.[43] Previous attempts at standing the patient have met with inconsistent results.[44] Functional electrical stimulation (FES) has been a novel mechanism for re-creating the mechanical stresses induced by ambulation. Chen et al[45] demonstrated that FES cycling temporarily was effective in increasing bone density. In stark contrast to Chen's results, Clark et al[46] found no beneficial effect of FES in improving bone mineral density.

The medical treatment of osteoporosis has become standard; however, its use to prevent SCI-induced osteoporosis is still being evaluated. Chen et al[47] demonstrated that the combined use of calcitriol with pamidronate decreased bony resorption after SCI. Other studies have also shown a decrease in postinjury resorption and hypercalcemia with the use of pamidronate.[48] A more recent study looked at the use of pamidronate alone to prevent osteoporosis in SCI patients.[49] The authors did not find any long-term therapeutic benefit with the use of pamidronate alone. Nance et al[50] found that the early use of pamidronate combined with ambulation within 6 months of injury prevented osteoporosis.

Pressure Ulcers (Table 14.3)

Pressure ulcers are the most common long-term complication following SCI.[51] The development and subsequent healing of pressure ulcers are determined by multiple factors, including the frequency of patient movement, immunologic conditions, and nutritional status. Areas at high risk for the development of pressure ulcers include trochanteric, sacral, ischial, and calcaneal tuberosities.

The National Pressure Ulcer Advisory Panel (NPUAP) has developed guidelines for both the prevention and treatment of pressure ulcers.[52] Patients should be put on a turning schedule, with no single position maintained for more than 2 hours to avoid tissue ischemia. High-risk areas in bed-bound patients should be examined on a daily basis. Specialty beds made of foam, air, gel, or water can be used to reduce focal compression. Newer rotating beds facilitate changes in patient position on a more frequent basis.

Treatment of pressure ulcers consists of removal of the pressure source, débridement of nonviable tissue, and establishment of a moist environment in which the tissue can heal. Modalities for débridement of necrotic tissue include surgical, mechanical, enzymatic, biologic, and ultrasound-assisted.[53] Frequently, a combination of multiple modalities is required. Negative pressure therapy has been shown to be effective for large, more advanced ulcers.[53]

Spasticity

The incidence of spasticity after SCI ranges from 25 to 67%.[54–57] Spasticity is a frequent cause of pain in patients with SCI, leading to joint contractures, loss of range of motion, and sleep impairment. Treatment with passive range of motion and stretching can minimize muscle spasm, but pharmacologic adjuvants are usually required. Fortunately, current oral pharmacologic agents are effective at treating spasticity.

Baclofen is the first-line agent in treating spasticity after SCI. If patients do not respond to oral baclofen, medications are added, including diazepam, dantrolene, gabapentin, and tizanidine. Clinical failure of these medications has led to the use of implantable baclofen pumps. A Cochrane review of pharmacologic treatments for spasticity demonstrated that there is very limited level I evidence to support the use of these medications.[58] Additional studies have been performed to assess the value of intrathecal pumps and botulinum toxin.[59] These compounds are used only in cases of failed oral pharmacologic management.

■ Rehabilitation (Table 14.4)

Rehabilitation of the SCI patient focuses on improving mobility, improving self-care ability, and reconditioning to improve exercise tolerance.

Self-Care

The techniques for improving self-care are well established. Areas of focus include bathing/grooming, nutritional management, medications, mobility/transfers/safety, skin/bladder/bowel management, and dressing. Patient evaluation through the Self-Care Assessment Tool (SCAT)

Table 14.3 Staging of Pressure Ulcers[93]

- Stage 1: Pressure-related alteration of intact skin whose indicators as compared with an adjacent or opposite area on the body may include the following: skin temperature (warmth or coolness), tissue consistency (firm or boggy), or sensation (pain, itching)

- Stage 2: Partial-thickness skin loss involving epidermis, dermis, or both. The ulcer is superficial and presents clinically as an abrasion, blister, or shallow crater.

- Stage 3: Full-thickness skin loss involving damage to, or necrosis of, subcutaneous tissue that may extend down to, but not through, underlying fascia. The ulcer presents clinically as a deep crater with or without undermining of the adjacent tissue.

- Stage 4: Full-thickness skin loss with extensive destruction, tissue necrosis, or damage to muscle, bone, or supporting structures (e.g., tendon, joint, or capsule). Undermining and sinus tracts also may be detected.

Table 14.4 Spinal Cord Injury Rehabilitation

Focus	Improve mobility, improve self-care ability, reconditioning
Self-care	• Techniques: use of adaptive equipment (splints, bed rails, transfer boards, and wheelchairs)
	• Progress evaluated through Self-Care Assessment Tool (SCAT)
	• Areas of focus: bathing/grooming, nutrition, medications, mobility, dressing, skin/bowel/bladder management
Exercise therapy	• Role: prevent joint contractures and improve mobility
	• Strengthen muscles with partial or no motor injury to compensate for what is lost
	• Passive range of motion to maintain joint mobility
	• Electrical stimulation and complex devices (Parastep system) show promise
	• Autonomic dysreflexia can be induced by exercise; treat immediately:
	• Position patient upright to decrease intracranial pressure
	• Administer vasodilators
	• Avoid beta-blockers
	• Strength conditioning limited to prevent fracture
	• Exercise can also induce hyperthermia due to thermal dysregulation
Exercise tolerance	• Programs tailored after assessing cardiac and pulmonary status
	• Combine strength with endurance training to improve cardiovascular function
	• Combine electrical stimulation with endurance training to prevent atrophy and improve glucose tolerance

can be used to follow the patient's progress through therapy.[60,61] Self-care focuses on the use of adaptive equipment, such as splints, bed rails, transfer boards, and wheelchairs. SCI patients work with occupational therapists to improve functionality.

Exercise Therapy

The role of exercise therapy is to prevent joint contractures and to improve patient mobility. Exercise is used to strengthen muscles with partial or no motor injury to better compensate for denervated muscles. Passive range-of-motion exercises maintain joint mobility for future function. Electrical stimulation of nonfunctional muscle groups has not been shown to have an effect on long-term function.[62] Complex devices such as the Parastep system have been developed incorporating functional electrical stimulation to promote ambulation.[63]

Autonomic dysreflexia can be induced by exercise or noxious stimuli. Practitioners should recognize this complication during exercise therapy and treat it immediately. Treatment includes positioning the patient upright to decrease intracranial pressure, administering vasodilators, and avoiding the use of beta-blockers.

Care must also be taken to avoid fractures in patients with SCI. Generalized osteopenia combined with spasticity puts patients at high risk for fracture. Strength conditioning should be limited to prevent this complication.

Spinal cord injury patients also have thermal dysregulation and can develop hyperthermia with excessive sweating.[11] Exercise therapies should be performed in cool areas, and the importance of rehydration should be emphasized.

Exercise Tolerance

Reconditioning the deconditioned SCI patient is challenging. Specific exercise therapies are similar to conditioning regimens used in normal individuals. Programs are tailored after assessing cardiovascular and pulmonary status. Strengthening exercises are combined with endurance training to improve cardiovascular status. Current research evaluates the use of electrical stimulation combined with endurance training to prevent muscular atrophy and improve glucose tolerance.[64–68]

■ Psychosocial Issues (Table 14.5)

Spinal cord injury not only affects patients physically but also affects their mental health and social interactions. Patients with SCI are more likely to suffer from depression. Rates of depression in SCI-affected patients range from 14 to 35%, with severe symptoms seen in 15% of patients.[69] Patients with depression are more likely to

Table 14.5 Psychosocial Issues of Spinal Cord Injury

Depression	• Rates of approximately 14 to 35% in SCI patients
	• More likely to develop decubitus ulcers and urinary tract infections (UTI)
	• Factors associated with increased risk of depression: greater severity of injury, less social support, lower level of education, history of substance abuse, lower functional ability
Suicide	• 7% of mortality after SCI injury
	• Most common: gunshot wounds, drowning, overdose
Return to work	• Rates increase with increased survival following SCI
	• 13 to 69% rate of employment
	• Education level prior to injury is predictive factor

have decubitus ulcers and UTIs.[70] Factors that have been associated with an increased risk of depression include greater severity of injury, less social support, lower level of education, history of substance abuse, and lower functional ability.[71] Suicide is one of the top preventable causes of death after SCI, and it accounts for up to 7% of mortality after SCI injury, with gunshot wounds, drowning, and overdose.[72]

As more people survive SCI, the rate of return to the work force is increasing. Rates of employment from previous studies vary from 13 to 69%, depending on location and the definition of employment.[73-76] Educational level before injury is one of the most predictive factors of returning to work after SCI.[77-80] People with previously lighter types of work are also more likely to return to work after SCI.[81]

Sexual Dysfunction (Table 14.6)

Sexual dysfunction after SCI involves neurologic, physical, and psychosocial issues. Two pathways for erection include the reflex pathway, which is based on cutaneous stimulation, and psychogenic pathways that incorporate

mental imagery, previous experiences, and senses of the patient. Parasympathetic innervation from the S2-S4 levels controls arteriovenous shunts in the corpora cavernosa to induce erection. The sympathetic centers responsible for ejaculation are located at the T11-L2 levels. Pharmacologic agents including sildenafil are effective at treating erectile dysfunction, allowing for functional erection in up to 80% of SCI patients.[82,83] Assistive devices such as rings, vacuum devices, and artificial penile prostheses can be used in addition to pharmacotherapy.

Electroejaculation and vibratory penile stimulation (VPS) have been used to assist in ejaculation. Electroejaculation works by placement of an electrode on the rectal wall near the prostate to stimulate contractions for ejaculation. VPS activates the ejaculatory reflex by vibratory stimulation of the frenulum.

In women, psychogenic and reflex stimulation influences vaginal lubrication. Women with lesions between C4 and C8 are able to have orgasms; however, the frequency is diminished, and the time to orgasm is prolonged. Peer counseling has also been shown to be beneficial for women for sexual function.[73] Finally, helping patients with other SCI-associated complications such as spasticity, bowel and

Table 14.6 Sexual Function Following Spinal Cord Injury

Pathways for erection	1. Reflex pathway: based on cutaneous stimulation
	2. Psychogenic pathway: mental imagery, previous experience, and senses
Parasympathetic innervation	S2-S4 levels; induces erection
Sympathetic innervation	T11-L2 levels; responsible for ejaculation
Pharmacologic agents	Sildenafil: functional erection in approximately 80% of SCI patients
Assistive devices	• Rings, vacuum devices, and artificial penile prostheses can be used
	• Electroejaculation and vibratory penile stimulation used to assist ejaculation
Women	• Lesion site between C4 and C8: can still have orgasms; frequency decreases, and time to orgasm is prolonged
	• Peer counseling and improving self-esteem are beneficial

Table 14.7 Prognosis

Recovery		• Dependent on rehabilitation team
		• Variable and dependent on return of muscular function and functional capacity
Timing of examination		• Delaying assessment until 72 hours after initial injury provides more information than immediate exam regarding long-term functional status
		• ASIA classification commonly used
SCI	Complete	• Literature inconclusive in regard to recovery
		• Past rate of recovery in lower extremities is approximately 2 to 15%
		• Fisher et al[92] study: no motor recovery in lower extremities in tetraplegics
		• Conversion from complete to incomplete rate is approximately 4 to 25%, occurring as late as 2.5 years after injury
	Incomplete	• Much better prognosis
		• 67% improve motor function > 3/5 one level below injury
		• 16% improve motor function two levels below injury
		• 3% improve motor function three levels below injury
		• Patients with initial strength of 1/5 or 2/5 regain functional strength 90% of time
		• In those with 0/5, this recovery drops to approximately 27%
		• Most neurologic improvement in tetraplegic occurs in first 6 to 9 months

bladder incontinence, and autonomic dysfunction will likely improve the self-esteem of both men and women, thereby improving sexual function and orgasm.

■ Prognosis (Table 14.7)

Recovery after acute SCI is largely dependent on the rehabilitation team. Various specialists plan for the future restoration of function and improvement of patients' activities of daily living. Understandably, patients want to know how much function they will be able to recover. Prognosis is variable and depends not only on return of muscular function but more importantly on functional capacity.

Timing of Examination for Prognosis

The initial examination after an acute SCI is not a good predictor of long-term prognosis.[84] Delaying assessment until 72 hours after the initial injury provides more information about the long-term functional status of the patient. The American Spinal Injury Association (ASIA) classification is commonly used and is reliable for determining the extent of SCI (**Table 14.8**).[85–88] The neurologic level of injury is the most caudal segment of the spinal cord with normal sensory and motor function on both sides of the body. The motor level is the segment most caudal with a functional muscle strength grade of 3/5. The

sensory level is the most caudal segment with normal sensation to pinprick and light touch. The other physical exam issue is "sacral sparing." Preservation of the most caudal sacral segment defines an incomplete SCI. Understandably, incomplete SCIs have a better long-term prognosis.

Complete Spinal Cord Injury

The literature is inconclusive with regard to determining recovery after complete SCI. Historic rates of motor recovery in the lower extremities after complete SCI range from 2 to 15%.[86,89–91] Fisher et al[92] reviewed SCI patients using the ASIA classification system and found no recovery of motor function in the lower extremities after complete SCI in tetraplegics. The issue of recovery is complicated by the very small percentage of patients who convert from complete to incomplete. The literature demonstrates a conversion rate between 4 and 25%, with conversion occurring as late as 2.5 years after injury.[86]

Incomplete Spinal Cord Injury

Incomplete SCI carries a much better prognosis with regard to neurologic recovery. Recent literature demonstrates that 67% of patients improve motor function to greater than 3/5 one level below the level of injury.[92] Only 16% of patients were able to restore function two levels caudal, and only 3% recovered function three levels caudal to the initial level of injury. Patients with initial strength

Table 14.8 ASIA Impairment Scale[88]

Classification		Definition
A	Complete:	No motor or sensory function is preserved in the sacral segments S4-S5
B	Incomplete:	Sensory but not motor function is preserved below the neurologic level and includes the sacral segments S4-S5
C	Incomplete:	Motor function is preserved below the neurologic level, and more than half of key muscles below the neurologic level have a muscle grade less than 3
D	Incomplete:	Motor function is preserved below the neurologic level, and at least half of key muscles below the neurologic level have a muscle grade of 3 or more
E	Normal:	Motor and sensory functions are normal

of 1/5 or 2/5 regain functional strength 90% of the time.[89,90] The number drastically decreases in muscle groups with an initial strength of 0/5, with the final functional strength achieved in 27% of cases.[90,91] Most of the neurologic improvement in the tetraplegic patient occurs in the first 6 to 9 months, with little change occurring 12 to 18 months after the injury.[89]

Prediction of Functional Capacity Based on the Level of the Motor Lesion (Table 14.9)

According to the practice guidelines of the Consortium of Spinal Cord Medicine,[29] patients with C1-C4 lesions require assistance in all activities of daily living (ADLs), turning in bed, and transfers. Patients with lesions at the C5 level have preserved elbow flexion. These patients may be able to perform some ADLs but still require assistance for transfers and movement in bed. C6 lesions, like C5 lesions, still require assistance, but patients have full rotator cuff function and wrist extension. Active wrist

extension is important because it allows patients to grasp objects. Patients with lesions at the C7 level have triceps function, which aids in transfers. Patients with C8 lesions and below typically are independent in transfers and ADLs and do not require assistance because of good upper extremity function.

Ambulation (Table 14.10)

The ability of patients with SCI to ambulate independently is a significant functional hurdle. Independent ambulation can have a major effect on depression and social integration. The prognosis for ambulation after complete SCI is dismal, with only 5% of patients recovering to a community ambulatory level.[90] On the other hand, after incomplete SCI resulting in paraplegia, up to 76% of patients ambulate at 2 years after the injury.[91] Intact proprioception also increases the likelihood of ambulation when compared with patients whose posterior columns have been injured.

Table 14.9 Prediction of Functional Capacity: Consortium of Spinal Cord Medicine Practice Guidelines

Lesion	Functional Capacity
C1-C4	Assistance in all activities of daily living
C5	Preserved elbow flexion; still requiring assistance for transfers and movement in bed
C6	Still require assistance; but wrist extension allows patients to grasp objects
C7	Triceps function, aiding in transfer
C8 and below	Independent in transfers and activities of daily living

Table 14.10 Ambulation

Independent ambulation	Can have major effect on depression and social integration
Prognosis	• Complete SCI: 5% recovery to community ambulatory level
	• Incomplete SCI: 76% recovery at 2 years after injury
Intact proprioception	Increased likelihood of ambulation

■ Conclusion

The management of patients with SCI is challenging for both the patients and the caregivers; however, it is possible for patients with SCI to function with independence.

A multidisciplinary approach is necessary to confront the many obstacles faced by SCI patients. As technologic improvements in neuroregeneration develop, SCI patients will continue to benefit and improve their quality of life after traumatic injury.

References

1. DeVivo MJ, Chen YY, Jackson AJ. Spinal Cord Injury: Facts and Figures at a Glance. Birmingham, AL: University of Alabama at Birmingham; 2006
2. DeVivo MJ, Black KJ, Stover SL. Causes of death during the first 12 years after spinal cord injury. Arch Phys Med Rehabil 1993;74: 248–254
3. Burns SP, Weaver FM, Parada JP, et al. Management of community-acquired pneumonia in persons with spinal cord injury. Spinal Cord 2004;42:450–458
4. Haisma JA, Bussmann JB, Stam HJ, et al. Changes in physical capacity during and after inpatient rehabilitation in subjects with a spinal cord injury. Arch Phys Med Rehabil 2006;87:741–748
5. Brooks D, O'Brien K, Geddes EL, Crowe J, Reid WD. Is inspiratory muscle training effective for individuals with cervical spinal cord injury? A qualitative systematic review. Clin Rehabil 2005;19: 237–246
6. Kang SW, Shin JC, Park CI, Moon JH, Rha DW, Cho DH. Relationship between inspiratory muscle strength and cough capacity in cervical spinal cord injured patients. Spinal Cord 2006;44:242–248
7. DiMarco AF, Kowalski KE, Geertman RT, Hromyak DR. Spinal cord stimulation: a new method to produce an effective cough in patients with spinal cord injury. Am J Respir Crit Care Med 2006; 173:1386–1389
8. Garshick E, Kelley A, Cohen SA, et al. A prospective assessment of mortality in chronic spinal cord injury. Spinal Cord 2005;43:408–416
9. Bauman WA, Spungen AM, Raza M, et al. Coronary artery disease: metabolic risk factors and latent disease in individuals with paraplegia. Mt Sinai J Med 1992;59:163–168
10. Schurch B, Knapp PA, Rossier AB. Autonomic hyperreflexia revisited. Urol Int 1997;58:148–152
11. Jacobs PL, Nash MS. Exercise recommendations for individuals with spinal cord injury. Sports Med 2004;34:727–751
12. Jones T, Ugalde V, Franks P, Zhou H, White RH. Venous thromboembolism after spinal cord injury: incidence, time course, and associated risk factors in 16,240 adults and children. Arch Phys Med Rehabil 2005;86:2240–2247
13. Green D, Hull RD, Mammen EF, Merli GJ, Weingarden SI, Yao JS. Deep vein thrombosis in spinal cord injury: summary and recommendations. Chest 1992;102(suppl):633S–635S
14. Deep venous thrombosis and thromboembolism in patients with cervical spinal cord injuries. Neurosurgery 2002;50(suppl):S73–S80
15. Consortium for Spinal Cord Medicine. Prevention of thromboembolism in spinal cord injury. J Spinal Cord Med 1997;20:259–283
16. Hebbeler SL, Marciniak CM, Crandall S, Chen D, Nussbaum S, Mendelewski S. Daily vs twice daily enoxaparin in the prevention of venous thromboembolic disorders during rehabilitation following acute spinal cord injury. J Spinal Cord Med 2004;27:236–240
17. Thumbikat P, Poonnoose PM, Balasubrahmaniam P, Ravichandran G, McClelland MR. A comparison of heparin/warfarin and enoxaparin thromboprophylaxis in spinal cord injury: the Sheffield experience. Spinal Cord 2002;40:416–420
18. Green D, Sullivan S, Simpson J, Soltysik RC, Yarnold PR. Evolving risk for thromboembolism in spinal cord injury (SPIRATE study). Am J Phys Med Rehabil 2005;84:420–422
19. Gaber TA. Significant reduction of the risk of venous thromboembolism in all long-term immobile patients a few months after the onset of immobility. Med Hypotheses 2005;64:1173–1176
20. van Kuijk AA, Geurts AC, van Kuppevelt HJ. Neurogenic heterotopic ossification in spinal cord injury. Spinal Cord 2002;40: 313–326
21. Banovac K. The effect of etidronate on late development of heterotopic ossification after spinal cord injury. J Spinal Cord Med 2000;23:40–44
22. Schuetz P, Mueller B, Christ-Crain M, Dick W, Haas H. Amino-bisphosphonates in heterotopic ossification: first experience in five consecutive cases. Spinal Cord 2005;43:604–610
23. Banovac K, Williams JM, Patrick LD, Levi A. Prevention of heterotopic ossification after spinal cord injury with COX-2 selective inhibitor (rofecoxib). Spinal Cord 2004;42:707–710
24. Banovac K, Williams JM, Patrick LD, Haniff YM. Prevention of heterotopic ossification after spinal cord injury with indomethacin. Spinal Cord 2001;39:370–374
25. Miyazato M, Sugaya K, Nishijima S, Kadekawa K, Ashimine S, Ogawa Y. Intrathecal or dietary glycine inhibits bladder and urethral activity in rats with spinal cord injury. J Urol 2005;174: 2397–2400
26. Mehta SS, Tophill PR. Memokath stents for the treatment of detrusor sphincter dyssynergia (DSD) in men with spinal cord injury: the Princess Royal Spinal Injuries Unit 10-year experience. Spinal Cord 2006;44:1–6
27. Patki P, Hamid R, Shah PJ, Craggs M. Long-term efficacy of AMS 800 artificial urinary sphincter in male patients with urodynamic stress incontinence due to spinal cord lesion. Spinal Cord 2006;44:297–300
28. Chen CY, Chuang TY, Tsai YA, et al. Loss of sympathetic coordination appears to delay gastrointestinal transit in patients with spinal cord injury. Dig Dis Sci 2004;49:738–743
29. Consortium for Spinal Cord Medicine. Outcomes Following Traumatic Spinal Cord Injury: Clinical Practice Guidelines for Health-Care Professionals. Washington, DC: Paralyzed Veterans of America; 1999
30. Correa GI, Rotter KP. Clinical evaluation and management of neurogenic bowel after spinal cord injury. Spinal Cord 2000;38: 301–308
31. Kojima Y, Nakagawa T, Katsui R, Fujii H, Nakajima Y, Takaki M. A 5-HT4 agonist, mosapride, enhances intrinsic rectorectal and rectoanal reflexes after removal of extrinsic nerves in guinea pigs. Am J Physiol Gastrointest Liver Physiol 2005;289:G351–G360

32. Andersen IS, Rijkhoff NJM, Vukovic A, Buntzen S, Djurhuus JC, Laurberg S. Anorectal motility responses to selective stimulation of the ventral sacral nerve roots in an experimental model. Br J Surg 2005;92:1513–1519

33. Chiarioni G, Ferri B, Morelli A, et al. Bio-feedback treatment of fecal incontinence: where are we, and where are we going? World J Gastroenterol 2005;11:4771–4775

34. Jiang SD, Dai LY, Jiang LS. Osteoporosis after spinal cord injury. Osteoporos Int 2006;17:180–192

35. Warden SJ, Bennell KL, Matthews B, Brown DJ, McMeeken JM, Wark JD. Quantitative ultrasound assessment of acute bone loss following spinal cord injury: a longitudinal pilot study. Osteoporos Int 2002;13:586–592

36. Lazo MG, Shirazi P, Sam M, Giobbie-Hurder A, Blacconiere MJ, Muppidi M. Osteoporosis and risk of fracture in men with spinal cord injury. Spinal Cord 2001;39:208–214

37. Vlychou M, Papadaki PJ, Zavras GM, et al. Paraplegia-related alterations of bone density in forearm and hip in Greek patients after spinal cord injury. Disabil Rehabil 2003;25:324–330

38. Garland DE, Adkins RH, Stewart CA, Ashford R, Vigil D. Regional osteoporosis in women who have a complete spinal cord injury. J Bone Joint Surg Am 2001;83:1195–1200

39. Frey-Rindova P, de Bruin ED, Stüssi E, Dambacher MA, Dietz V. Bone mineral density in upper and lower extremities during 12 months after spinal cord injury measured by peripheral quantitative computed tomography. Spinal Cord 2000;38:26–32

40. de Bruin ED, Dietz V, Dambacher MA, Stüssi E. Longitudinal changes in bone in men with spinal cord injury. Clin Rehabil 2000;14:145–152

41. Dauty M, Perrouin Verbe B, Maugars Y, Dubois C, Mathe JF. Supralesional and sublesional bone mineral density in spinal cord-injured patients. Bone 2000;27:305–309

42. Jones LM, Legge M, Goulding A. Intensive exercise may preserve bone mass of the upper limbs in spinal cord injured males but does not retard demineralisation of the lower body. Spinal Cord 2002;40:230–235

43. Eser P, Frotzler A, Zehnder Y, Schiessl H, Denoth J. Assessment of anthropometric, systemic, and lifestyle factors influencing bone status in the legs of spinal cord injured individuals. Osteoporos Int 2005;16:26–34

44. Kunkel CF, Scremin AM, Eisenberg B, Garcia JF, Roberts S, Martinez S. Effect of "standing" on spasticity, contracture, and osteoporosis in paralyzed males. Arch Phys Med Rehabil 1993;74: 73–78

45. Chen SC, Lai CH, Chan WP, Huang MH, Tsai HW, Chen JJ. Increases in bone mineral density after functional electrical stimulation cycling exercises in spinal cord injured patients. Disabil Rehabil 2005;27:1337–1341

46. Clark JM, Jelbart M, Rischbieth H, et al. Physiological effects of lower extremity functional electrical stimulation in early spinal cord injury: lack of efficacy to prevent bone loss. Spinal Cord 2007; 45:78–85

47. Chen B, Mechanick JI, Nierman DM, Stein A. Combined calcitriol-pamidronate therapy for bone hyperresorption in spinal cord injury. J Spinal Cord Med 2001;24:235–240

48. Massagli TL, Cardenas DD. Immobilization hypercalcemia treatment with pamidronate disodium after spinal cord injury. Arch Phys Med Rehabil 1999;80:998–1000

49. Bauman WA, Wecht JM, Kirshblum S, et al. Effect of pamidronate administration on bone in patients with acute spinal cord injury. J Rehabil Res Dev 2005;42:305–313

50. Nance PW, Schryvers O, Leslie W, Ludwig S, Krahn J, Uebelhart D. Intravenous pamidronate attenuates bone density loss after acute spinal cord injury. Arch Phys Med Rehabil 1999;80:243–251

51. McKinley WO, Jackson AB, Cardenas DD, DeVivo MJ. Long-term medical complications after traumatic spinal cord injury: a regional model systems analysis. Arch Phys Med Rehabil 1999;80: 1402–1410

52. National Pressure Ulcer Advisory Panel (NPUAP). Statement on Pressure Ulcer Prevention, 1992

53. Niezgoda JA, Mendez-Eastman S. The effective management of pressure ulcers. Adv Skin Wound Care 2006;19(suppl 1):3–15

54. Johnson RL, Gerhart KA, McCray J, Menconi JC, Whiteneck GG. Secondary conditions following spinal cord injury in a population-based sample. Spinal Cord 1998;36:45–50

55. Maynard FM, Karunas RS, Waring WP III. Epidemiology of spasticity following traumatic spinal cord injury. Arch Phys Med Rehabil 1990;71:566–569

56. Walter JS, Sacks J, Othman R, et al. A database of self-reported secondary medical problems among VA spinal cord injury patients: its role in clinical care and management. J Rehabil Res Dev 2002;39:53–61

57. Noreau L, Proulx P, Gagnon L, Drolet M, Laramée MT. Secondary impairments after spinal cord injury: a population-based study. Am J Phys Med Rehabil 2000;79:526–535

58. Taricco M, Adone R, Pagliacci C, Telaro E. Pharmacological interventions for spasticity following spinal cord injury: results of a Cochrane systematic review. Eura Medicophys 2006;42:5–15

59. Simpson DM. Clinical trials of botulinum toxin in the treatment of spasticity. Muscle Nerve Suppl 1997;6:S169–S175

60. Boss BJ, Barlow D, McFarland SM, Sasser L. A self-care assessment tool (SCAT) for persons with a spinal cord injury: an expanded abstract. Axone 1996;17:66–67

61. Boss BJ, Pecanty L, McFarland SM, Sasser L. Self-care competence among persons with spinal cord injury. SCI Nurs 1995;12:48–53

62. Dobkin BH. Do electrically stimulated sensory inputs and movements lead to long-term plasticity and rehabilitation gains? Curr Opin Neurol 2003;16:685–691

63. Spadone R, Merati G, Bertocchi E, et al. Energy consumption of locomotion with orthosis versus Parastep-assisted gait: a single case study. Spinal Cord 2003;41:97–104

64. Mahoney ET, Bickel CS, Elder C, et al. Changes in skeletal muscle size and glucose tolerance with electrically stimulated resistance training in subjects with chronic spinal cord injury. Arch Phys Med Rehabil 2005;86:1502–1504

65. Phillips SM, Stewart BG, Mahoney DJ. Body-weight-support treadmill training improves blood glucose regulation in persons with incomplete spinal cord injury. J Appl Physiol 2004;97:716–724

66. Jeon JY, Weiss CB, Steadward RD, et al. Improved glucose tolerance and insulin sensitivity after electrical stimulation-assisted cycling in people with spinal cord injury. Spinal Cord 2002;40:110–117

67. Mohr T, Dela F, Handberg A, et al. Insulin action and long-term electrically induced training in individuals with spinal cord injuries. Med Sci Sports Exerc 2001;33:1247–1252

68. Chilibeck PD, Bell G, Jeon J, et al. Functional electrical stimulation exercise increases GLUT-1 and GLUT-4 in paralyzed skeletal muscle. Metabolism 1999;48:1409–1413

69. Krause JS, Kemp B, Coker J. Depression after spinal cord injury: relation to gender, ethnicity, aging, and socioeconomic indicators. Arch Phys Med Rehabil 2000;81:1099–1109

70. Elliott TR, Frank RG. Depression following spinal cord injury. Arch Phys Med Rehabil 1996;77:816–823

71. Martz E, Livneh H, Priebe M, Wuermser LA, Ottomanelli L. Predictors of psychosocial adaptation among people with spinal cord injury or disorder. Arch Phys Med Rehabil 2005;86: 1182–1192

72. Soden RJ, Walsh J, Middleton JW, Craven ML, Rutkowski SB, Yeo JD. Causes of death after spinal cord injury. Spinal Cord 2000; 38:604–610

73. Forsythe E, Horsewell JE. Sexual rehabilitation of women with a spinal cord injury. Spinal Cord 2006;44:234–241

74. De Vivo MJ, Richards JS, Stover SL, Go BK. Spinal cord injury: rehabilitation adds life to years. West J Med 1991;154: 602–606

75. Hess DW, Ripley DL, Mckinley WO, Tewksbury M. Predictors for return to work after spinal cord injury: a 3-year multicenter analysis. Arch Phys Med Rehabil 2000;81:359–363

76. Krause JS. Adjustment after spinal cord injury: a 9-year longitudinal study. Arch Phys Med Rehabil 1997;78:651–657

77. Ville I, Ravaud JF. Work, non-work and consequent satisfaction after spinal cord injury. Int J Rehabil Res 1996;19:241–252

78. DeVivo MJ, Rutt RD, Stover SL, Fine PR. Employment after spinal cord injury. Arch Phys Med Rehabil 1987;68:494–498

79. Krause JS, Sternberg M, Maides J, Lottes S. Employment after spinal cord injury: differences related to geographic region, gender, and race. Arch Phys Med Rehabil 1998;79:615–624

80. Krause JS, Anson CA. Employment after spinal cord injury: relation to selected participant characteristics. Arch Phys Med Rehabil 1996;77:737–743

81. Tomassen PC, Post MW, van Asbeck FW. Return to work after spinal cord injury. Spinal Cord 2000;38:51–55

82. Deforge D, Blackmer J, Garritty C, et al. Male erectile dysfunction following spinal cord injury: a systematic review. Spinal Cord 2006;44:465–473

83. Langtry HD, Markham A. Sildenafil: a review of its use in erectile dysfunction. Drugs 1999;57:967–989

84. Brown PJ, Marino RJ, Herbison GJ, Ditunno JF Jr. The 72-hour examination as a predictor of recovery in motor complete quadriplegia. Arch Phys Med Rehabil 1991;72:546–548

85. Waters RL, Adkins RH, Yakura JS. Definition of complete spinal cord injury. Paraplegia 1991;29:573–581

86. Kirshblum SC, O'Connor KC. Predicting neurologic recovery in traumatic cervical spinal cord injury. Arch Phys Med Rehabil 1998;79:1456–1466

87. Potter PJ, Hsieh J. Predicting neurologic recovery in SCI. Arch Phys Med Rehabil 1999;80:474

88. American Spinal Injury Association (ASIA). International Standards for Neurological Classification of Spinal Cord Injury. 6th ed. Chicago: ASIA; 2000

89. Waters RL, Adkins RH, Yakura JS, Sie I. Motor and sensory recovery following complete tetraplegia. Arch Phys Med Rehabil 1993;74:242–247

90. Waters RL, Yakura JS, Adkins RH, Sie I. Recovery following complete paraplegia. Arch Phys Med Rehabil 1992;73:784–789

91. Waters RL, Adkins RH, Yakura JS, Sie I. Motor and sensory recovery following incomplete paraplegia. Arch Phys Med Rehabil 1994;75:67–72

92. Fisher CG, Noonan VK, Smith DE, Wing PC, Dvorak MF, Kwon BK. Motor recovery, functional status, and health-related quality of life in patients with complete spinal cord injuries. Spine 2005;30:2200–2207

93. National Pressure Ulcer Advisory Panel (NPUAP). NPUAP Staging Report, 1994

15 Socioeconomics of Spinal Injuries

Rob D. Dickerman, Michael O'Malley, and Jack E. Zigler

The annual incidence of spinal cord injuries (SCIs) in the United States is approximately 40 cases per 1 million population, resulting in 11,000 new cases per year.[1] The costs to the patient, family, and society are staggering, with the lifetime costs for a tetraplegic patient injured at age 25 years closely approximating $3 million.[2] According to the Centers for Disease Control and Prevention (CDC), SCIs cost the nation an estimated $9.7 billion each year. Pressure sores alone, a common secondary condition among people with SCI, cost an estimated $1.2 billion.[3] As stated by Formal et al,[4] economic costs of SCI are high, as seen in charges that can amount to approximately $350,000 for those with high tetraplegia in the first year alone. To break it down further, medical costs for the average SCI average $200,000 in the first year and $25,000 each year thereafter. Societal costs remain very high, as life expectancy rates increase, with direct costs amounting to $2.7 billion and indirect costs at $3.7 billion.[5] Several studies were conducted in the 1990s on the direct and indirect costs of SCI to the patient and society, with varying results and estimations.[6,7] The main source of spinal cord injury data in the United States is the National Spinal Cord Injury Statistical Center (NSCISC). Since 1989, NSPISC has collected data on SCI patients from the 18 regional Model Spinal Cord Injury Care Systems located throughout the United States the NSCISC collects on injury severity, hospitalization and inpatient rehabilitation period, postdischarge rehabilitation, and mortality. This chapter reviews the costs, to both the patient and society, of SCI in the United States and Canada.

■ SCI Financial Costs

Both the acute and rehabilitation care stages for the SCI patient place a significant financial strain on society due to the "intensive resources" needed for patient management.[8] In addition, life expectancy postinjury continues to increase, further increasing the financial burden that is associated with continued care of an SCI patient. To achieve some perspective of this cost of care, insight on the care and rehabilitation programs set in place at the time of, and following, patient assessment is necessary.[9] Rehabilitation consists of certain objectives, including but not limited to maximizing patient medical and functional outcomes, as well as educating both patient and family on the current situation and what is required of them during the long road ahead. This can only be accomplished via initial and continuing patient assessment by a team of physicians, therapists, psychologists, social workers, and case managers. Realistic functional outcomes must also be predicted and discussed. Only then can the patient, family, and rehabilitation team begin to work on attaining these functional goals.

With regard to the education and information needs of SCI patients and their families, Burkell et al[10] state that self-directed care is an integral aspect of health for those living with a chronic illness or disability. Not only is it important to realize that one's health care needs change over time, but studies have shown that the need for information regarding prevention, identification, and treatment of SCI actually increases with time. Thus, the comprehensive education that patients and families receive during initial contact with the health care team must be carried over, and must evolve with the patients' course of care. The timely and precise nature of information delivery remains a significant challenge. Internet use is becoming more common, but the most used information source remains periodicals (journals, newsletters, etc.). Advances in information accessibility could significantly decrease SCI costs, as many of the common complications, such as pressure sores and urinary tract infections, can be avoided given appropriate self-care measures.[10]

The severity of spinal cord injuries varies, as does the cost of care for each patient. Complete SCI refers to those injuries resulting in complete loss of motor and sensory function below the site of injury. Patients with incomplete SCI retain some function below the level of injury, whether it is sensory, motor, or both.[3] Those with more severe injuries generally require more health and rehabilitation services.[10] **Table 15.1** lists the levels of functional dependence on others, as well as the need for assistive devices, wheelchairs, and specialized cars, all of which add to the burden of cost for these patients.

■ The Role of Modern Technology

Technologic advancements have enhanced the functional capabilities of patients, but not without a cost. Assistive devices, orthotics, surgical reconstruction, and functional electrical stimulation (FES) may all play a role.[10] The dawning of the 21st century saw the design of various interfaces allowing computer influence on neuronal function. These human–machine interfaces present the

Table 15.1 Spinal Cord Injury Variations

C1-C3 tetraplegia	• Long-term mechanical ventilatory support
	• Head, neck, possibly shoulder mobility
	• Dependent on others for rest of mobility and self-care
	• Swallowing and phonation preserved
C1-C4 tetraplegia	• Same as above, except injury at C4 level generally does not require mechanical ventilation
	• Communicate via assistive technology (e.g., environmental control units)
C5 tetraplegia	• Functional elbow flexion
	• Eat and groom independently with assistive devices
	• Require assistance for most self-care
C6 tetraplegia	• Addition of functional wrist extension and passive thumb adduction on index finger during wrist extension
	• Functional independence with assistive devices for feeding, grooming, bathing, bed mobility
	• Can assist with bladder and bowel program
	• Manual or power wheelchair use
C7 tetraplegia	• Highest level of injury where one can still live independently
	• Functional independence in most things requiring upper body, and independence with use of assistive devices for lower extremities
	• Can write, type, answer phone, use computer
C8 tetraplegia	• Functional finger flexion resulting in increased grasp
	• Functionally independent
	• Can drive in specialized car with hand controls
Thoracic paraplegia	• Innervation and function of all upper extremities
	• Functionally independent at wheelchair level
	• Can also drive specialized car
Lumbar paraplegia	• Functionally independent for all mobility, self-care, bladder and bowel skills
	• Like thoracic, may need advanced wheelchair training
	• Drive specialized car

tantalizing possibility of a decrease in disabilities and an increase in functional independence.[11] At a significant cost to the patient, neuroprosthetics that utilize electrical stimulation to nerves and muscular motor units can now be purchased. These may enable certain movements that the uninjured, healthy individual may take for granted, such as emptying of the bladder.[11] Devices for functional neuromuscular stimulation (FNS), which is also referred to as FES, have been developed to promote functional movements of otherwise paralyzed muscles.[11] These advances, however, have surfaced in the face of various roadblocks, involving disputes with regulatory agencies over efficacy and safety issues, cost-benefit analysis, and limited markets.[11]

In a study by Jack Edwards, 470 individuals with SCIs were enrolled in upright mobility programs, which involved the use of a reciprocal gait orthosis (RGO). These individuals could walk distances of over 300 m at speeds of 0.2 to 0.5 m/s. In addition, a distance of 0.6 km could be achieved without having to sit down. Incidence of pain, spasms, and urinary and respiratory tract infections were all decreased.[12]

Michael Keith examined the results following implantation of the Freehand (NeuroControl Corp., Cleveland, Ohio) neuroprosthesis, which attempts to re-create hand motion in tetraplegics. At the time of the study, approximately 200 neuroprosthetics had been implanted. Compared with their preoperative state, patient independence was improved by an average of 85%.[12]

Cotler et al[13] assessed the beneficial role of orthotics used in patients with closed cervical spine dislocations. Two populations were examined: patients using orthotics with previous nonoperative treatment, and those patients using orthotics with previous operative treatment. Better outcomes were seen in those treated operatively at an early time. Approximately 64% of those treated nonoperatively sustained a redisplacement of their dislocation. The study showed an average financial savings of $18,407 in those treated operatively.

■ Spinal Cord Injury Studies

Several studies examined the socioeconomic costs related to SCI. Dryden et al[14] followed 233 patients suffering an SCI in Canada for 6 years from the date of injury. Patients were matched with a group of 1165 randomly selected patients from the general population for age, gender, and region of residence and were followed for 6 years. Costs were calculated from central databases and included health care use, hospitalizations, physician contacts, long-term care admissions, home health care services, and secondary complications. Results demonstrated that SCI patients were rehospitalized 2.6 times more often, and when hospitalized the SCI patients required an average of 3.3 more days. SCI patients contacted physicians 2.7 more times and required 30 times more hours on home health care. Of the medical complications suffered by SCI patients, almost 48% suffered urinary tract infections, 34% pneumonia, 28% depression, and 20% decubitus ulcers (**Table 15.2**). The study demonstrated the magnitude of long-term posttraumatic secondary care often required by SCI patients and its associated costs.

In 2003 a large systematic review was performed analyzing the costs and effectiveness of surgical spinal fixation for SCI and delayed versus immediate surgical referral to an SCI unit.[15] Sixty-eight studies on spinal fixation versus no spinal fixation were reviewed and suggested benefits of spinal fixation surgery. Of the 68 studies, only four were performed in specific spinal injury units, and in these centers there were no benefits demonstrated with spinal fixation. There were 28 retrospective observational studies reviewed on the benefits of referral to a spinal injury unit, which suggested that referral to a spinal injury unit did improve overall neurologic outcomes. Authors went on to recommend that primary research involving audits of selected hospital records be commissioned and published. In addition, future research should include full economic evaluations alongside randomized controlled studies, which can then consider the costs of implementing certain treatments in SCI.

DeVivo[6] performed a cross-sectional multicenter study to estimate the direct costs of each cause of spinal cord injury. The purpose was to compare random samples of 227 new injuries and 508 patients postinjury ranging from 2 to 16 years. Prospective data collected for 1 year included emergency medical services, hospitalizations, home health care, equipment, supplies, medications, environmental modifications, physician and outpatient services, nursing homes, household assistance, vocational rehabilitation, and miscellaneous items. The injury types were categorized and first-year costs compared along with recurring annual costs and projected lifetime costs. Motor vehicle accidents averaged $233,947 (annual recurrence $33,439, lifetime $969,659), violence $217,868 ($17,275, $613,345), sports $296,643 ($27,488, $950,973), and falls $185,019 ($26,238, $630,453). The leading cause of SCI in sports is diving (66%) (**Table 15.3**). Males comprise 82% of SCI patients, and 57% are in the age range of 16 to 30 years at the time of injury.

The direct costs were then calculated based on the approximately 11,000 cases of SCI per year, 2% discount rate—a discount function $f(t)$ specifying the present value of a unit payment time t in the future—survival data from the National Spinal Cord Injury Statistical Center, and the incidence of each type of SCI.[2] Thus, motor vehicle accidents are 36% of all SCIs and cost the United States approximately $3.48 billion; violence 30%, $1.81 billion; falls 20%, $1.28 billion; and sports 7.0%, $694 million. The study demonstrated that

Table 15.2 Dryden Study of Spinal Cord Injury Patients Versus Non–Spinal Cord Injury Patients

SCI patient characteristics	• Rehospitalized 2.6 times more often
	• Required a length of stay averaging 3.3 days longer
	• Contacted physicians 2.7 more times
	• Required 30 times more hours on home health care
Medical complications suffered by SCI patients	• 48% urinary tract infections
	• 34% pneumonia
	• 28% depression
	• 20% decubitus ulcers

Table 15.3 Direct Costs for Each Cause of Spinal Cord Injury

Cause	Average First-Year Costs	Annual Recurring Costs	Lifetime Costs
Vehicle accidents	$233,947	$33,439	$969,659
Violence	$217,868	$17,275	$613,345
Sports	$296,643	$27,488	$950,973
Falls	$185,019	$26,238	$630,453

Source: From Devivo MJ. Causes and costs of spinal cord injury in the Unites States. Spinal Cord 1997;35:809–813.

total direct costs to the United States would approximate $7.7 billion based on 1995 income. These costs were not isolated to the health care industry. For example, because motor vehicle accidents are the leading cause of SCI in patients, the automotive industry remains very involved in researching ways to better safeguard vehicles, in the hopes of minimizing SCI to their occupants. Everything from vehicle rollover to the more commonly seen accident types resulting in SCI have been studied.[16]

Regarding the role of violence in SCI, gunshot wounds are currently the second leading cause of spinal cord injury in the United States Concomitant injuries or complications accompanying gunshot wounds often increase patient morbidity as well. McKinley et al[17] studied a patient base of 217, over a 5-year period, admitted to a hospital due to traumatic SCI. Of these hospital admissions, a total of 49 cases involved gunshot-related events. Common medical complications accompanying these cases included pain (54%), infections (40%), pneumothorax (24%), nonspinal fractures (22%), colonic perforation (17%), cerebrospinal fluid leak (10%), and retroperitoneal hematoma (10%) (**Table 15.4**). This study revealed that complete SCI and paraplegia were the most common injury types in gunshot-related SCI. It is also important to note that although patients with these injuries had lengths of hospital stays similar to nonviolent SCI, there seemed to be a specific population base more at risk for the violence-related SCI, that being a younger, non-Caucasian, unmarried, and unemployed adult population.

More recent studies have focused on direct and indirect costs. Dryden et al[18] in 2005 focused on the direct

costs in Canada of SCI attributed to trauma. Patients were classified as complete SCI or incomplete SCI. Data were compared from centralized health databases for first-year costs and subsequent annual costs for 5 years. These costs included hospitalizations, physician services, home care, and long-term care. First-year costs for complete SCI were $121,600 and for incomplete SCI were $42,100. Subsequent annual costs for 5 years averaged $5400 for complete and $2800 for incomplete (**Table 15.5**). As expected, the study demonstrated that complete SCI patients accrue greater total costs, and the first-year costs for taking care of complete and incomplete SCI patients is substantial.

In comparison to direct costs of care in SCI patients data from the United States in 2004, high tetraplegics' first-year costs were estimated to be $683,000 and each subsequent year $122,334; for low tetraplegics, these costs are $441,025 and $50,110; for paraplegics, $249,549 and $25,934; and for incompletes, $201,273 and $14,106. These drastic differences are due to the bundling of so-called direct costs. The direct costs in this study included hospitalizations, physician services, home health care attendants, durable medical equipment, home modifications, medications, medical supplies, and transportation (**Table 15.5**).[2]

■ Direct Psychological and Sociologic Effects

To date, there are numerous studies demonstrating that SCI patients suffer higher lifetime unemployment rates, significant income losses, reduced life expectancy, long-term health care requirements and costs, significant pain and suffering, reduced likelihood to marry or remain married, and an alarmingly high suicide rate at almost five times greater than that of the general United States population.[19] The suicide rate does not significantly change beyond the fifth year after injury. DeVivo[19] found that suicide was the leading cause of death in SCI for complete paraplegics and the second leading cause for incomplete paraplegics. Self-inflicted gunshot was the most common route chosen for suicide (**Table 15.6**).

Employment rates on SCI patients, as determined by the National Spinal Cord Injury Association, are 61% at the

Table 15.4 Complications Associated with Gunshot Wound–Induced Spinal Cord Injury

Pain	54%
Infections	40%
Pneumothorax	24%
Nonspinal fractures	22%
Colonic perforation	17%
Cerebrospinal fluid leak	10%
Retroperitoneal hematoma	10%

Table 15.5 Comparing Costs of Complete Versus Incomplete Spinal Cord Injury

Dryden et al[18] Study: Canada 2005

	First-Year Costs	**Subsequent 5-Year Annual Costs**
Complete SCI	$121,600	$5400
Incomplete SCI	$42,100	$2800
Costs include:	Hospitalizations, physician services, home care, and long-term care	

NSCISC Statistics[2]: United States 2006

	First-Year Costs	**Subsequent Annual Costs**
High tetraplegics	$683,000	$122,334
Low tetraplegics	$441,025	$50,110
Paraplegia	$249,549	$25,934
Incomplete SCI	$201,273	$14,106
Costs include:	Hospitalizations, physician services, home health care attendants, durable medical equipment, home modifications, medications, medical supplies, and transportation	

Abbreviation: NSCISC, National Spinal Cord Injury Statistical Center.

time of injury and 13.6% by the end of the first year after injury.[2] Due to advances in SCI research, an increasing number of SCI patients are returning to work, with 30% of quadriplegics and 40% of paraplegics eventually returning to work. Overall unemployment averages approximately 50% for SCI patients in the 20 years following the injury.

Among other social effects of SCI is sexual dysfunction. The high incidence of erectile dysfunction following traumatic SCI can have a considerable effect on the quality of life of patients and their significant other. There are treatment options available for these patients, including sildenafil administration, intracavernous injections of papaverine/alprostadil (Caverject), alprostadil/papaverine/

Table 15.6 Direct Psychological and Socioeconomic Effects of Spinal Cord Injury

Psychological	• Depression
	• Reduced life expectancy
	• Significant pain and suffering
	• Reduced likelihood to marry or remain married
	• Higher suicide rate*
Socioeconomic	• Higher lifetime unemployment rates
	• Significant income losses
	• Long-term health care requirements and costs

* It is important to note that the suicide rate for SCI patients was five times that of the general population, with gunshot being the most common route.

phentolamine ("triple mix"), transurethral suppository medicated urethral system for erections (MUSE), surgically implanted prosthetic devices, and vacuum erection devices.[20] Cost-effective analysis has shown that sildenafil was the most economically sensible treatment when compared with surgically implanted prosthetic devices, MUSE, and Caverject.[20] Basic statistical studies have also demonstrated that SCI patients who are single at the time of injury are more likely to remain single than an age-matched non-SCI person. In addition, those SCI patients who are married at the time of injury have a divorce rate of almost 20% in the first 5 years postinjury, while the age-matched comparison calculations found a rate of 11% for a non-SCI person.[2]

Spinal cord injury patients experience continuing medical problems requiring lifetime medical care and medical expenses. The average SCI patient spends 79 days in the hospital after the injury, and first-year costs and added living expenses directly attributable to SCI vary substantially by the severity of the injury.

■ Indirect Psychological and Sociologic Effects

Costs of SCI impacts a larger portion of the population than just the patients themselves and are not always reflected in dollars. Weitzenkamp et al[21] performed an interesting study on the social impact to the spouse of the SCI patient. Social demographics, health concerns, depression tests, perceived stress scales, and life satisfaction indices were analyzed. Spouses of SCI patients ($n = 124$)

Table 15.7 Common Psychological Effects of Spinal Cord Injury: The "4 D's"

1. Depression	25 to 45% of SCI patients suffer from some form of depression
2. Dependency	Increased dependence on others for everyday tasks and self-care
3. Drug addiction	Increased use of narcotics and alcohol in SCI patients
4. Divorce	20% divorce rate of SCI patients compared with 11% for non-SCI individuals

Table 15.8 Risk of Death Due to Respiratory Disease, the Leading Cause of Death in Spinal Cord Injury Patients

Ages	Risk Ratio of Death Due to Respiratory Disease
31–45	4.87 times greater risk
46–60	19.04 times greater risk
61 and older	45.98 times greater risk

were tested, all of whom had been with an SCI patient for 23 or more years. Interestingly, spouses of SCI patients had a more depressive affect ($p < .001$) than did their partners with SCI. There were no differences in perceived stress scales between the spouses and SCI patients. However, when spouses were categorized into caregiving and noncaregiving, the caregiving spouses demonstrated significantly more stress than their SCI partners and noncaregiving spouses ($p = .005$). Conclusions were that spouses of SCI patients who perform a caregiving role suffer significantly more stress and depression than their partners with SCI or the spouses who are not caregivers.[19]

Christian[22] discussed the most common psychological issues that are seen in those suffering from SCIs. In his book, he referred to the work of Joyce Fichtenbaum, PhD, and Steven Kirschblum, MD, and their identification of the "4 D's" (**Table 15.7**): depression, dependency, drug addiction, and divorce; 25 to 45% of those suffering from SCI experience a certain level of depression following their injury. This can have several manifestations, from loss of appetite or decreased attention, to suicidal tendencies. An increased dependency on the health care team is frequently observed. It is very important that patients learn to maximize all of their functional capabilities before giving in to complete dependence on others. Increases in drug and alcohol abuse have also been seen. This tendency should be addressed as soon as possible.

■ Long-Term Disability Costs and Longevity

When discussing life expectancy in SCI, one must consider the five types of SCI: ventilator dependent, high tetraplegic, low tetraplegic, paraplegic, and incomplete. In general, the least severe forms of SCI have a life span decrease of only approximately 10%, varying to almost a

70% reduction in life expectancy for the most severe form (ventilator dependent) of SCI.[2]

Diseases of the respiratory system were the leading cause of death (71% of these were cases of pneumonia). Supporting evidence can be seen in a study by Frankel et al,[23] showing that the cause of death in the period 1973 to 1990 in a sample population of 226 patients was pneumonia, influenza, or other respiratory diseases in 76 patients (34%). The study also showed that SCI patients between the ages of 31 and 45 were 4.87 times more likely to die from respiratory problems than those under the age of 30. This risk ratio quadruples to 19.04 for those between the ages of 46 and 60, and further increases to 45.98 for those 61 or older, which stands as the group most vulnerable to death from respiratory disease (**Table 15.8**). These infections arise mainly due to weakened respiratory muscles and difficulty removing secretions, which then tend to build up in the lungs, predisposing an individual with SCI to subsequent infection.[22] The diaphragm is the most important muscle involved in respiration and is innervated by the phrenic nerve (C3-C5). The abdominal muscles, which have T6 and L1 innervation, can also become important in the breathing process, especially in forced expiration and inspiration, or if there is phrenic nerve dysfunction.[22] High and midlevel cervical spinal cord injuries can result in paralysis of the diaphragm and a subsequent increased longevity of mechanical ventilator dependence. Proper ventilator management is necessary and involves the constant monitoring of inspiratory and expiratory muscles, aspiration, clearing of secretions, potential lung parenchyma injury, bronchoconstriction, and nutrition. Phrenic nerve conduction studies can be made to assess the possibility of nerve recovery.[24]

Heart disease ranked as the second most common cause of death in SCI; however, these were often unexplained heart attacks (55%). Although some recent studies have actually shown that for long-term SCI, morbidity and mortality from causes related to the cardiovascular system, particularly coronary artery disease, have surpassed those from renal and pulmonary conditions, most authors still consider it the second leading cause of death.[25] Underlying risk factors in the SCI patient include a sedentary lifestyle and decreased physical activity, hyperlipidemia, obesity, and diabetes (**Table 15.9**). Furthermore, the disturbance of normal autonomic

Table 15.9 Risk Factors of Cardiovascular Disease in Spinal Cord Injury Patients

Low HDL, high total cholesterol, high LDL	Blood pressure abnormalities
High C-reactive protein	Deep vein thrombosis, thromboembolic events
High prevalence of obesity	Rhythm disturbances (bradyarrhythmias, decrease in heart rate variability)
High rate of smoking	Diabetes, metabolic syndrome
Sedentary lifestyle	Decrease in cardiovascular response to exercise

Abbreviations: HDL, high-density lipoprotein; LDL, low-density lipoprotein.

cardiovascular control seen in SCI patients puts these individuals at risk.[25] These effects are more commonly seen in injuries occurring at or above the T6 level of the spinal cord.[22] Abnormalities are seen in blood pressure, heart rate variability, arrhythmias, and a decreased cardiovascular response to exercise, limiting one's ability to perform physical activity. Hypotension is commonly seen in SCI patients as the combination of lower leg paralysis and gravity results in blood pooling below the waist, thus limiting venous return to the heart. In the attempt to move, such as getting out of a wheelchair, dizziness due to orthostatic hypotension is a common side effect.[22] Tetraplegics experience a 16% higher risk of all cardiovascular disease, whereas paraplegia corresponds with a 70% higher risk of developing coronary artery disease. All the factors present in **Table 15.2** play a role in determining the care and treatment of SCI patients, which then determines the cost of treatment for each individual. With these factors present, these patients can no longer be treated strictly as SCI patients.

The third leading cause of death was bacterial infection and parasitic diseases. Most of these patients had septicemia (93%) and usually had decubitus ulcers (discussed in more detail later in the chapter) and urinary tract or respiratory infections. Urinary tract infections are a common development in those with SCI because the bladder may not be emptying completely, or simply may not be emptying frequently enough. The bladder itself then essentially becomes a prime location for infection. It is also not uncommon to resort to the use of catheters to drain the bladder, which always presents the risk of introducing infection during insertion. It has also been shown that untreated urinary infections can then predispose the patient to other adverse health problems, such as pyelonephritis, septicemia, and kidney stones. Education provided to the patient and family pertaining to this risk of infection and the importance of self-monitoring is very important in the prevention of these complications.[26] Hypertensive heart disease and suicide competed for the fourth and fifth leading causes of death in multiple studies.

The value of a life is an actively researched and highly controversial area in the socioeconomic literature, and a survey in 1993 concluded that the results cluster in the $3 million to $7 million range.[27] Federal agencies are currently required to use $5.8 million as the value of life.[28]

The value per year of life remaining averages $180,000 in 1986 dollars.[29] Moore and Viscusi's[29] results, when combined with three other studies, provide one estimate of the value of reduced life expectancy due to SCI.[12] For example, a low tetraplegic SCI incurred by a 40-year-old (who survives the first year after injury) would reduce life expectancy by 14 years, and at $180,000 per year, the value of the lost years is $2,520,000 in 1986 dollars. Recent research by the NSCISC has found that the cumulative 20-year survival rate for patients with spinal cord injury was approximately 71% (**Table 15.10**).[2]

Unemployment leads to elevations in indirect costs, which include lost wages, fringe benefits, and productivity. The average SCI patient loses $57,000 annually, which by estimation of the total number of SCI patients and annual losses equals approximately $16 billion to $26 billion per year.[2]

■ Initial Hospitalization Costs

Mean days hospitalized in the SCI care system's acute and rehab units are greater for persons with tetraplegia than for those with paraplegia (**Table 15.11**). In most years, the difference in acute care length of stay between persons with tetraplegia and those with paraplegia is relatively small, whereas differences in rehabilitation length of stay are substantial. Mean days hospitalized in the acute care unit are usually greater for patients with neurologically

Table 15.10 The "Value of Life"

- A 1993 survey concluded the value of life is $3 million to $7 million

- Federal agencies are currently required to use $5.8 million for the value of life

- The value per year of life remaining averages $180,000 in 1986 dollars

- A low tetraplegic SCI incurred by a 40-year-old who survives the first year after injury would reduce life expectancy by 14 years, and at $180,000 per year, the value of the lost years is $2,520,000 in 1986 dollars

- Recent 20-year survival rate for SCI patients has reached 71%

Table 15.11 Mean Days Hospitalized in Spinal Cord Injury Care System

Acute care facility	
Neurologically complete tetraplegia	• 1982: 46 days
	• 1997: 16 days
Neurologically incomplete paraplegia	• 1973 and 1982: 29 days
	• 1999: 11 days
Rehab facility	
Neurologically complete tetraplegia	• 1975: 165 days
	• 2002: 59 days
Neurologically incomplete paraplegia	• 1975: 90 days
	• 2001: 30 days

complete cervical injuries than for patients with neurologically incomplete cervical injuries. Mean days hospitalized in the system's acute care unit for persons with neurologically complete tetraplegia ranged from 46 in 1982 to 16 in 1997, whereas for those with neurologically incomplete paraplegia, the comparable range was from 29 days in 1973 and 1982 to 11 days in 1999. Mean days hospitalized in the rehab unit are greatest for patients with neurologically complete injuries. Mean days hospitalized in the system's rehab unit for persons with neurologically complete tetraplegia ranged from 165 in 1975 to 59 in 2002, and for those with neurologically incomplete paraplegia, the comparable range was from 90 days in 1975 to 30 days in 2001.[2]

In constant 2003 dollars, mean total system charges (**Table 15.12**) increased from $150,328 during 1973 and 1974 to $236,136 in 1991 and 1992. This increase most likely reflects the trend toward improved survival of more severely injured persons at the scene of the injury who subsequently require greater intensity of service (such as mechanical ventilation) despite declining rehabilitation lengths of stay. Since 1992, mean total system charges decreased to only $206,176 in 2002 but increased again to $254,161 in 2003.[2]

Table 15.12 Total Mean Charges for Care (2003 dollars)

Year	Total Mean Charges
1973–1974	$150,328
1991–1992	$236,136
2002	$206,176
2003	$254,161

■ Post–Spinal Cord Injury Complications/Rehospitalizations

The most frequent complication is pressure (decubitus) ulcers observed during the annual examination, beginning at 15% in the first postinjury year and steadily increasing thereafter. Due to immobility and the fact that these patients have no feeling of pressure or pain below the level of injury, they often fail to shift their weight to relieve the pressure. In addition, skin care, irritation, and nutritional deficiency can play an integral role in the development of these pressure sores. Once again, education and information access and delivery are in the forefront for prevention. Although they may appear superficial, untreated sores can progress to a state of massive infection and even to necrosis of the skin and underlying tissues. This infection can ultimately involve the bone.[26] Even though aggressive early intervention, followed by discharge to a rehabilitation facility, is ideal, the average stay prior to transfer was 32.7 days.[8] In a study by Fielingsdorf and Dunn,[8] a 2-week goal for transfer was established, and only 40% of the SCI patients met this goal. This followed significant delays in admission due to the distances involved and limited bed availability; 50% of the patients were admitted on either the day of injury or the day following, whereas 67% were admitted within 2 days of the date of injury. These delays have a significant impact on morbidity, as seen by the incidence rates of pressure sores of 11% upon admission to the unit. Another 11% then develop these sores during their stay in the rehab facility. It is important that adjustments be made to ensure resource allocation to this area to reduce pressure ulcer incidence, or else it will remain a significant problem in prolonging hospital stay and adding greatly to the cost of care.

The next most common complication was pneumonia, which ranged from 2.5 to 3.9% over time. For those patients rehospitalized, the average length of stay was relatively constant over time (26 days in the first postinjury year and 20 days in the 25th year). Diseases of the genitourinary system were the leading cause of rehospitalization during postinjury years 1, 10, 15, 25, and 30, whereas diseases of the skin were the most common cause of rehospitalization during postinjury years 5 and 20. Circulatory, respiratory, digestive, and musculoskeletal diseases and conditions were also relatively common causes of rehospitalization.[2]

■ Past, Present, and Futu Moving Forward

In 1970, the first regional SCI system Phoenix, Arizona.[5] By the early 1990s, were receiving government funding.

rehabilitation programs were eventually established: free-standing rehab clinics and rehab units within acute care facilities. Although the latter type provides the opportunity of a continuum of care, from emergency medical services to acute inpatient rehabilitation, very few clinics have used this continuum.[5] Thus, they have not seen the many benefits that can result in establishing an SCI program that provides acute care, rehab, and therapeutic services all at the same location. These benefits include, but are not limited to, fewer postinjury complications (e.g., decubitus ulcers) for those admitted less than 24 hours from injury, decreased costs of acute care for patients admitted within this 24-hour window (a reported $5000 savings in 1992), and shorter rehab length of stays.[5] However, this type of clinic may clash with the evolving SCI program structure that has deviated from the fee-for-service reimbursement system to a Medicare-based prospective payment system.

The area of SCI remains a highly attractive field for research due to an overwhelming clinical need for prevention and effective therapy.[30] Previous clinical trials need to be examined to reveal and correct any inadequacies.

The incorporation of new trial designs discovered in other fields, such as cancer research, that are applicable to SCI studies can also be examined.[30] Continued improvements in SCI clinical trials, such as the use of randomized prospective controlled trials, adoption of a uniform clinical grading system, and development of other dependable outcome measures, facilitate conducting better, more efficient trials. By way of these changes, possible improvements can be made in the quality of care and cost-effectiveness of treatment plans for SCI patients.

With the exception of the Veterans Affairs system, most SCI programs involve long-term care at outpatient clinics, following discharge from an acute care facility. Follow-up care involves annual checkups, but little effort is made to provide primary care services.[5] It should be obvious that such a fragmented system results in clinical outcomes that are less than ideal, at a much greater overall cost. If the future of SCI care remains in outpatient therapy clinics, then primary care services must be provided, allowing both the initial access to rehab services and a study of the long-term health care needs of patients within this system.

References

1. Webster B, Giunti G, Young A, Pransky G, Nesathurai S. Work-related tetraplegia: cause of injury and annual medical costs. Spinal Cord 2004;42:240–247
2. The National Spinal Cord Injury Statistical Center, University of Alabama at Birmingham, 2006
3. American Association of Neurological Surgeons. Spinal cord injury. http://www.neurosurgerytoday.org/what/patient_e/spinal.asp; 2005
4. Formal C, Ditunno JF, Benzel EC. Fundamentals, techniques, and expectations of the rehabilitation process. In: Tator CH, Benzel EC, eds. Contemporary Management of Spinal Cord Injury: From Impact to Rehabilitation. Parke Ridge, IL: AANS Publications Committee; 1995:297–302
5. Waring WP III, Maiman DJ. The spinal cord injury unit in the new millennium. In: Tator CH, Benzel EC, eds. Contemporary Management of Spinal Cord Injury: From Impact to Rehabilitation. Parke Ridge, IL: AANS Publications Committee; 1995:303–310
6. DeVivo MJ. Causes and costs of spinal cord injury in the United States. Spinal Cord 1997;35:809–813
7. Berkowitz M. Assessing the socioeconomic impact of improved treatment of head and spinal cord injuries. J Emerg Med 1993;11:63–67
8. Fielingsdorf K, Dunn RN. Cervical spine injury outcome—a review of 101 cases treated in a tertiary referral unit. S Afr Med J 2007;97:203–207
9. McKinley W, Silver TM, Santos KG, Pai AB. Functional outcomes per level of spinal cord injury. eMedicine (online from WebMD): http://www.emedicine.com/pmr/topic183.htm#sectionapproximately c1-c4,_or_high,_tetraplegia; 2006
10. Burkell JA, Wolfe DL, Potter PJ, Jutai JW. Information needs and information sources of individuals living with spinal cord injury. Health Info Libr J 2006;23:257–265
11. Dobkin MD, Bruce H. The Clinical Science of Neurologic Rehabilitation. New York: Oxford University Press; 2003
12. Johnston L. Human spinal cord injury: new and emerging approaches to treatment. Spinal Cord 2001;39:609–613
13. Cotler HB, Cotler JM, Alden ME, Sparks G, Biggs CA. The medical and economic impact of closed cervical spine dislocations. Spine 1990;15:448–452
14. Dryden DM, Saunders LD, Rowe BH, et al. Utilization of health services following spinal cord injury: a 6-year follow-up study. Spinal Cord 2004;42:513–525
15. Bagnall AM, Jones L, Richardson G, Duffy S, Riemsma R. Effectiveness and cost-effectiveness of acute hospital-based spinal cord injuries services: systematic review. Health Technol Assess 2003;7:1–92
16. O'Connor PJ, Brown D. Relative risk of spinal cord injury in road crashes involving seriously injured occupants of light passenger vehicles. Accid Anal Prev 2006;38:1081–1086
17. McKinley WO, Johns JS, Musgrove JJ. Clinical presentations, medical complications, and functional outcomes of individuals with gunshot wound-induced spinal cord injury. Am J Phys Med Rehabil 1999;78:102–107
18. Dryden DM, Saunders LD, Jacobs P, et al. Direct health care costs after traumatic spinal cord injury. J Trauma 2005;59:443–449
19. DeVivo MJ. Suicide following spinal cord injury. Paraplegia 1991;29:620–627
20. Mittmann N, Craven BC, Gordon M, et al. Erectile dysfunction in spinal cord injury: a cost-utility analysis. J Rehabil Med 2005;37:358–364
21. Weitzenkamp DA, Gerhart KA, Charlifue SW, Whiteneck GG, Savic G. Spouses of spinal cord injury survivors: the added impact of caregiving. Arch Phys Med Rehabil 1997;78:822–827
22. Christian A. Living with Spinal Cord Injury: A Wellness Approach. New York: Demos Medical Publishing; 2004
23. Frankel HL, Coll JR, Charlifue SW, et al. Long-term survival in spinal cord injury: a fifty year investigation. Spinal Cord 1998;36:266–274

24. Strakowski JA, Pease WS, Johnson EW. Phrenic nerve stimulation in the evaluation of ventilator-dependent individuals with C4- and C5-level spinal cord injury. Am J Phys Med Rehabil 2007;86: 153–157

25. Myers J, Lee M, Kiratli J. Cardiovascular disease in spinal cord injury: an overview of prevalence, risk, evaluation, and management. Am J Phys Med Rehabil 2007;86:142–152

26. Falvo D. Medical and Psychological Aspects of Chronic Illness and Disability. Sudbury, MA: Jones and Bartlett; 2005

27. Viscusi WK. The value of risks to life and health. J Econ Lit 1993;31:1912–1946

28. Peterson CH. Business and Government. 4th ed. New York: Harper & Row; 1996

29. Moore MJ, Viscusi WK. Compensation Mechanisms for Job Risks. Princeton, NJ: Princeton University Press; 1990

30. Tator CH. Review of treatment trials in human spinal cord injury: issues, difficulties, and recommendations. Neurosurgery 2006; 59:957–987

16 Quality of Life, Professionalism, and Research Ethics in the Treatment of Spinal Injuries

Paul J. Ford

The ethical challenges in neurotrauma compose a vast array of intertwined issues and topics. In many ways the division between the ethics of brain trauma and spine trauma are arbitrary and artificial. Hence, a discussion of ethics addresses the type of ethics problems faced, with an emphasis on either brain trauma or spine trauma. This chapter addresses issues of research ethics, innovative therapies, conflicts of interest, and quality of life. In *Neurotrauma and Critical Care of the Brain*,[1] the ethics chapter focused on explaining a basic ethics framework for making difficult decisions, and it applied that framework to several end-of-life questions. This ethics model explicitly described ethical dilemmas as situations where something morally is lost to preserve another morally important element. For example, the resolution of an ethical dilemma might require putting a patient's cognitive function at risk to save the patient's life. Or the resolution of an ethical dilemma might require allowing a patient to die to respect the patient's religious belief, a quality-of-life judgment, or an avoidance of undue suffering. In *Neurotrauma and Critical Care of the Brain* we also discussed life and death decisions, including withdrawing/withholding lifesaving therapy, vulnerable patient populations, and formal decision-making documents in the context of neurotrauma. Those topics provided a basic primer for standard ethical issues. However, ethical dilemmas faced by neurosurgeons extend well beyond end-of-life decisions. The ethics of surgery become particularly interesting when discussing spine trauma and research.

This chapter extends the ethics discussions from *Neurotrauma and Critical Care of the Brain* by exploring ethics through the issues of research, conflicts of interest, and quality of life. A moral imperative of medicine dictates that a patient's entire course of treatment and care be considered from the initial trauma through long-term treatment. Although it is easiest to swoop in to perform a function-saving or life-saving surgery, certain circumstances require careful consideration of the long-term consequences of rescue therapy. This may involve balancing considerations of patient goals, professional responsibility not to harm, and responsible stewardship of limited resources. Often, these situations involve a professional judgment that a surgery should not move forward because of surgical limitations and poor outcomes. Hence, a surgery may not constitute best practice. Conversely, patients and surrogates may be unable to fully understand the short-term suffering needed during recovery for the achievement of long-term goals. The patient or surrogate may want to withhold medically indicated surgery that is in the patient's best interest. In both cases difficult conversations with patients or surrogates may be necessary to accomplish a good outcome. These conversations may require some persuasion that attempts to avoid moving to coercion. The level of appropriate persuasion varies by many factors and should always be done in an open and honest way (**Table 16.1**).

Adding to this milieu of practice, physicians have a moral imperative to continually search for better ways to care for patients. This imperative requires a balance between the principles of avoiding doing unnecessary harm to patients while attempting to gain knowledge that will help other patients. This constitutes the justification for well-reasoned research. In undertaking research, a patient-subject should be valued and not used only as a means toward the goal of gaining knowledge. Although this ideal sounds easy, it can be lost in the myriad of obligations and well-intentioned regulations found in the current practice of research.

Table 16.1 Appropriate Persuasion

Patients rely on physicians to guide them in medical decisions
Always persuade in an open and honest way
Always respect dignity
Time-dependent decisions may justify more persuasion. (particularly when there is a very high likelihood of life, significant function, or preservation)
Patients are permitted to make informed decisions that appear harmful to their interests
Any "deal" struck should be honored later or not offered in the first place
Stronger levels of persuasion are permissible in clinical cases than in research

Finally, surgeons derive their livelihood from the treatment of patients. This creates a need to balance sustainable personal lives, to continue helping patients, to maximize the good for future patients, and to remain accessible to those in greatest medical need. The tasks become even more difficult in the research endeavor when collaborations with funding agencies, both governmental and industry, exist by necessity. Conflicts of interests and commitment challenge the integrity of both research and treatment. A special subset of conflicting commitments involves the care of athletes in the context of contracting as a team surgeon. The following discussion expands on the basic issues of research ethics, quality of life in the aftermath of traumatic injury, and conflicting interests/commitments. These issues can be used as a foundation for thinking through particularly challenging ethical circumstances in spine surgery. An important theme throughout this chapter is the importance of transparency undertaken in a prospective and honest manner.

■ Research Ethics

There exists a positive obligation in health care to provide patients with the best possible care based on scientific evidence. Although this obligation applies equally to surgery, creating an appropriate evidence base for surgical treatment poses several challenges. Although we strive toward class I evidence as proof of the effectiveness of therapies, many times we must settle for less than this. Choosing a treatment course that does not have the highest degree of scientific support is an example of giving up one valued thing to preserve another (i.e., an ethical choice). We might settle for using a therapy with lesser proof (**Table 16.2**) in procedures in which it is unethical to randomize a patient to a sham surgery or ones in which proper double-blind procedures are impossible. Although there continues to be a lively debate about the ethical appropriateness of randomized controlled trials in spine surgery, there are at least some procedures that do not fit well into this model.[2,3] Practical considerations that could make careful study difficult

Table 16.2 Reasons Surgeries Might Not Be Tested in Controlled Trial

Impossible to double blind
Unethical to undertake sham surgery
Standard therapy is effective
Lack of equipoise with standard therapy
Available "off label" so patients will not enroll
Lack of "consentable" subject
Lack of resources

include patients refusing to enter a study because of the off-label availability of the procedure or there being a lack of sufficient "consentable" subjects to enroll in the study. Performing a procedure for clinical purposes and not undertaking it for research is an ethical choice of partially giving up the principle of treating on the basis of best knowledge in favor of attempting to help a particular patient right now. The converse is also true, that withholding a potentially effective therapy because it lacks sufficiently strong evidence values avoiding harm for a patient because of unknown outcomes at the expense of not potentially helping that patient by withholding the intervention. **Table 16.3** presents one way of evaluating the strengths and weaknesses of attempting or withholding a procedure for which we have less than the best knowledge. For the time being these types of procedures could be labeled as "innovative" or "off-label." Clearly there is a wide spectrum of levels of knowledge available that influence how to properly balance these considerations of harm, benefit, and scientific advancement of treatment. We discuss the ethics of innovation in later sections. Because the surgical profession has an imperative to further our knowledge about treating patients, it is important to understand ethical considerations in developing research protocols that will pass strong ethical scrutiny by review boards, journals, scientific peers, and the general population.

Table 16.3 Balancing Values in Choosing Unproven Therapy (Innovation)

Values (Risked/Preserved)	Attempting Innovation	Withholding Innovation
Practice on best evidence	Risk	Preserve
Provide active benefit	Preserve	Risk
Avoid active harm	Risk	Preserve
Career advancement	Risk/preserve	Neutral
Use of valuable resources	Potentially risk	Potentially preserve
Advancement of knowledge	Preserve	Neutral

Table 16.4 Protection of Human Subjects

Based on "natural law" that consent is normally required (independent of the country)
Helsinki accord and Belmont Report provide articulation of important principles
Ethics review boards (IRB, REB, etc.) required prospectively
Data and safety monitoring boards (DSMBs) may be required
Subject advocate may be helpful in risky research
Incarcerated and involuntarily committed have special protections
Children require special protections as well as permission from parents/guardians
Regulations do not guarantee ethical trials, remain researcher's responsibility

Research abuses in the 20th century, such as the Nazi medical experiments and the American Tuskegee syphilis study, gave rise to an increased attention to research ethics.[4,5] Neurosurgery has equally had well-documented challenges in its development of therapeutic interventions.[6] Important research ethics codes arose out of the Belmont Report and the Declaration of Helsinki that today provide the elements by which research protocols are ethically judged.[7,8] These include discussions about basic ethical principles to be preserved during research as well as an articulation of special protections needed for subject populations. Given the past abuses, most countries have review boards focused on protecting the rights and welfare of human subjects (**Table 16.4**). These boards operate under various names, such as institutional review boards (IRBs) for the protection of human subjects and research ethics boards (REBs), depending on the country. Although there are many differences between these boards, many common threads flow through them all, including that the boards must prospectively approve research protocols and that informed consent is expected whenever possible. In addition, these review boards may require a data and safety monitoring board (DSMB) or a patient advocate for riskier interventions. Increasingly, peer-reviewed scientific journals require documentation of prospective ethics reviews of research protocols before publishing research results. These codes also address the obligation of physicians to study, with proper oversight, new techniques and procedures prior to implementing them as a standard of care.

The informed consent process has become the hallmark for good research practice. Review boards spend most of their time reviewing informed consent issues. Unfortunately, many review boards focus on the completeness of consent forms rather than focusing on the process by which patient-subjects enter into a research study. More important than a subject having a completed consent form, it is more ethically important that the subject understand and agree to be part of the research study. Further, although the consent form may highlight ethical gaps in a research protocol, there may be ethical standards not met in the protocol that would not show up in the consent form. With this trend toward consent forms and bureaucracy, researchers must not assume that because a review board has passed their protocol that the protocol comports with the highest ethical standards. As researchers develop studies, there must be a full recognition of what is being put at stake and who is risking themselves, that is, what values are being sacrificed and preserved. A simple rule of thumb is for researchers to ask if they would enroll one of their loved ones in the trial they are designing. If the answer is no, researchers should attempt to find a better protocol structure. The informed consent process is only one of many important elements of an ethically robust research plan.

As hallmarks of good research, subjects are expected to provide clear, informed consent, be advised of all alternatives, not be unduly influenced by incentives, and have the ability to withdraw from the research protocol at any time. The voluntary nature of participation plays a prominent role in research ethics. Any researcher dealing with a research ethics board, such as an IRB or REB, will recognize the attention paid to voluntary subject recruitment. As we will see, studying spinal trauma in an emergency setting provides further challenges in informed consent and voluntariness because of the innate pressures and constraints of emergency research. Finally, the balance between fair subject compensation and effective encouragement for research participation must be balanced with an avoidance of coercing patients into research trials. In each case there must be a valuing of the patient-subject first as a patient and then as a subject (**Table 16.5**).

The issue of withdrawal of consent for participation in a protocol presents a difficulty in the case of spine surgery for at least two reasons (**Table 16.6**). First, clinical research on trauma patients is always intertwined with clinical treatment. Although a patient can revoke consent very easily for the research component of an intervention plan, it can be more difficult to revoke consent for a treatment that shows some efficacy. When a surgeon

Table 16.5 Special Ethical Challenges in Emergency Trauma Research

Time constraints do not allow for best informed consent
Emergencies are unavoidably coercive situations
The role of compensation for participation is unclear
High level of review necessary to justify research without consent

Table 16.6 Revoking Consent for Clinical Research in Spine Trauma

Revoke consent harder for continued treatment than for continued research participation
Patients cannot obligate surgeon to harm by removing implants
Patients prospectively informed of distinct research and treatment components
Subjects can remove themselves from study at any time
Clinician obligated to advocate for best treatment course
Need informed revocation of consent when serious risks involved
Clinician/researcher may have conflicting role (see **Table 16.8**)

Table 16.7 Veracity and Transparency in Research

Subjects informed clearly of study purpose
Researcher must discloses all conflicts of interest and obligation (see **Table 16.11**)
Deception only when no alternative
Disclose to subject that there might be deception
Inform subject of all alternatives, including receiving therapy off study
Subjects informed as early as possible about the entire protocol

believes that continued follow-up care is necessary for a patient's recovery, there is an obligation for the surgeon to assist and influence the patient in making a choice consistent with patient goals. This influence goes contrary to the general understanding in research that no person should be pressured into continuing in a research protocol. However, for the patient's doctor, there is an obligation to advocate for the best plan of care. Second, withdrawing from a surgical protocol may involve a request to remove implanted material or to reverse a procedure. Although patients never have a positive right to ask a surgeon to harm them, which reversing or removing implants might do, these situations ought to be addressed ahead of time in the protocol and during the consent process so that there is no misunderstanding about what revocation means. The protocol should be explicit about whether a patient-subject needs to revoke informed consent or have an informed revocation of consent.[9] Simply, can a patient-subject completely withdraw from a protocol without question, or does the patient-subject need to meet the same standard of consent for revocation as he or she did for the original consent? Both the potential benefit of a procedure and the practical harm of revocation need careful ethical evaluation as researchers set a standard for withdrawal from a clinical research protocol.

Beyond voluntariness, informed consent for research places a premium on veracity and transparency (**Table 16.7**). Subjects need to be informed clearly about the study's purpose and the particulars involved in the research procedures. Further, they should be told of any significant potential conflicts of interest or conflicts of commitments that exist for the research team and institution. If a protocol involves any type of deception, such as a placebo, the researcher is expected to inform the subject to the degree possible without interfering with the protocol. Transparency also necessitates informing the patient or surrogate of all potential therapeutic alternatives. For the sake of enrollment, a researcher is not permitted to exclude mentioning other treatment options or the availability of the treatment outside the research protocol. This latter point is important when the researcher has a vested interest in completing a research study. The patient needs to know if the intervention is available without the challenges of being a subject in a research study. All aspects of the trial and a subject's choices should be made apparent as early in the process as possible.

As the above discussion points out, research protocols necessitate a shift in values away from a wholly patient-centered model, as described in *Neurotrauma and Critical Care of the Brain*. Contemporary clinical research balances a patient-centered model with a scientific model of inquiry. The most interesting research ethics questions arise in the context of clinical trials where some component of the research is intended to improve the patient's condition. In such situations, the clinician/researcher must take into account both the patient's well-being and the success of the research protocol for the benefit of other patients who may find themselves in similar situations. The divided focus causes a shift in values. These are outlined in **Table 16.8**. The interventional plan becomes more rigid and standardized in the shift from patient care to research protocol. The researcher's primary interest lies in the benefit of future patients through gaining scientific knowledge that is generalizable and repeatable. It is in the researcher's interest to have subjects complete the protocol and to share the information through publication and presentation. The clinician values confidentiality of information, avoidance of harm for an individual patient, benefiting the patient maximally, and using professional judgment to decide the best for the patient. Clearly, values can come into conflict when the surgeon acts as both clinician and researcher. No matter who acts as clinician and researcher, a balance of interests and goals must be maintained in a way that respects the patient-subject.

Table 16.8 Shift in Values from Clinician to Researcher

Values	Clinician	Researcher
Treatment plan aimed at	Individual	Uniform
Benefit to	Patient	Patient group in future
Knowledge	Professional judgment	Scientific knowledge
Protection	Avoid harm of patient	Protection of subjects
Information use	Confidentiality	Publish information
Role	Advocating for patient	Generalizability/repeatability
Influence	Patient to healthier life	Subject to complete protocol

■ Emergency, Surrogate, and Research Advanced Directives for Consent

The ideal for research involves careful informed consent from the patient to participate as a research subject. However, the questions remain open in neurotrauma cases as to who should decide enrollment in clinical trials and what, if any, special protections are necessary for patient-subjects.[10] Generally, neurotrauma patients are young adults who prior to the trauma were competent individuals. Further, much of the neurotrauma research is undertaken in an emergency setting, where even for competent patients, the stressed environment does not lend itself to careful, well-reasoned decision making. In many ways these patients may be considered vulnerable and in need of special protections, given the stresses of the situation and the potential for the injury to have affected their judgment.[11] A good voluntary informed consent for most spine trauma research protocols may not be possible even for those patients who retain sufficient decision-making capacity. In reality, the majority of neurotrauma patients are not decisionally capable of parsing a complex ethics review board consent form. If the patient is unable to provide informed consent, the task of finding a way to ethically undertake research becomes more complex. The underlying value of informed consent involves respect for patients' values and patients' ability to control their bodies. The question is whether the value of informed consent

from the patient can be trumped by other values, such as the need to improve therapy for similar patients, or a therapeutic privilege invoked by a clinician/researcher.

There are those who believe that such emergency research can be done without consent as long as there is careful oversight and advocacy. In the United States the federal regulations allow for a waiver or exception to informed consent in certain circumstance. The most difficult condition for this exception involves a requirement to consult with the "community" before beginning recruitment into a protocol like this. Knowing who the "community" is and getting a consensus regarding what should be done have become intractable problems with which many have struggled.[12] Simply bypassing consent can set a dangerous precedent that constantly needs a counterbalance.

In general, there are no specific guidelines, in most regulations or ethics, for allowing proxy consent for research in adults,[13] although for clinical purposes, when patients cannot consent for themselves, most often there is a reliance on the closest family members to guide surgeons in treatment. When clinical research offers a substantial potential benefit for the patient, this practice of getting consent from a surrogate has strong ethical support. Because the consent is for a potential therapeutic benefit, the surrogate would first use a substituted judgment, then a best interest standard, and finally a reasonable treatment standard as discussed in *Neurotrauma and Critical Care of the Brain.* **Table 16.9**, reprinted

Table 16.9 Proxy Decision-Making Models

	Strengths	Weaknesses	When to Apply
Substituted judgment	Most direct expression of patient	Prior wishes about a therapy may not be relevant to current context	Patient wishes known
Best interest	Respect for the unique individual	Difficult to apply to individual therapeutic choices	Patient values known
Reasonable treatment	Often based on standard practices	Does not account well for individual desires and goals	Little known patient values and wishes

from *Neurotrauma and Critical Care of the Brain* highlights these standards. However, because few people discuss their wishes to be a research subject, the substituted judgment model may not be possible. Further, when the research is unrelated to a potential benefit, an informal surrogate decision maker may not be an acceptable solution either. This leaves open a great deal of ethical and legal uncertainty. The most important ethical principle in this context is that patients who cannot consent for themselves should not be used for research out of simple convenience and should garner some benefit as an individual or group from the research being performed.

In the *Neurotrauma and Critical Care of the Brain* we discussed the challenges of advanced directives in the clinical care context. As noted, the success of these documents in clinical settings has been somewhat limited in providing useful guidance in end-of-life decision making. In spite of this, there have been attempts to apply this concept of advance directive to the research world so that patient-subjects could agree to be research subjects prior to being decisionally incapacitated. This is conceived as a means to allow clinical research directed toward benefiting the subject and generating knowledge to benefit future patients without relying either on a surrogate decision maker or a waiver of informed consent. However, the likelihood of these directives actually being used by patients appears to be small.[14,15] Further, the applicability of the directive to any particular research protocol would be limited given the inability to foresee the specific details of the research and the unexpected nature of traumatic injuries.

■ Innovative Therapy

There is a gap between the initial conceptualization of an intervention and the actual development of a research protocol. This gap, usually referred to as innovation, may involve a procedure not yet ready for a formalized research project. Also, there are cases where no other therapy is available and the particular patient circumstances

are rare enough that no research is even planned. The set of activities referred to as innovative is not a single type of activity, but rather a variety of activities grouped by exclusionary definition as not fitting into standard or research practice. Bernstein and Bampoe[16] demarcate at least five different types of innovation, all of which may require different levels of oversight. Four of these categories are those undertakings that compose a new procedure to all surgeons, an amendment of a standard procedure, a unique combination of established procedures, and a procedure new to a particular neurosurgeon. Each activity invokes different meanings of innovation and might require anything from informal peer review to IRB oversight. Although each surgeon may practice medicine based on expertise, good practice often benefits from collegial review. A review can make for robust practice and perhaps even have a positive influence on risk management and can be undertaken formally or informally. In cases where significant harm may be done to a patient-subject and a research ethics board will not provide review, a multidisciplinary review by experts is well advised.

For the sake of the ethics framework we have been discussing, **Table 16.10** is a comparison of the differences in values in providing standard clinical, innovative, and research treatments. It is clear that innovation presents an interesting blend between clinical practice and clinical research. The question marks in the table represent areas for which there is no clear consensus. Of particular note is the question of how to properly provide oversight for innovative practice that both protects patients from harm and allows patients to potentially benefit from innovative procedures.

■ Conflicts of Interest and Commitment: Research and Practice

Numerous studies have been undertaken to prove the influence of financial ties and inducement on research results.[17–19] The literature appears to show that the clinical

Table 16.10 Comparison of Value Elements in Treatment, Innovation, and Clinical Research

	Treatment	Innovation	Clinical Research
Consent given by	MD/patient/proxy	MD/patient/proxy	Researcher/subject with IRB consent form
Withdrawal given by	MD/patient consultation	MD/patient consultation	Simple subject request
Standardization	Flexible	Flexible	Rigid
Focus of intervention	Individual	Individual/future group	Future group/individual
Selection of intervention	Patient/MD	MD/patient	Randomized (placebo?)
Oversight of intervention	Medical board	Medical board/FDA?/institution?	IRB/FDA?
Primary benefit	Patient	Patient	Future patients

and research practice of physicians can be negatively manipulated by industry. Apart from the actual influence on science and practice, simply the appearance of a conflict can negatively affect patient trust and thus negatively affect clinical practice.[20] However, in many neurosurgical research endeavors, a collaborative relationship with industry is both beneficial and necessary.[21] In such cases, transparency is the most important step toward managing those financial conflicts of interest. Prospectively full disclosing the interests to patients and research subjects now constitutes best practices for both research and clinical practice. Although these disclosures may not change actual surgical practice, they provide patients with a full understanding on which they can make a judgment.

Financial interests are not the only potential conflicts that influences research and practice. A conflict of commitment or obligation can be equally influential for surgeons. A surgeon's career and commitment to an institution may deeply influence the choices in treatment options that could disproportionately sway clinical judgment. More importantly, in academic centers a balance between the duty to train new neurosurgeons and the duty to help particular patients may come into conflict.[22] The degree to which a surgeon oversees a trainee must be balanced against the need for a trainee to work independently. This balance occurs in the context of providing patients with the best surgical procedure. A suboptimal procedure should never be undertaken simply for the sake of training. This would be an inappropriate balance of the trainee's need to take part in a particular procedure against providing the best care for a patient. Further, inviting industry representatives to be present in the operating room may present a negative influence on practice and should be carefully evaluated and disclosed to patients.[23] Although conflicts of interest and commitment are unavoidable, as a whole they comprise a need for explicit balancing of values. Each potential conflict must be actively managed by emphasizing transparency, honesty, and careful reflection. In all types of conflicting interests, the individual patient-subject's safety and benefit must be weighed most heavily (**Table 16.11**).

■ Spine Injury and Sports

The choices faced by a surgeon, patient, and sports teams are complex when an athlete incurs a traumatic spine or brain injury (**Table 16.12**). Although there are many professions for which traumatic injury can be career ending, the factors of celebrity, money, and conflicting obligations make treating athletes a rich paradigm in which to discuss ethics. Perhaps the clearest sets of challenges exist in the professional arena, particularly in a sport such as American football. The American football season is short, the forces of impact large, and the financial stakes high for athletes and teams. Although there are guidelines emerging as to when to allow an athlete to compete in the context of a spine injury, the decision always must be made on an individual basis in collaboration with the patient.[24] At first these choices may appear to be simply scientific/medical judgments. However, confounding factors influence whether a player actually returns to the field to play in a game. These include the patient's willingness to risk health for other gains (fame, fortune, or ego), a surgeon's willingness to open himself or the patient to risk, and a team's interest in putting its "human capital" at risk. As recognized widely, medical specialists employed by professional sports teams have competing commitments to those who pay for their services via a contractual agreement related to the treatment and evaluation of players and to the players themselves as patients.[25] Further, as with treating any celebrity, there are ethical challenges in properly masking the identity of these patients if they are to be presented for educational purposes. For instance, if the 2006 starting quarterback for the Indianapolis Colts were to be evaluated for spine surgery,

Table 16.11 Conflicts of Interest, Commitment, and Obligation

Financial conflicts receive most attention
Industry ties, both financial and personal, can negatively influence
No such thing as a "free lunch"
Conflict of commitment between teaching, research, clinical, care, and career
However, industry collaboration necessary for furthering better patient care
Manage through transparency, oversight, and rescue self from selected activities

Table 16.12 Team Doctor's Commitments

Values	To Athlete	To Team
Medical disclosure	Full	Degree agreed upon prospectively
Conflict disclosure	Prospectively	Prospectively
Financial influence	Very little	Contracted
Vulnerable	Often	Never
Deception	Never	Never? (to protect the vulnerable)
Paternalism	Sometimes	Advocate of patients

that descriptor uniquely describes one easily identifiable person. If the results are important to report, then consent should be attained from such a person before presenting the information. Again, there exists a great potential for secondary gain for the surgeon through being known as the treating physician for a famous athlete that must be carefully evaluated. This provides another example of the intricacies of balancing the various commitments and interests that every practicing surgeon has. **Table 16.12** summarizes some of the competing types of commitments involved in being a team surgeon where the surgeon is both the athlete's doctor and a contracted professional for the team. Perhaps the most difficult situation involves the case where an injury could be career ending and a player asks that this not be disclosed to a team because of contract negotiations. In line with the theme of this entire chapter, prospective transparency of commitments is the ethically best way to set up a consulting role well before a dilemma arises. By informing the athlete of an obligation to the team and informing the team of your limits of obligation to them, many of the dilemmas can be avoided. The triad of physician, team, and patient constitutes a very difficult ethical area.

■ Quality of Life, Depression, and Patients with Paralysis

Spine trauma poses several interesting challenges in quality of life decisions related to paralysis (**Table 16.13**). Because contemporary society places great importance on independence, many perceive a life of paralysis as not being worth living. Further, many who suffer traumatic spine injury are young and of limited means to prepare themselves for life after a severe spinal injury. There have been many studies documenting high levels of grief and depression for this population.[26] It is not uncommon for there to be suicidal ideation in this population. Further, a very lively discussion exists regarding whether disabled patients have a right to die or whether there are built-in biases against those with disabilities in society.[27] This context sets up a very difficult dynamic for the health care team. Surgeries become futile if a patient plans to simply forfeit her life in the near future through withdrawal of a life-sustaining intervention such as artificial nutrition or a ventilator. Further, surgeries in this context might actually cause more suffering for no good benefit if life is limited. However, allowing someone to die before he or she fully experiences life with paralysis does an injustice to the patient in that it may be premised on inappropriate stereotypes about quality of life. Patients need sufficient time to allow for a realignment of values. Good ethics rely on decisions consistent with both short- and long-term goals of patients. Given that we know the

Table 16.13 Ethical Challenges in Paralysis

High rates of depression, grief, and suicidal ideation early in course
Many retain capacity to consent that needs to be respected
Surgeon expected to act in the patient's long-term goals and values
Patient needs to know/experience life of paralysis to fully appreciate
Surgical intervention may be futile if there is a plan to withdraw other life-sustaining therapies
Goals of care should always be to improve quality of life

transitory nature of grief for many patients who lose function, we would be ill-advised to take a patient's request for being allowed to die without a very careful evaluation of long-term goals and a consistent expression over time. Although patients have a right to bodily integrity, surgeons have an obligation to preserve function and life that is consistent with a patient's long-term goals. These considerations should also carefully determine whether patient problems arise from the social circumstances that could be changed rather than from the inherent nature of being paralyzed.[28] Finally, the very injuries the patients have suffered may deeply influence the way in which their minds work. This may raise many challenges in the cooperation of patients with the rehabilitation that is necessary for good outcomes.[29] The goal of care should always be an improved quality of life, and debate continues about the successful matching of medical interventions and goals.[28] These considerations require a fine balance that involves careful discussion and consideration.

■ Conclusion

In the various stages of treatment for spinal trauma patients, ethical dilemmas can appear. These may manifest themselves in innovation, research, or standard treatments. Careful reflection on what is lost and gained through various decisions should be integrated into best practice. One must go beyond simply giving a description of risks and benefits to patients for them to make an "autonomous" decision. This idealized view of practice does not match real-world practice where patients look to surgeons to act in their best interest in tragic circumstances. That trust does not give license to simply ignore patient wishes and values. It provides a greater responsibility to carefully evaluate the personal costs and to recognize the limits of practice.

References

1. Jallo J, Vacarro AR. Neurotrauma and Critical Care of the Spine New York: Thieme Medical Publishers, 2008

2. Carey TS. Randomized controlled trials in surgery: an essential component of scientific progress. Spine 1999;24:2553–2555

3. Winter RB. The prospective, randomized, controlled clinical trial in spine surgery: fact or fiction? Spine 1999;24:2550–2552

4. Cohen BC. The ethics of using medical data from Nazi experiments. Virtual Jewish Library. http://www.jewishvirtuallibrary.org/jsource/Judaism/naziexp.html#1

5. Cave E, Holm S. Milgram and Tuskegee—paradigm research projects in bioethics. Health Care Anal 2003;11:27–40

6. Ford PJ, Henderson J. Neuroethics in the operating room: functional neurosurgical interventions. In: Illes J, ed. Neuroethics: Defining the Issues in Theory, Practice and Policy. New York: Oxford University Press; 2005:213–228

7. The Belmont Report. Ethical Principles and Guidelines for the Protection of Human Subjects or Research. Report of the National Commission for the Protection of Human Subjects of Biomedical and Behavioral Research, 1979

8. Declaration of Helsinki. Ethical Principles for Medical Research Involving Human Subjects, General Assembly, Washington, 2004. http://www.wma.net/e/policy/b3.htm

9. Ford PJ. Neurosurgical implants: clinical protocol considerations. Camb Q Healthc Ethics 2007;16:308–311

10. Pape TL, Jaffe NO, Savage T, Collins E, Warden D. Unresolved legal and ethical issues in research of adults with severe traumatic brain injury: analysis of an ongoing protocol. J Rehabil Res Dev 2004;41:155–174

11. Schmidt TA, Salo D, Hughes JA, et al; SAEM Ethics Committee. Confronting the ethical challenges to informed consent in emergency medicine research. Acad Emerg Med 2004;11:1082–1089

12. Blixen CE, Agich GJ. Related stroke patients' preferences and values about emergency research. J Med Ethics 2005;31:608–611

13. Kim SY, Appelbaum PS, Jeste DV, Olin JT. Proxy and surrogate consent in geriatric neuropsychiatric research: update and recommendations. Am J Psychiatry 2004;161:797–806

14. Muthappan P, Forster H, Wendler D. Research advance directives: protection or obstacle? Am J Psychiatry 2005;162:2389–2391

15. Stocking CB, Hougham GW, Danner DD, Patterson MB, Whitehouse PJ, Sachs GA. Speaking of research advance directives: planning for future research participation. Neurology 2006;66:1361–1366

16. Bernstein M, Bampoe J. Surgical innovation or surgical evolution: an ethical and practical guide to handling novel neurosurgical procedures. J Neurosurg 2004;100:2–7

17. Bhandari M, Busse JW, Jackowski D, et al. Association between industry funding and statistically significant pro-industry findings in medical and surgical randomized trials. CMAJ 2004;170:477–480

18. Fenton JJ, Mirza SK, Lahad A, Stern BD, Deyo RA. Variation in reported safety of lumbar interbody fusion: influence of industrial sponsorship and other study characteristics. Spine 2007;32:471–480

19. Okike K, Kocher MS, Mehlman CT, Bhandari M. Conflict of interest in orthopaedic research. An association between findings and funding in scientific presentations. J Bone Joint Surg Am 2007;89:608–613

20. Mirza SK. Accountability of the accused: facing public perceptions about financial conflicts of interest in spine surgery. Spine J 2004;4:491–494

21. Fins JJ, Schachter M. Investigators, industry, and the heuristic device: ethics, patent law, and clinical innovation. Account Res 2001;8:219–233

22. Bernstein M. Surgical teaching: how should neurosurgeons handle the conflict of duty to today's patients with the duty to tomorrow's? Br J Neurosurg 2003;17:121–123

23. Moskowitz S, Ford PJ. Ethical issues associated with health care industry representatives in the operating room. SpineLine 2006;4:8–40

24. Maroon JC, Bailes JE. Athletes with cervical spine injury. Spine 1996;21:2294–2299

25. Tucker AM. Ethics and the professional team physician. Clin Sports Med 2004;23:227–241

26. de Carvalho SA, Andrade MJ, Tavares MA, de Freitas JL. Spinal cord injury and psychological response. Gen Hosp Psychiatry 1998;20:353–359

27. Gill CJ. Depression in the context of disability and the "right to die." Theor Med Bioeth 2004;25:171–198

28. Jennings B. Traumatic brain injury and the goals of care: the ordeal of reminding. Hastings Cent Rep 2006;36:29–37

29. Levenson JL, Hamric AB. Ethical dilemmas in the treatment of patients following traumatic brain injury. Psychiatr Med 1989;7:59–71

Index

Note: Page numbers followed by *f* and *t* indicate figures and tables, respectively.